HEALTH CARE SYSTEM AND HOSPITAL ADMINISTRATION

5

PRIMARY/RURAL HEALTH CARE

HEALTH CARE SYSTEM AND HOSPITAL ADMINISTRATION

5

PRIMARY/RURAL HEALTH CARE

DR. S.L. GOEL

Professor of Public Administration (Retd.),
Panjab University, Chandigarh
Editor, Indian Journal of Public Administration, IIPA, New Delhi
Former Member, UGC, Former Member Distance Education Council
Former Member All India Board of Management, AICTE
Member, Executive Council, IIPA, New Delhi.
Former Vice-President, IIPA, New Delhi.
Emeritus Fellow, University Grants Commission
Former Director, State Bank of India (Local Board) Chandigarh
Former Director, National Horticulture Board, Ministry of Agriculture,
Government of India, New Delhi.

DEEP & DEEP PUBLICATIONS PVT. LTD.

F-159, Rajouri Garden, New Delhi-110027

HEALTH CARE SYSTEM AND HOSPITAL ADMINISTRATION
Vol. 5—Primary/Rural Health Care

ISBN 978-81-8450-195-7 (Vol. 5)
ISBN 978-81-8450-198-8 (Set)

Typeset by S.S. COMPOSERS
3190, Mohindra Park, Shakur Basti, Delhi-110034.

Printed in India at MAYUR ENTERPRISES
WZ Plot No. 3, Gujjar Market, Tihar Village, New Delhi-110018.

Published by DEEP & DEEP PUBLICATIONS PVT. LTD.
F-159, Rajouri Garden, New Delhi-110027.
Phones: 25435369, 25440916
E-mail: ddpbooks@yahoo.co.in • ddpubs@gmail.com
Showroom:
2/13, Ansari Road, Daryaganj, New Delhi-110002 • Telefax: 23245122

Contents

	Preface	vii
1.	Administration of Primary/Rural Health Care	1
2.	National Rural Health Mission (NRHM)	38
3.	Inter-Sectoral Co-ordination for Health Promotion	73
4.	Community Participation and Health Development	90
5.	Financial Administration for Primary Health Care	125
6.	Personnel Administration for Primary Health Care	136
7.	Appropriate Technology and Research for Primary Health Care	150
8.	Trained Birth Attendants (TBAs)	164
9.	Community Health Centres	174
10.	Organisation and Working of Primary Health Centres	206
11.	Organisation and Working of Sub-Centres	249
12.	Working of Primary Health Care—A Case Study of Punjab	280
	Annexures	
	I. Declaration of Alma-Ata	307
	II. Alma-Ata Recommendations	311
	Bibliography	322
	Index	325

Preface

11th Five Year Plan stresses on the improving governance. All our efforts to achieve rapid and inclusive development will only bear fruit if we can ensure good governance both in the implementation of public programme and in governments interaction with the ordinary citizens. Corruption is now seen to be endemic in all spheres of life and this problem needs to be urgently redressed. Better design of projects, implementation mechanisms and procedures can reduce the scope for corruption. Much more needs to be done by both the Centre and the States to lessen the discretionary power of government, ensure greater transparency and accountability, and create awareness among citizens. The Right to Information Act empowers the people to demand improved governance, and as government we must be ready to respond to this demand.

The Crisis in Rural Health Care an article in *Economic Times,* dated January 24, 2008 by Arvind Panagariya, a non-resident Professor at Columbia University and Senior Fellow at Brookings Institution laments and says while the dilapidated state of infrastructure and poor supply of drugs and equipment are partly to blame, the primary culprit is the rampant absenteeism at rural health centers.

Rural health care in India faces a crisis unmatched by any other sector of the economy. To mention just one dramatic fact, rural medical practitioner (RMP), who provides 80% of outpatient care, have no formal qualifications for it. They sometimes lack even a high-school diploma.

Despite this elaborate network of facilities, only 20% of those seeking outpatient services and 45% of those seeking indoor treatment avail of public services. While the dilapidated state of infrastructure and poor supply of drugs and equipment are partly to blame, the primary culprit is the rampant absenteeism. Nationwide average absentee rate is 40%.

The employees are paid by the state, with the local officials having no authority over them. Not surprisingly, many medical officers visit the PHC infrequently and run parallel private practice in the nearby town. ANMS are frequently unavailable for childbirths even if the mother is willing to come to PHC. Though PHCs are supposed to be free, most of them informally charge a fee. Under these circumstances, even many among the poor have concluded in favour of private services.

Sadly, public health services have done poorly even along the income distribution dimension. According to a 2001 study, the poorest 20% of the population captures only 10% of public health subsidy compared with 30% by richest 20%. The share in the subsidy rises monotonically as we move from the bottom 20%. The justification for the government provision of health services on income distribution grounds does not find support in the data.

To make improvements in the delivery of health services, atleast three reforms are urgently required. First, it is time to accept the fact that the government has at best limited capability to deliver health services and that a radical shift in strategy that gives the poor greater opportunity to choose between private and public providers is needed. This can best be accomplished by providing the poor cash transfers for out-patient care and insurance for in-patient care. Once this is done, a competitive price must be charged for services provided at public facilities as well. The government should invest in public facilities only in health to reach regions where private providers may not emerge.

Second, the government must introduce up to one-year long training courses for practitioners engaged in treating routine illness. This would be in line with the National Health Policy, 2002, which envisages a role for paramedics along the lines of nurse practitioners in the United States. The existing RMPs may be given priority in the provision of such training with the goal being replacement of all RMPs by qualified nurse practitioners.

Finally, there is urgent need for accelerating the growth of MBBS graduates to replace unqualified "doctors" who operate in both urban and rural areas. Taking into account the evolution of medical colleges and assuming that doctors remain active 30 years after receiving their degrees, there are at the most 650,000 doctors in India today. With a population of 1.1 billion, this implies approximately 1,700 people per doctor. In comparison, there are just 400 people per doctor in the United States and 220 in Israel. Whereas private colleges and institutes in engineering, computer applications and business fields have mushroomed in response to demand, the same has not happened in the medical field.

The dynamics of having a large population being sustained on a comparatively low resource base has several disturbing repercussions. Over the last few decades, while India has made significant progress in the areas of poverty eradication, improvement of literacy rates and health standards, etc., there still remains a disparity between India and the rest of the world on various social development indicators. The Human Development Report (HDR-2001) places India at the 115th position in the world as judged by the Human Development Indicator (HDI). India's HDI was estimated at 52.9. In comparison, the average HDI of all other developing countries was 64.5. On other parameters such as infant mortality, literacy rates, access to amenities, etc. though there has been a distinct improvement over the last couple of decades, India's performance relative to the other developing countries in the world has been less than satisfactory.

Indicators given below points to indicate that the challenge before the nation in terms of improving the basic factors that provide a decent quality of life to its populace is rather onerous.

India's Human Development Indicators

- Infant mortality—72 per thousand live births.
- Literacy rates—65.2%.
- Households with access to safe drinking water—62.3%.
- Households with access to proper sanitation facilities—49.32%.
- Households with electricity connection—42.37%.
- Households with electricity, safe drinking water and proper sanitation facilities—16.1%.
- Households with permanent houses—41.61%.
- Households with semi-permanent houses—30.95%.
- Households with temporary shelters—27.44%.

It was held that health is best pursued as part of development. Development implies social progress and not only economic progress, since its principal aim is to improve the quality of life. Health, economic and social development are thus intimately interlinked. Indeed, health development, which is universally valued by all people should be used as a power lever for social and economic development. "Without health, life has little quality, for even if health is not everything, without it the rest is nothing." (Mahler)

That health is a universal and fundamental human right and its attainment is an essential social goal; that the just distribution of health resources is as important as their quantity and quality.

To reach a more equitable distribution of health resources, it is necessary to pay greater attention to those least served, the social periphery, the disease-ridden majority. The guiding principle should be the greatest health benefit to the greatest number of people at the lowest cost.

In 1977, the World Health Assembly decided that the main social target of governments and WHO should be "the attainment by all the citizens of the world by the year 2000 of a level of health that will permit them to lead a socially and economically productive life." In 1978, a conference held in Alma-Ata, USSR, declared that primary health care was the key to attaining this target (sponsored by WHO and UNICEF). Health for All is a process, leading to progressive improvement in the health of people.

- Essential health care.
- Made accessible to everyone in the community.
- At a cost the country and community can afford.
- With methods that are practical, scientifically sound and socially acceptable.
- Everyone should be involved in it.
- Related sectors should be involved in it in addition to the health sector.
- At the very least, it should include:

1. Education of the community on health problems prevalent and on methods preventing and controlling them.
2. Promotion of adequate supply of food and proper nutrition.
3. Sufficient safe water and basic sanitation.
4. Maternal and Child Health Care, including family planning.
5. Prevention and control of locally endemic diseases.
6. Immunization against the main infectious diseases.
7. Appropriate treatment of common diseases and injuries.
8. Provision of essential drugs.

As it will be seen from the above definition, the primary health care approach is based on certain principles such as:

1. *Accessible*: Covering all both rural and urban.
2. *Affordable*: To be maintained and sustained, thus promoting self-reliance
3. *Appropriate technology*: This does not mean primitive technology. Oral Dehydration Therapy (ORT) for prevention of dehyradation is an example of advanced technology, simpler, cheaper and more effective than the intravenous approach.
4. Involvement/participation of the individual and the community.
5. Intersectoral action for health and overall social development.
6. Emphasis on promotive and preventive aspect in addition to curative aspects.

The realization of health goals and objectives, therefore, requires that the primary health care as defined above needs to be translated into action. Health service infrastructure at the primary level needs to be reoriented to take new roles in line with primary health care approach.

As primary health care approach is people-oriented approach, thus the organisation of health care starts with the people, individuals and families, and communities. These need to be connected with the health facilities at primary level, secondary level, and tertiary level with effective system of referral.

(a) Primary health care level

This level starts with individuals/families to the first health facility. Health personnel work closely with other sectoral personnel and with the community to support the provision of the essential health care for all the community. This is the most important level of health system. It is the foundation of health care in a country. It is the first line in health development.

(b) Secondary level of health care

This level cares for people requiring specialized services, not available at the primary health care level. It serves as referral for the primary health level. It should also provide support for the primary level.

(c) Tertiary level of health care

This level is more specialized, with more trained personnel and more sophisticated diagnostic and therapeutic technology. It provides care to those in need for more specialized services. It is usually located at university hospitals at national level and regional levels.

Primary health care concept is very different and broader from the idea of treating the sick (medical care). In medical care approach, the focus is on doctors, drugs, dispensaries/hospitals, diagnostic technology, to treat disease or persons after they become sick. On the other hand, health care approach strives to promote health, prevent disease in the population, with their participation, in addition to caring for the sick. The medical care approach keeps the process of sickness on-going, while in health care approach effort is made to stop the cycle of disease, and promotion of health through attention to the individual/family lifestyle and environmental factors.

The functioning of Primary Health Care System is not doing well. Even the Ninth Five Year Plan (1997-2002) has admitted it and enlisted a number of factors responsible for inefficient functioning:

1. Persistent gaps in manpower and infrastructure especially at the primary health care level.
2. Sub-optimal functioning of the infrastructure; poor referral services.
3. Plethora of hospitals not having appropriate manpower, diagnostic and therapeutic services and drugs, in Government, voluntary and private sector.
4. Massive interstate/inter-district differences in performance as assessed by health and demography indices; availability and utilisation of services are poorest in the most needy states/districts.
5. Sub-optimal intersectoral coordination.
6. Increasing dual disease burden of communicable and non-communicable diseases because of ongoing demographic, lifestyle and environmental transitions.
7. Technological advances which widen the spectrum of possible interventions.
8. Increasing awareness and expectations of the population regarding health care services.
9. Escalating costs of health care, ever widening gaps between what is possible and what the individual or the country can afford.

Shortfall in Health Personnel—All India

For the existing Infrastructure	*Required (R)*	*Sanctioned (S)*	*In Position*	*Vacant (S-P)*	*Shortfall (R-P)*
Multipurpose workers (Female) ANM at Sub-Centre and PHCs	167657	162772	149695	13126 (8.06%)	18318 (10.93%)
Health Workers (Male)/ MPWs (M) at Sub-Centres	144998	94924	655111	29437 (31.1%)	7421 (51.53%)
Health Assistant (Female) LHV at PHCs	22669	19874	17107	2871 (12.99%)	5941 (26.21%)
Health Assistants (Male) at PHCs	22669	24207	18223	5984 (24.72%)	7169 (31.62%)
Doctors at PHCs	22669	27927	22273	5801 (20.77%)	1793 (7.91%)
Total Specialist at CHCs	15640	9071	3979	4681 (51.60%)	9413 (60.19%)
Radiographers at CHCs	3910	2400	1782	620 (25.83%)	1330 (34.02%)
Pharmacists at PHCs and CHCs	26579	22816	18419	4445 (19.48%)	4389 (16.51%)
Lab Technicians at PHCs and CHCs	26579	15143	12351	2792 (18.44%)	9509 (35.78%)

Source : Bulletin of Rural Health Statistics in India, Special Revised Edition, MOHFW, GOI, 2006.

At the time of Independence, Health Care Services were mainly urban-centered and hospital-based. Realising the importance of creating a functional Primary Health Care infrastructure, national norms for the primary health care infrastructure were drawn up. These take into account the population, population density and terrain. At the national level the total number of functional Sub-Centres and the PHCs nearly meets the set norms. However, there are marked disparities at the State and District level. It is a matter of concern that many of the districts with poor health indices do not have adequate health infrastructure. There is considerable backlog in terms of construction of the buildings for sub-centres, PHCs and Community Head Centres.

Some States have adopted innovative measures including mobilisation of local resources to clear this backlog. Taking cognizance of the widening disparities among the States in the availability of Basic Minimum Service (BMS), the Conference of the Chief Ministers in July 1996, recommended that Additional Central Assistance (ACA) may be provided to the states for correcting the existing gaps in the provision of seven Basic Minimum Services (BMS). The modalities of implementation of the programme are discussed in detail in the section on Basic Minimum Services. Of these, access to primary health care, safe drinking water and primary education were given higher priority with the mandate that universal access to these services is to be achieved by 2000 A.D. There is an urgent need to encourage involvement of the people's representatives, voluntary organisations and the people themselves in these activities.

The term "primary" has acquired a variety of connotations, some of them technical (referring to the first contact with the health system, or the first level of care, or simple treatments that could be delivered by relatively untrained providers, or interventions acting on primary causes of disease) and some political (depending on multi-sectoral implications for policy) help explain why there is no one model of primary care, and why it has been difficult to follow the successful examples of the countries or states that provided the first evidence that a substantial improvement in health could be achieved at affordable cost. There was a substantial effort in many countries to train and use community health workers who could deliver basic, cost-effective services in simple rural facilities to populations that previously had little or no access to modern care. In India, for example, such workers were trained and placed in over 1,000,000 health posts, intended to serve nearly two-thirds of the population.

Despite these efforts, many such programmes were eventually considered at least partial failures. Funding was inadequate, the workers had little time to spend on prevention and community out-reach; their training and equipment were insufficient for the problems they confronted; and quality of care was often so poor as to be characterised as "primitive" rather than "primary", particularly when primary care was limited to the poor and to only the simplest services. Referral systems, which are unique to health services and necessary to their proper performance, have proved particularly difficult to operate adequately. Lower level services were often poorly utilized, and patients who could do so commonly bypassed the lower levels of the system to go directly to hospitals. Partly in consequence, countries continued to invest in tertiary, urban-based centres.

Need for this Book

The question arises as to how we can develop the administrative skill and capability along with the professional competence among the personnel responsible for health care administration? This can be made possible by two methods. The first is to incorporate the teaching and research of health care administration in the syllabus of under-graduate and post-graduate medical education. The second method is to impart training to the personnel already engaged in health care administration, especially through executive development programmes. A few steps have been taken in this direction, such as the setting up of the National Institute of Health and Family Welfare for the training of personnel in health and family welfare administration; starting of diploma courses in health and hospital administration; starting a distance education programme in health and hospital management by NIHFW; arranging seminars on various aspects of administration, etc.

The success of these methods depend upon the availability of well-prepared literature in health care administration based on the researches and case studies. The literature in this form is non-existent. Most of the available literature relating to the health care administration has tended to be historical or broadly descriptive. In a publication from Pittsburgh University, it has been affirmed that "In health administration, there are few theoreticians, few training centres, few books, and an absolute dearth of strict scientific investigations."

Whatever scanty literature is available on Health Care Administration is in the context of the developed world and hence totally unsuited to the different political, social, economic and cultural milieu of the developing world. Conventional health practices designed on the basis of Western models have proved inappropriate and beyond the capacity of the developing world. Why has Health Care Administration literature not been developed for such a long time? A contributory factor in this regard has been the dichotomy between Public Health and Medical Care specialists and social scientists. Both worked in their narrow grooves without benefiting each other. Fortunately, in recent years this dichotomy has been disappearing progressively. Even in the WHO, there has been a growing consciousness that the social scientists have an increasing role to play in regard to the formulation of curative, preventive, promotive and rehabilitative health policies and programmes, along with the medical scientists to solve the complex health care problems of a rapidly increasing population. A healthy trend is emerging wherein some health administrators are feeling interested in learning the social sciences relevant and useful to the understanding of their field. Some of the social scientists are feeling motivated to analyse the whole process of health care administration to help these experts in finding solutions to various problems outside their domain. Encouraged by such trends, the author has written earlier three books on Health Care Administration, three volumes on Hospital Administration followed by Four Volumes in Hospital Administration and a book on Family Planning Administration and Beyond. In addition, the author guided 10 students from India and abroad for successfully completing their Doctoral Research.

To be effective, any strategy dealing with the problem of poverty has to simultaneously tackle a number of social sector issues such as health care, literacy, empowerment of women, and improved governance. Accordingly, the Government of India has launched a number of initiatives in a variety of social sectors backed by substantial investments.

Improvement in the health status of the population has been one of the major thrust areas in social development programmes of the country. This was to be achieved through improving the access to and utilization of Health, Family Welfare and Nutrition Services with special focus on underserved and underprivileged segments of the population. Technological improvements and increased access to health care have resulted in a steep fall in mortality but the diseases burden due to communicable diseases, non-communicable diseases and nutritional problems continue to be high. Despite the fact that norms for creation of health care infrastructure and manpower are similar throughout the country, there remain substantial inter-state/inter-district variations in availability and utilization of health care services and health indices of the population.

The 10th Five Year Plan focused on the re-organisation and restructuring of existing health care infrastructure, including the infrastructure for delivering indigenous system of medicine and health care services at primary, secondary and tertiary care levels so that they have the responsibility of serving populations residing in a well defined geographical area and have appropriate referral linkages with each other. All the above-mentioned programmes are implemented in collaboration with state governments, local self-governments and civil society.

The 10th Plan aimed at providing essential primary health care, particularly to the underprivileged and underserved segments of our population. It also sought to devolve responsibilities and funds for health care to PRIs. However, progress towards these objectives has been slow and the 10th Plan targets on MMR and IMR have been missed. Accessibility remains a major issue especially in areas where habitations are scattered and women and children continue to die en route to hospitals. Rural health care in most states is marked by absenteeism of doctors/health providers, low levels of skills, shortage of medicines, inadequate supervision/monitoring and callous attitudes. There are neither rewards for service providers nor punishments for defaulters. As a result, health outcomes in India are adverse compared to bordering countries like Sri Lanka as well as countries of South East Asia like China and Vietnam.

To improve the primary health care system, the 11th Plan will first pay emphasis on integrated district health plans and second, on block specific health plans. These plans will ensure involvement of all health-related sectors and emphasise partnership with NGOs. The NRHM has already been launched to ensure quality health care in rural areas. The next step should be to extend this to make it a Sarva Swasthya Abhiyan that also covers the health needs of the urban poor, particularly the slum-dwellers by investing in high calibre health professionals and appropriate technology

Besides reducing the burden and the level of risk of existing, growing and emerging diseases, the 11th Plan will also take care of the special needs of people living with AIDS, in particular the women. The 11th Plan will recognise the feminine face of HIV and accord it the highest priority.

The 11th Plan will continue to advocate fertility regulation through voluntary and informed consent. The Plan will address the special health care needs of the elderly, especially those who are economically and socially vulnerable

A seven year National Rural Health Mission (NRHM), which spans the duration of the 11th Plan, has been launched to address infirmities and problems across rural primary health care. Converging the public health approach with primary health care has been one of the primary objectives of this mission. Another objective is to genuinely empower and support Panchayati Raj Institutions to manage, administer and be accountable for health services at community levels. Supervision of health sub-centres by gram panchayats will improve attendance of staff, motivate appropriate quality of care and provide constant feedback on patient satisfaction. The NRHM will also converge the management of health delivery across all systems of medicine (including ISM) at primary health care levels.

Eleventh Five Year Plan, 2007-2012, Vol. II observes that: Five Planks of the NRHM, The Mission is expected to address the gaps in the provision of effective health care to rural population with a special focus on 18 States, which have weak public health indicators and/or weak infrastructure.

The Mission is a shift away from the vertical health and family welfare programmes to a new architecture of all inclusive health development in which societies under different programmes will be merged and resources pooled at the district level.

The Mission aims at the effective integration of health concerns with determinants of health like safe drinking water, sanitation, and nutrition through integrated District Plans for Health. There is a provision for flexible funds so that the States can utilize them in the areas they feel are important.

The Mission provides for appointment of ASHA in each village and strengthening of the public health infrastructure, including outreach through mobile clinics. It emphasizes involvement of the non-profit sector, especially in the under-served areas. It also aims at flexibility at the local level by providing for untied funds.

The Mission, in its supplementary strategies, aims at fostering PPPs; improving equity and reducing out of pocket expenses introducing effective risk-pooling mechanisms and social health insurance; and taking advantage of local health traditions.

Eleventh Five Year Plan, 2007-2012, Vol. II observes features of Sarva Swasthya Abhiyan as:

- NRHM has been launched for meeting health needs of all age groups and to reduce disease burden across rural India.
- NUHM will be launched to meet the unmet needs of the urban population (28.6 crore in 2001 and 35.7 crore in 2011). As per the 2001 Census, 4.26 crore lived in urban slums spread over 640 towns and cities. The number is growing.

- NUHM based on health insurance and PPP will provide integrated health service delivery to the urban poor. Initially, the focus will be aligned with NRHM and existing urban schemes.
- Besides, Sarva Swasthya Abhiyan aims for inclusive growth by finding solutions for strengthening health services and focusing on neglected areas and groups.

India has its own well developed indigenous systems of health care like Ayurveda, Yoga, Siddha, Unani, etc, along with diverse ecosystem specific, local health traditions. These traditional systems could be used to complement the allopathic system, as they could be more useful in certain areas of curative/preventive health care. This would enhance the quality and outreach of public health services, which are currently unable to meet the health needs of our people. However, care would have to be taken to ensure that we do not substitute the allopathic system of health care in areas like immunization, etc. where it has no alternative.

The present volume 5 out of total 7 volumes deal with Primary/Rural Health Care. Chapter 1 discusses the meaning, nature and features of Primary/Rural Health Care Administration. Chapter 2 discusses the newly developed National/Rural health mission and its potentialities. Chapter 3 examines the relationship between health and other sectors of social and economic development that is inter-sectoral development. Chapter 4 deals with the role of community participation in health care and development. Chapter 5 examines the role of Appropriate Technology and Research for primary health care. Chapters 6 and 7 examine the Financial and Personnel for Primary/Rural Health Care. Chapter 8 deals with TBA and Chapters 9, 10 and 11 deal with working of Community Health Centre, Primary Health Centres and Sub-Centres. Chapter 12 discusses the working of Primary Health Centre in Punjab. All the chapters are supplements with charts, tables and case studies.

What is needed is to lay emphasis on emerging and thrust areas to keep the medical science knowledge and delivery of health services as per the needs of the people. It is hoped that this book on "Health Care System and Hospital Administration—Primary/Rural Health Care" would make a modest contribution to the knowledge and existing literature on this expanding field. Besides, this would help the academicians, national health officials, public health administrations, medical research workers and the policy-makers and planners in the proper understanding of health care delivery system. I will consider my labour well rewarded if the findings of the study are translated to provide decent health care to the millions of people living in rural areas, urban slums and tribal areas. Comments and suggestions from the readers would always be welcome.

Chandigarh S.L. GOEL

1

CHAPTER

Administration of Primary/Rural Health Care

Primary Health Care is essential both for developed and developing countries. Alastair Andusen visualises this need when he rightly says,[1] people who live in most of the world's industrialized countries tend to take their health services as much for granted as the water that comes from the tap, the electricity that gives them light at the press of a switch, or the public transport that gets them to work or school. (See Chart 1.1)

For the less privileged countries, a health service is far from being one of the accepted facts of life. It tends to concentrate on urban areas and caters in particular to the healthy sections of the big cities. Frequently, in these countries, the rural masses are deprived of adequate health care.

Gururaj Mutalik in his article, "The Challenge of PHC" in the *World Health*, Oct. 1980 observed that Primary Health Care—the vital key for attainment of our goal—has two essential dimensions. First and foremost, it is an upward movement of the community towards a better quality of life for its members, primarily through its own efforts but of course with assistance from the government's developmental activities in various sectors. Secondly, primary health care is also the ultimate extension of the health care services to the hearth and home of every member of the community. The whole, in this regard, is truly larger than the sum of these two parts. It is only when these two fundamental facets are woven into an inextricably interlinked process that this magic key can unlock the doors towards better health.

C. Madhavan Nair, Chairman, Indian Space Research Organisation, Chairman, Space Commission and Secretary to Government of India, Department of Space, Bangalore delivered the Convocation Address at the Seventh Convocation of Sri Ramachandra Medical College and Research Institute (Deemed University) on March 29, 2005. He said, "Altruistic

CHART 1.1

Community Health Centre (CHC)
A 30 bed Hospital/Referral Unit for 4 PHCs with Specialised Services

↑

Primary Health Centre (PHC)
A Referral Unit for 6 Sub-Centres
4-6 bed manned with a Medical Officer In-charge and 14 subordinate paramedical staff

↑

Sub-Centre (SC)
Most peripheral contact point between Primary Health Care System and Community manned with one MPW(F)/ANM and One MPW(M)

service is the hallmark of any profession, more so for medicine. You will agree with me that the doctors practice their profession today in a different environment compared to earlier years. Health Care itself has become a commodity today and hospitals are run as business houses, emphasizing often values such as profit, competition, responsibility to stockholders, and services driven by the market forces. Technologies and economics intrude very prominently into the sanctum sanctorum of medicine, threatening the very personal relations between the doctors and the patients. The corporate transformation of medicine inadvertently challenges many of the ideals embedded in the Hippocratic Oath, the tough-stone of your profession for over 2500 years. Obviously, an enlightened medical leadership is essential for preserving the professionalism and ensuring a delicate balance between the purely financial considerations needed to run the institutions and the professional ethics and values emphasized in the medical profession. Your profession's values ultimately must become the anchor that holds to the holy profession of medicine." Excerpts

PRIMARY HEALTH CARE MUST PROVIDE ESSENTIAL PUBLIC HEALTH

Lack of proper utilization of Resources

The International Conference on Primary Health Care, held in Amla-Ata in 1978, had called for a radical change in both the content and design of health services. This was primarily aimed at fostering equity in health services through primary health care, leading to the goal of health for All by the year 2000.

In 1988, ten year after Alma-Ata, it was decided to review developments since Alma-Ata and the prospects for the year 2000 and beyond. The meeting was held in Riga, the capital of the Latvian Republic of the USSR, in March 1988.

Alma-Ata: Reaffirmed at Riga

- Maintaining health for all as a permanent goal of all nations upto and beyond the year 2000.
- Renewing and strengthening strategies for health for all.
- Intensifying social and political strategies for health for all.
- Intensifying social and political action for health for all.
- Developing and mobilizing leadership for health for all.
- Empowering people.
- Making inetersectoral collaboration a force for health for all.
- Strengthening district health systems based on primary health care.
- Planning, preparing and supporting health personnel for health for all.
- Ensuring the development and rational use of science and appropriate technology.
- Overcoming problems that continue to resist solution.

Declaration on Health Development: This historic "Declaration" was adopted by the Ministers of Health of the South-East Asia Region at their Fifteenth Meeting, held in Bangkok, Thailand from 26-29 August, 1997.

The Preamble to the Declaration reads:

> "We, the Member-States of the South-East Asia Region of WHO, take note of the developments in our Region since the social goal of 'health for all', with primary health care as the key approach, was first adopted by the Member-States of WHO two decades ago. Envisaging the scenarios as we move into the next century, recognizing the challenges that lie ahead, as well as the aspirations of our people, we now state our deepest concerns and unstining commitment in this Declaration on Health Developments in our Region. We affirm our unwavering commitment to ensure access to health care to all. Guided by strong political will, we pledge to take action and responsibility to ensure Health for All by mobilizing All for Health. Through collective leadership, we resolve to strengthen the character of the health sector, and to enhance national capacity and Regional solidarity to further this aim. We declare that we will make relentless efforts to realize our people's aspirations."[1]

The International Conference on Primary Health Care was held from 6-12 Sept. 1978 at Alma-Ata, USSR. It was a truly historic landmark as it heralded a new era in health. The Conference adopted various recommendations and the Declaration of Alma-Ata. The Declaration spelt out health in the social and economic contexts, and declared that primary health care was the key to attaining the target of health for all by the year 2000 in a spirit of social justice.

Roots of Primary Health Care

The concept of primary health care for rural populations can be traced back to 1937 when the League of Nations Health Organisation convened an Inter-governmental Conference of Far-Eastern Countries on Rural Hygiene in Bandung, Indonesia. The recommendations made at the conference foreshadowed those made at the International Conference on Primary Health Care at Alma-Ata nearly 40 years later.

The concept of primary health care was at first essentially an expansion of the ideas contained in the concept of basic health services. But it was the Alma-Ata Conference that broadened this concept to encompass a philosophy which went beyond the provision of the first-contact health services. It also provided a political dimension to primary health care. The principles of the PHC philosophy are equity, community involvement, appropriate technology and a multi-sectoral approach.[2]

Alastair Andersen further gives a detailed definition of Primary Health Care[3]: Primary Health Care integrates at the community level all the elements necessary to make an impact on the health status of the people. It calls for measures that are simple and effective in terms of costs, technique and organisation, that are easily accessible, and that improve living conditions. It should use available local resources including manpower, material and funds generated within the community itself as well as strictly essential resources allocated by the government. It should be fully integrated with the national health system and with the other sectors involved in community development—agriculture, education, public works, housing, communications.

Primary health care activities should be carried out by trained health auxiliaries and should reflect real problems and community concerns, and should be based on practicable, modern, scientific knowledge and health technology, as well as accepted and proven traditional healing practices. The treatment of everyday minor injuries, advice and instruction to pregnant and nursing mothers, childhood immunization against common infectious diseases, provision of safe water supplies, building of latrines and waste disposal systems-all these come within the purview of primary health care. At the same time, a higher echelon of medical care should be available to which serious or dubious cases can be referred.

A. NEED, MEANING AND SCOPE OF PRIMARY HEALTH CARE

Need for providing Primary Health Care with Special Emphasis on the Preventive, Promotion and Rehabilitation Aspects

Presently, despite the constraints of resources, there is disproportionate emphasis on the establishment of curative centres—

dispensaries, hospitals, institutions for specialist treatment—the large majority of which are located in the urban areas of the country. The vast majority of those seeking medical relief have to travel long distance to the nearest curative centre, seeking relief for ailments which could have been readily and effectively handled at community level. Also, for want of a well-established referral system, those seeking curative care have the tendency to visit various specialist centres, thus further contributing to congestions, duplication of efforts and consequential waste of resources. To put an end to the existing all-round unsatisfactory situation, it is urgently necessary to restructure the health services within the following broad approach:

1. To provide, within a phased, time-bound programme, a well-dispersed network of comprehensive primary health care services, integrally linked within the extension and health education approach which takes into account the fact that a large majority of health functions can be effectively handled and resolved by the people themselves, with the organised support of volunteers, auxiliaries, paramedicos and adequately trained multi-purpose workers of various grades of skill and competence, of both sexes. There are a large number of private, voluntary organisations active in the health field all over the country. Their services and support would require to be utilized and intermixed with the governmental efforts in an integrated manner.
2. To be effective, the establishment of the primary health care approach would involve large scale transfer of knowledge, simple skills and technologies to Health Volunteers, selected by the communities and enjoying their confidence. The functioning of the front-line workers, selected by the community would require to be related to definitive action plans for the translation of medical and health knowledge into practical action, involving the use of simple and inexpensive interventions which can be readily implemented by persons who have undergone short periods of training. The quality of training of these health guides/workers would be of crucial importance to the success of this approach.
3. The success of the decentralised primary health care system would depend vitally on the organised building-up of individual self-reliance and effective community participation, on the provision of organised, back-up support of the secondary and tertiary levels of the health care services, providing adequate logistical and technical assistance.
4. The decentralisation of services would require the establishment of a well worked out referral system to provide adequate expertise at the various levels of the organisational set-up nearest to the community, depending upon the actual needs and

problems of the area, and thus ensure against the continuation of the existing rush towards the curative centres in the urban areas. The effective establishment of the referral system would also ensure the optimal utilisation of expertise at the higher levels of the hierarchical structure. This approach would not only lead to the progressive improvement of comprehensive health care services at the primary level but also provide for timely attention being available to those in need of urgent specialist care, whether they live in the rural or the urban areas.

5. To ensure that the approach to health care does not merely constitute a collection of disparate health interventions but consists of an integrated package of services seeking to tackle the entire range of poor health conditions, on a broad front, it is necessary to establish a nation-wide chain of sanitary-*cum*-epidemiological stations. The location and functioning of these stations may be between the primary and secondary levels of the hierarchical structure, depending upon the local situations and other relevant consideration. Each such station would require to have suitably trained staff equipped to identify, plan and provide preventive, promotive and mental health care services. It would be beneficial, depending upon the local situations, to establish such stations at the Primary Health Centres. The district health organisation should have, as an integral part of its set-up, a well organised epidemiological unit to coordinate and superintend the functioning of the field stations. These stations would participate in the integrated action plans to eradicate and control diseases, besides tackling specific local environmental health problems. In the urban agglomerations, the municipal and local authorities should be equipped to perform similar functions, being supported with adequate resources and expertise, to effectively deal with local preventable public health problems. The aforesaid approach should be implemented and extended through community participation and contributions, in whatever form possible, to achieve meaningful results within a time-bound programme.
6. The location of curative centres should be related to the populations they serve, keeping in view the densities of population, distances, topography, transport connections. These centres should function within the recommended referral system, the gamut of general specialties required to deal with the local disease patterns being provided as near to the community as reliable, at the secondary level of the hierarchical organisation. The concept of domiciliary care and the field-camps approach should be utilised to the fullest extent, to reduce the pressures on these centres, socially in efforts relating to the control and eradication of blindness, tuberculosis, leprosy,

etc. To maximise the unilisation of available resources, new and additional curative centres should be established only in exceptional cases, the basic attempt being towards the upgradation of existing facilities, at selected locations, the guiding principle being to provide specialists services as near to the beneficiaries as may be possible, within a well-planned network. Expenditure should be reduced through the fullest possible use of cheap locally available building materials, resort to appropriate architectural designs and engineering concepts and by economical investment in the purchase of machineries and equipment, ensuring against avoidable duplication of such acquisitions. It is also necessary to devise effective mechanisms for the repair, maintenance and proper upkeep of all bio-medical equipments to secure their maximum utilisation.

7. With a view to reducing governmental expenditure and fully utilising untapped resources, planned programmes may be devised related to the local requirements and potentials, to encourage the establishment of practice by professional, increased investment by non-governmental agencies in establishing curative centres and by offering organized logistical, financial and technical support to voluntary agencies active in the health field.
8. While the major focus of attention in restructuring the existing governmental health organisations would relate to establishing comprehensive primary health care and public health services, within an integrated referral system, planned attention would also require to be devoted to the establishment of centres equipped to provide speciality and super-speciality services, through a well dispersed network of centres, to ensure that the present and future requirements of specialist treatment are adequately available within the country. To reduce governmental expenditures involved in the establishment of such centres, planned efforts should be made to encourage private investments in such fields so that the majority of such centres, within the governmental set-up, can provide adequate care and treatment to those entitled to free care, the affluent sectors being looked after by the paying clinics. Care would also require to be taken to ensure the appropriate dispersal of such centres, to remove the existing regional imbalances and to provide services within the reach of all, whether residing in the rural or the urban areas.
9. Special, well-coordinated programmes should be launched to provide mental health care as well as medical care and the physical and social rehabilitation of those who are mentally retarded, deaf, dumb, blind, physically disabled, infirm and the aged. Also, suitably organised programmes would require to be

launched to ensure against the prevention of various disabilities.

10. In the establishment of the re-organised services, the first priority should be accorded to provide services to those residing in the tribal, hilly and backward areas as well as to endemic disease affected populations and the vulnerable sections of the society.
11. In the re-organised health service scheme, efforts should be made to ensure adequate mobility of personnel, at all levels of functiong.
12. In the various approaches, set out in (1) to (11) above, organized efforts would require to be made to fully utilise and assist in the enlargement of the services being provided by private voluntary organisations active in the health field. In this context, planning, encouragement and support would also require to be afforded to fresh voluntary efforts, specially those which seek to serve the needs of the rural areas and the urban slums.

According to Dr. Manuel Carballo, "Rural communities the world over have tended to share a common predicament, namely that relative to urban areas they have been underserved and, in many respects, have experienced a quality of life and health inferior to that found in large towns and cities. In terms of overall national investment directed towards them or of the self-development they have been encouraged to generate, rural areas have historically been at a disadvantage and have enjoyed less well developed communication infrastructures, educational facilities and health-related services.[4]

It appears that the benefits of modern medicine would accrue to only a small population. The Regional Director of South-East Asia Region affirmed that most of the governments in the Region recognise that despite every effort to extend the provision of basic health services to the population, during the last three decades. The achievements have not been impressive. In view of this situation, systematic health planning and country health programming have, in some countries, resulted in the formulation of primary health care projects as integral part of the basic health services.[5]

Thus, the health care administration in developing countries has failed to meet the minimum health care needs of its people.

Dr. N.R.E. Fendall has nicely explained the shortfalls of health care system: "If I were asked to compose an epitaph on medicine throughout the twentieth century, it would read: brilliant in its discoveries, superb in its technological breakthrough but woefully inept in its application to those most in need. Medicine will be judged, not in its vast and rapid accumulation of knowledge *per se* but on its trusteeship of that knowledge. We are now experienced and all that remains is the problem of translating what is common knowledge and routine medicine and hence practice, to the world. The implementation gap must be closed."[6]

The basic question which needs to be answered is: What model of administration on health care can meet the health care needs of all the people in the developing world? What are the constituents of such a model? Past experience has amply made clear that by adoption and uncritical transfer of the model health systems from the developed to the developing world, the basic health needs of the people in the developing world cannot be fulfiled. Henry R. Labouisse, Executive Director of UNICEF, vehemently held while submitting to the First International Conference on Primary Health Care, "The developing countries have come to realise that the conventional approach inherited from industrialised countries was hopelessly inappropriate when it came to meet, within a reasonable period of time, the health care needs of these vast populations. And the industrialised countries themselves after making spectacular advances in the field of medicine and building up services with expensive facilities, sophisticated technology and highly specialised personnel, are now finding themselves burdened with ruinous medical care systems with which they are unable to provide proper health protection to their own very numerous people. So, there has to be change everywhere."

It has been recognised and accepted that the health care services, which exist in most parts of the world, have not been meeting the basic needs of very large groups of the population, especially in the developing countries.

Urban Primary Health Care

Urban health is not better than rural health as far as the poor are concerned. Disaggregated health indices show that the health of the urban poor (in the sums and scattered through the towns and cities) is often worse. There is need for comprehensive health care, especially in the slums, where the people do not have social support, which is present in the rural areas.

Meaning and Strategy

The most effective and acceptable form of health system for the people in the developing world has to be evolved by the community itself. Development is indigenous to each society and builds primarily on a country's resources, mainly land and people. Each country must develop its own model for social fulfilment. This will enlarge the capacity of individuals and communities to create and innovate. The mobilisation of the energies and resources of the people, especially the rural poor themselves, emerges as the key factor in increasing their productivity and self-reliance. Such mobilisation assumes the formation, adaptation and strengthening of community structures. Since each country differs from others in its resources and needs, the concept of Country Health Programme (CHP) must be practised by every country. It is a pragmatic approach, which tailors the services precisely to the national situation. In his Preface to the Annual Report for 1975, Dr. Mahler said that, "Such programming is a long-term process, not a one-time intensive planning effort. In order to attain the systematic development of health programmes and services, countries that have not already done so well need to set-up permanent mechanism for formulating health policies and translating these policies into operational programmes.

This implies a continuing process of planning, implementing, monitoring, controlling, evaluating and replanning—a truly new approach for most countries and the need for appropriate mechanism to launch the venture and maintain its dynamism which will continue for the foreseeable future. Community Health Programming would give high priority to the needs of the underserved. Thus, the developing countries must design their own health care delivery models to provide primary health care to all its people. Let us now define the meaning and essential features of such care, commonly known as Primary Health Care.

Nature of Primary Health Care

The WHO defined Primary Health Care as "essential health care made universally accessible to individuals and families in the community by means acceptable to them through their full participation and at a cost that the community and country can afford. It forms an integral part both of the country's health system of which it is the nucleus and of the overall social and economic development of the community."[7]

The first International Conference on Primary Health Care defined it as "essential health care based on scientifically sound and socially acceptable methods and technology made universally acceptable to individuals and families in the community through their full participation and at a cost that the community and country can afford to maintain at every stage of their development in a spirit of self-reliance and self-determination." There are many different ways of defining primary health care. The 28th *World Health* Assembly accepted the working definition of primary health care. According to this definition, primary health care is taken to mean, health approach which integrates at the community level all the elements necessary to make an impact upon the state of health of the people. Such an approach should be an integral part of the national health care system. It is an expression or response to the fundamental human needs of how a person can know of and be assisted in the actions required to live a healthy life and where a person can go if he or she needs relief from pain or suffering. A response to such needs must be a series of simple and effective measures in terms of cost, technique and organisation which are easily accessible to the people in need and which assist in improving the living conditions of individuals, families and communities. These include preventive; promotive, curative and rehabilitative health measures and community development activities.[8]

WHO's former Director General, urged to give thrust to Primary Health Care. To quote him:

"WHO is proposing a simple yet dynamic approach to health, a powerful strategy to intensity and move forward the integration of health care, disease prevention and rehabilitation. It is based on an inclusive vision of health, comprising the individual, the family, community and the environment, in which families serve as entry points for health promotion, disease prevention and care.[9]

In short, we can say that primary health care is an approach which integrates at the community level all the elements necessary to make an impact upon the health status of the people. Primary Health Care should not be understood as primitive care. It uses simple administrative structures, procedures and operates—within the community but "it is an essential first level in a scale of services and is in no way inferior." It is providing the benefits of modern medicine to the community through better methods based upon the socio-economic conditions prevalent in each country. It was mentioned by a delegate from Switzerland—"To wish to promote primary health services does not signify the establishment of two parallel or juxtaposed systems of which one is for the poor and the other, the classic system, more complex, more sophisticated, is reserved for the rich. The goal is to set-up a system where primary health care forms the base of a structure accessible to all, upon which other levels of care can be grafted and can develop." Gururaj Mutalik in his article, "The Challenge of PHC" rightly says that Primary Health Care—the vital key for attainment of our goal—has two essential dimensions. First and foremost, it is an upward movement of the community towards a better quality of life for its members, primarily through its own efforts but of course with assistance from the government's developmental activities in various sectors. Secondly, primary health care is also the ultimate extension of the health care services to the health and home of every member of the community. The whole, in this regard, is truly larger than the sum of these two parts. It is only when these two fundamental facets are woven into an inextricably interlinked process that this magic key can unlock the doors towards better health. The spread of primary health care that is seen in the countries of the South-East Asia Region today is indeed very encouraging.

Jagdambi Prasad Yadav, in his presidential address delivered at the Twentieth Convocation of IIPI (Bombay, 15 July, 1978), defined the philosophy of the Primary Health Care as: "The philosophy of the community health workers' scheme is to place people's health in people's hand. It is well-known that in most parts of rural India even rudimentary public health facilities are lacking from times immemorial. The CHW's scheme is designed to take health care to door-steps of people. It is hoped that the community health workers will bridge the gap between rural community and health care-preventive, promotional and curative."

Speaking on the new health policy, Shri Morarji Desai, former Prime Minister of India, said: "Whatever development we want to do in the country depends upon the capacity of the people to do their work efficiently and to go on increasing their productive capacity in any field of work, that they can take up. And if this is to be done, health becomes a very primary condition. Unless a person enjoys fairly good health, it will not be possible for him to do work efficiently. It is, therefore, necessary for us to see that the people of the country are enabled to maintain their health in a fairly good manner, so that they are able to follow their work and profession efficiently and live also a healthy life."

Essentials

1. Primary Health should be shaped around the lifestyles of the people to be served.
2. The local people should be actively involved in planning health care so that it suits their needs and priorities.
3. The health care offered should make maximum use of community resources.
4. Primary Health Care should not only deal with the prevention and cure of disease but also promote health, in the community, in the family and in the individual.
5. All health interventions should take place in or as near as possible to the patient's home and be carried out by the worker most simply (but adequately) trained to give the treatment in question.
6. Other services, in particular supplies, supervision and referral and technical support, should be designed to support the needs at the local level.
7. Comprehensiveness—Primary Health Centre has to be comprehensive. It has to include
   - A School health
   - Health Education and its promotion
   - Promotion of nutrition
   - Adequate supply of safe water
   - Basic sanitation
   - Maternal and child care and family welfare services
   - Immunisation against the major infectious diseases
   - Prevention and control of the locally endemic diseases
   - Appropriate treatment for common diseases in injuries
   - Use of Indigenous system of Health

PRINCIPLES (See Chart 1.2)

Prim ary Health Care is part of human development in social, educational and economic spheres. It rests on the following 8 principles:

I. Equitable Distribution

Health services should be available to all sections of the society with

CHART 1.2

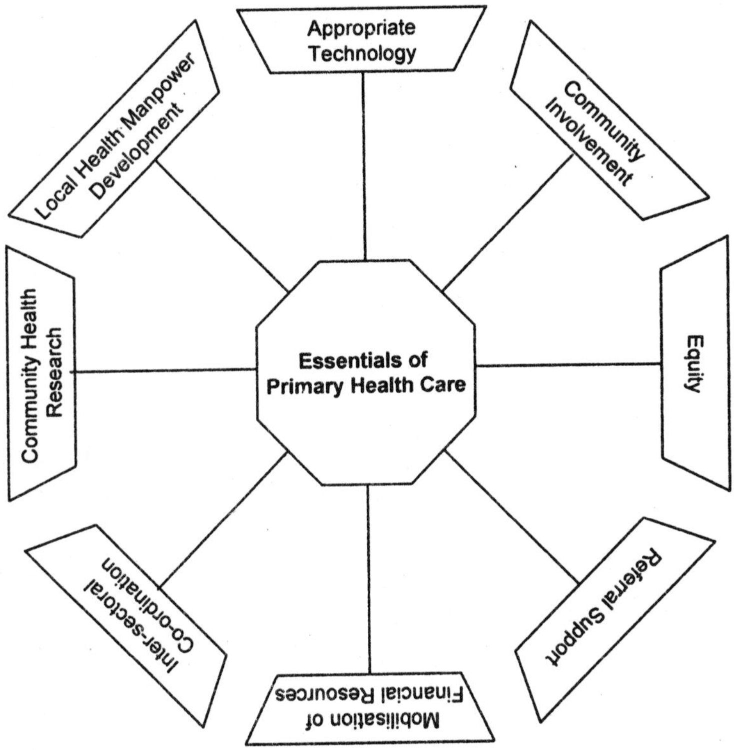

special attention to the needy and vulnerable groups. Primary Health Care aims at correcting urban-rural imbalance and bringing health services as near to people's homes as possible. It should be supported by higher level of health care to which the needy can be referred.

2. Community Involvement

The involvement of individuals, families and communities in promotion of their own health and welfare, including self-care, is an essential ingredient of Primary Health Care. The community should participate in the planning, implementation and maintenance of health services. The active role of communities in the development process is essential. The negative image of patients and communities passively receiving health care judged appropriate by others, having no voice in assessing their heath needs, planning for services, and providing and evaluating services is bleak indeed. Fundamental to the development process is the involvement of the people who are most affected. At least two strong factors are at work here. One is the importance of respect for the people, human dignity and trustful sharing. The other is that often the critical determinants of health or illness are in the hands of the community,

CHART 1.3

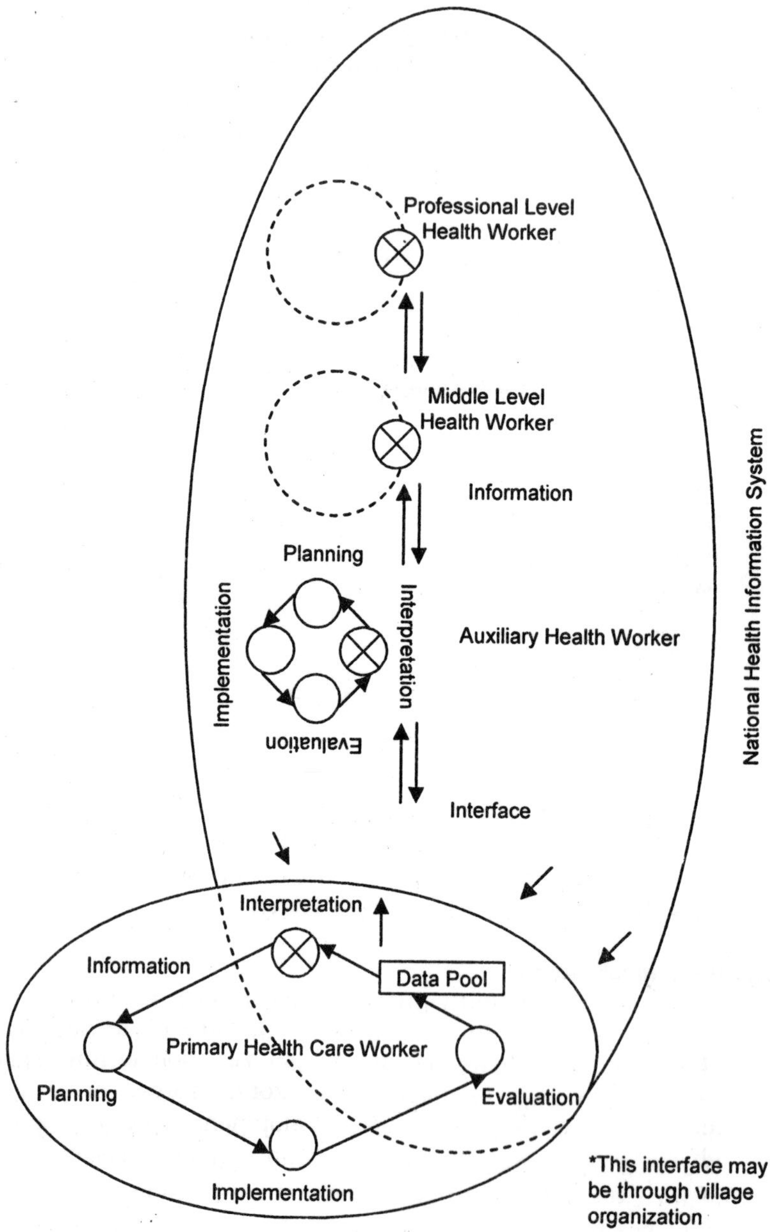

both in understanding the nature of the problems and participating in finding solutions to those problems. To ignore these two major contributions to be made by the community is to miss the essential resource for health and development.

Examples of community participation include village development committees, mothers' clubs, village drug cooperatives, village funds for nutrition, community-based health insurance schemes and health care schemes. The community-based approach is also being developed to address emerging problems such as health for the elderly and home care for persons with chronic degenerative diseases. These innovations are being shared among the Member-States in the Region.

The involvement of health-related sectors is facilitated when the community is mobilized. To mention some examples, the Basic Minimum Needs approach of Thailand involves four major sectors (health, local government, education and agriculture). In Indonesia, the Family Welfare Movement's cadres are volunteers who play important roles in health, women and family development. The involvement of district administrators in Bhutan has been instrumental in the promotion of anti-smoking environment and in the development of a model village approach, which seeks to improve the village environment, including water supply, sanitation, housing and roads. The mandating of rural development committees in India, with men and women elected by the rural community (Panchayati Raj) through a constitutional amendment, is expected to lead to enhanced community participation in development, including health.[10]

3. Multi-Sectoral Approach

One of the basic tenets of Primary Health Care is that full health cannot be provided by the health sector alone. It requires the joint efforts of the health sector and other health-related sectors. Primary Health Care should be set in context of integrated development to include health, housing, transport, water and sanitation, nutrition, agriculture, education, community development including women's development.

The role of education in health development, including family planning, cannot be overemphasized. The literacy rate, in particular the functional literacy rate of women, is cardinal to health development. Health is so much in the hands of women that female literacy rate becomes crucial. Likewise, the education of children is important. As with growth, so with education, it is the length of time that improved rates of literacy have prevailed that makes a difference. There is much variation in this regard amongst the countries of the Region. The horizontal spread of primary education seems more critical for health development than the vertical spread of higher education to selected population segments. For example, the success of clean water and environmental sanitation is critically dependent upon education in the hygienic use of water and appropriate disposal of wastes.

Health professionals often lack familiarity with the methods and tools which could predict health futures, and lack the skills needed to establish linkages with other sectors. A major challenge for them is to extend their horizons and pursue health as an achievable social goal.

Since medicine alone cannot deal with ill-health caused by adverse socio-economic conditions, there is a need to involve professionals of other health-related sectors such as health economists and social scientists to provide other missing but vital inputs, necessary for health planning and health development. Such inputs would also provide health planners with the vision and understanding on the ongoing demographic, social and political changes and make them responsive to such changes.

In other words, for a clear vision of the future, it is imperative that health issues in Region are viewed holistically, that is, in the context not merely of epidemiological trends and forecasts, but also within the cultures and attitudes prevailing among administrators, professionals and health workers.

4. Appropriate Technology

This does not mean cheap, primitive technology for the poor. It calls for scientifically sound materials and methods that are socially acceptable, directed against relevant health problems. The examples are domiciliary treatment as against sanatorium treatment for Tuberculosis patients, sputum examination for mass Tuberculosis Screening, immunisation by the health workers through outreach sessions, ORS, simple weighing scales, growth monitoring cares, collection of blood smear for malaria control programme.

Science should be accorded a central role in health development. The scientific capacity of developing countries should be seen as essential components of international health development.

First, it must be recognized that science and health technology have an irreplaceable role in advancing health and human development. Here is where both developed and developing countries must join hands in using scientific skills to advance understanding of problems as they exist in local settings or as they move across national boundaries. Science and the sciences—basic, clinical, public health, social, economic, information—have an essential place in the processes related to health development.

Second, science should play a crucial role in advancing the equitable pursuit of health development, by providing appropriate, affordable user-friendly technological applications at the peripheral level of health care so that improvements can be achieved even in the face of continued scarcity of resources. For example, the analyses of health determinants and distribution of burden of disease make it possible to define differential needs for health care and to monitor progress in responding to those needs—steps that are at the heart of equity-oriented and rights-oriented approaches to health.

Third, there is a need to bridge the gaps between research and policy-makers. Mechanisms of cooperation should be further developed and partnerships built between researchers and health managers, so that priority projects maybe supported and results implemented in more efficient and cost-effective ways. It is important to recognize the frequently-found gaps between research and policy-making that are imperative to close if the rigorous thinking of science is to bear on the socially and developmentally sensitive processes of policy-making. Too often, researchers and policy-makers come from widely diverse personal and professional backgrounds and have difficulty entering into a true sharing relationship that is crucial to overcoming threats to health and well-being. Any form of partnership must be built sensitively and insistently, or the benefits of science risk being lost to societal needs.

Fourth, science serves the essential role of broadening understanding of what is meant by health and illness, and what the parameters are or should be of pursuing health for all. Evidence-based or research-based thinking and decision-making should have prominent place in efforts to advance health development. For example, recent understandings of mental health as a disease burden seen in the form of morbidity have led to the appreciation of a much greater prevalence, whereas it had tended to be overlooked when measured mainly in terms of mortality. In order to promote evidence-based medical and public health practice, knowledge and skills in ramdomized clinical trials must be developed. This is an area that needs to be promoted widely in the Region to promote science-based public health.

Fifth, research needs to be open to the participation of those who might be affected by the research and its findings. This means considering the use of research methodologies such as action research and participatory research in situations where both the research and the participants would benefit. Clearly, there would have to be close interactions and a spirit of sharing between the subjects and the experienced researchers.

Sixth, a growing challenge to science exists in the massive poverty settings of Asia, where development failures loom as both determinants of illness and impediments to solutions, where traditional technology-centred health interventions are rendered ineffective, and where risk factors for morbidity and mortality are immersed in social, economic and environmental complexity. The science-based approaches need to discern risk factors in relation to specific vulnerable groups, and also to guide the search for interventions that have the possibility of countering mortality-enhancing features of the poverty-setting.

Seventh, the twenty-first century will be characterized by expansion and improvement of service delivery systems. Unless current constraints in delivery of services are corrected, introduction of new technologies will do little to expand utilization. Each new technology introduced must be user-friendly and an appropriate balance between new methods and service delivery contexts has to be established. There are many gaps which still need to be bridged through research between product development and its incorporation in the service sector. Inter-personal dynamics between users and providers also need to be taken into account. Technology driven approaches must consider that their effective functioning would depend upon the strengths and weaknesses of existing systems.

Eighth, this should be a widely shared effort, across the Region and internationally, and the building of the scientific capacities of developing countries should be seen as an essential component of the international pursuit of health development. Science lays out the guidelines, indicators and measures by which we can monitor and evaluate our pursuit of health-for-all. It is of major importance that the elements of health for all strategies, including equity, be constructed on scientifically sound and socially sensitive concepts, and that the indicators for measuring progress in pursuit of health for all be widely accepted by the communities of scientists and policy-makers.[11]

5. Prevention of Disease and Promotion of Health

This is the basic strategy of Primary Health Care. All activities use this strategy as it is cost effective to prevent diseases than to treat the same.

6. Development of Effective Referral Support

There is a need to develop proper referral support of secondary and tertiary levels.

7. Medical and Health Services Research including innovative approaches

Innovative approaches in the following areas aimed at responding to the socio-economic and political changes and epidemiological transitions that are taking place will be needed: How to sustain the commitment to PHC and HFA principles? How to reorient health systems (health care reform)? How to intensify efforts to increase managerial capabilities? What are the innovative measures needed to respond to the transition: moving from quantity to quality, health for the underserved or underprivileged, improving the shape of human resources for health, partnerships in health development, community actions for health, health system research?

Considering the vast numbers of people in India the majority live in rural areas but with an expanding proportion in urban settings, the need for networks of health services developed as close as possible to these populations and adapted to their changing needs is a challenging priority. Meanwhile, change will inevitably come in the ways health services are planned, financed and managed, and new approaches to health care reform will be undenaken in various countries. Countries in the Region will want to be aware of these approaches and be prepared to test and possibly absorb those that could be useful to them.

Health sector reforms should take place as sustained process of fundamental change in the context of health policy and health institutional arrangements. They are not sequential, nor incremental processes. The main areas of reform are: (1) reorienting and restructuring of ministries of health, including publicly-financed and organized services; (2) broadening the health financing options; (3) improving the performance of civil service, including decentralization, and (4) expanding partnerships. Thus, it may be said that it is essential to develop a new framework for public health action to have a long-term perspective, and to strengthen national capabilities, infrastructure and technologies which can be sustained with available resources.

8. Health Manpower Development

Primary health care requires development and mobilisation of resources, especially trained medical staff. Dynamic linkages between planning, production and utilization of health personnel are essential. Imbedded within such systems are pathways for leadership development.

Too often, the training of health personnel follows a pattern of yesterday's view of health care, or even of only the clinical care, and falls seriously short of meeting today's and tomorrow's requirement for personnel who can lead or participate in effective health services responding to people's needs.

9. Availability of Medicine

Primary Health Care can only be truly effective if even the most remote health can rely on receiving the regular supply supplies of affordable drugs of good quality and if health workers are trained in their use of medicines are not available at the health centre, people lose confidence in the whole system and will seek other remedies, usually from sources unqualified to diagnose or prescribe.

Muthu Subramanian in his article "Bridging the Gaps" in the *World Health* March, 1995—outlines four priorities for international action. These are as follows:

- Allocating resources to support those countries and population groups where the minimum levels set by the global targets for Health for all by the year 2000 have not yet been reached. Low-income, severely indebted, least developed countries, mostly in Sub-Saharan Africa, should be the focus of an intensive campaign for international funding and technical support to establish and sustain an effective health infrastructure, particularly at the community level.
- Improving labour productivity by enhancing the health of the work-force and of school children (the potential workforce) while ensuring that the poor, particularly families with young children and the elderly, have access to primary health care. Special initiatives should be launched to improve the status of women.
- Improving equity of access to health and not merely to health care as the basis for public health policy for the future. Long-term strategies should address simultaneously the emerging double burden of diseases and conditions in the developing world, and increased efforts must be made to mobilize contributions from other sectors such as education, agriculture and the environment for achieving better health for all.

- Strengthening the capabilities of Member-States in epidemiological surveillance and emergency management in the context of sustainable development.

An article in the *World Health,* May-June 1992 indicates that communities and individuals have always been concerned with their health and participated in health activities. During the 20th century such participation has become more effective through the creation of voluntary organisations at local, national and international levels. People are also much better informed about health matters. The policy, adopted at the conference on Primary Health Care in Alma-Ata in 1978, of involving communities in health development in a more organized way has accelerated this trend. Thus, in 1992 the World Health Organisation could report that most countries consider community involvement in health not only a political necessity but also an important mechanism for planning, implementing and evaluating health programmes.

Health matters are frequently discussed in local communities (1). In many countries these communities are represented in health councils and hospital boards, and students participate in school health committees. Health is also a popular theme in newspapers, magazines, radio and television.

Health posts and health centres are often built by communities which provide voluntary labour (2) and materials. It is important that the construction plans should be coordinated with the Government, since the community will expect the Government to cover the staff salaries and the cost of drugs, equipment, transport and so on.

People influence health policies through consumer associations and other groups such as patient groups. Recently some of the most active pressure groups have been concerned with the deterioration of environment (3).

Community health workers, who are selected and often paid by their local communities, provide the needed health care (4); in many parts of the world they are the only permanent health workers in villages. Many non-governmental organisations also provide health care, as well as support to patients and their families, home care, and other services through volunteers.

Environmental sanitation has traditionally been a field where male volunteers have done much of the work; they install water pumps (5), construct small swere systems, and maintain and repair them. Women have become increasingly involved in such activities as repairing and maintaining handpumps.

Most health care is provided by the family, particularly the mothers. Increasingly, fathers and other family members are becoming involved in such activities as rehabilitation of the handicapped (6) Family members can also give oral rehydration for diarrhea, take care of the sick and the elderly, and provide many other services.

Elements

In 1978, WHO identified eight elements of Primary Health Care:

1. Promotion of food supplies and proper nutrition.
2. Education about health problems and their control.
3. Safe water supply.
4. Basic sanitation.
5. Mother and child health including family planning.
6. Immunisation against infectious diseases and injuries.
7. Prevention and control of locally endemic diseases.
8. Treatment of common diseases and injuries.

Alma Ata Declaration (1978)

In the International Conference on Primary Health Care, jointly organized by the WHO and UNICEF in Alma Ata, USSR in September 1978, fundamental principles of health development were enunciated and a declaration was made which was endorsed by the 30th World Health Assembly (1977). This is popularly known as Health for All (HFA) and it is to be achieved through primary health care approach in a spirit of social justice and as a part of overall development. (See Appendices I and III for Alma Ata Declaration and Alma Ata Recommendations).

Basic Concepts: Parameters for Assessment of Primary Health Care (Chart 1.4)

1. Availability of Health Services

The availability of health services is taken to mean the physical presence of a health service provider, who constitutes a primary entry point to the health service system, either providing the service directly, or providing referral to another health care provider at an appropriate facility level.

2. Accessibility of Health Services

"Accessibility" is taken to mean the composite of the characteristics of health services, which facilitate or obstruct their utilization by potential consumers. Accessibility also incorporates such factors as the availability of needed drugs and supplies; affordable costs to consumers who seek and receive services, including service cost, transportation cost, and cost in time, and social factors relating to the consumer provider interaction, such as the service provider's attitude towards and rapport with consumers.

3.. Acceptability and Acceptance of Health Services

The proof of accessibility and acceptability of health services is "acceptance" of health services, that is the actual utilization of health services or the expressed demand for services by consumers. W.A. Hassouna in his article, "A Strategy against poverty", says that in most

CHART 1.4

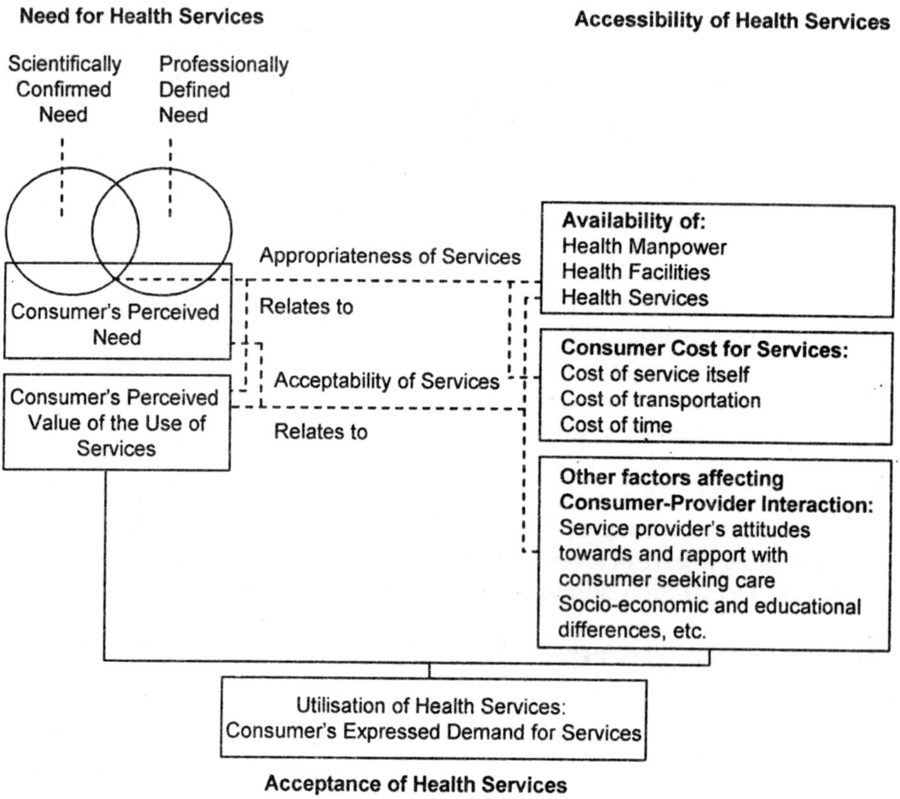

developing and some developed countries, governments have been the major providers of preventive and curative health care. These services used to be accessible to the poor since they were provided without charge. But the unprecedented escalation of the cost of health services in the last ten years and the adoption of economic reforms which usually resulted in sizeable reductions of allocations for health services have greatly reduced the access of the poor to government health services. Such reforms have affected curative more than preventive care since many governments provide the latter free or at minimal cost.

Several ways have been adopted in various countries to increase access to health services, all of which are aimed at reducing the patient's economic burden. Unfortunately, most of the approaches, such as health insurance and cost-sharing, are geared to helping middle-income groups rather than the poor, who cannot afford to pay insurance premiums or even reduced fees, and in many cases will not have the cash to pay for health services when they are seriously sick. It seems clear that what is needed is a system that ensures for the poor a reasonable access to health services with a minimal economic burden. This could be done by including specific health benefits within a compulsory social insurance system or making available interest-free loans from group savings to be used in case of sickness.

Certainly, increasing access to health services as a strategy for poverty alleviation should be dealt with in a comprehensive manner that takes into account physical, social, cultural and economic factors. The ultimate aim should be to put "reasonable quality of care" at an affordable cost within the reach of the poor, rather than offering low quality of care at cheaper prices.

We must, however, be clear that Health for all does not mean that in the year 2000, nobody will be sick or disabled nor does it mean that in the year 2000, doctors and nurses will provide medical care for every body in the world. It does mean that health begins at home, in schools, and in working places. It does mean that the people will use better approaches than they do now for preventing diseases and reducing unavoidable illness and disability and better ways of growing up, growing old, and dying, gracefully.

B. GENERAL PRINCIPLES OF PRIMARY HEALTH CARE DEVELOPMENT

(1) Increasing involvement of the community in all aspects of programmmg.
(2) Adaptation of local health service personnel to Primary Health Care.
(3) The closer links of health with general development.
(4) Need of national resources and political will to support Primary Health Care.

1. Participation: It Means Self-motion[12]

It gives the ordinary citizen a chance to show his willingness to carry out constructive public work and to demonstrate his good citizenship by other means than periodically exercising his right to vote.[13] It means the full involvement of the community in the planning, implementation and control of Primary Health Care, People's involvement has to be understood in the following four senses:

(i) Participation and decision-making, such as in the identification, development priorities and planning of development programmes, projects and activities;
(ii) Participation in monitoring and evaluation of development programmes and projects;
(iii) Participation in implementation of development programmes and projects; and
(iv) Participation in sharing the benefits of development.[14]

Such participation can be mobilised if the community is properly educated. This education would help them pinpoint the obstacles to development. In the field of health. this would enable them to diagnose their health problems and to deal with their problems in the most effective way. When the community is enlightened, every man and woman would become a sacred teacher. Man's energy is the most powerful tool of health and socio-economic development.[15] "It does not tally with reality to view the political and administrative environment solely in terms of a Central Government acting upon an inert periphery."[16] According to Professor Ramalingaswami, Ex-Director General ICMR:

> "An indigenous health system based on community health derived personnel is needed in which the services are economical, acceptable, continuous and belong to the people."[17]

Community participation must not become an amorphous and abstract slogan like all other socio-political entities; a community comprises different and often conflicting interests. Community participation will only have real meaning when a democratic and genuinely participatory system prevails, political power must be in the hands of the people and not in those of interested groups, such as local chiefs and property holders. The poor individually cannot stand up or speak up for their rights and privileges and remain meek spectators in the development process. So, participation by the majority is possible only if they are mobilised. Mobilisation should be done tactfully. To gain the confidence of the poor, we must guard against the strong opposition by the power group in the village.

2. Adaptation of Local Health Service Personnel to Primary Health Care and their Utilisation

The Primary Health Care envisages the provision of health care through trained personnel indigenous to the community. This worker is chosen from the village and by the village and trained to deliver elementary integrated health service. Such workers properly trained through well-designed short-term courses can provide effective, acceptable and inexpensive health care to the community. According to WHO: "Primary Health Care is likely to be most effective if it employs means that are understood and accepted by the community and applied by community health workers at a cost the community and the country can afford. These community health workers, including traditional practitioners where applicable, will function best if they are properly trained socially and technically to respond to the community's expressed health needs. The skills that community health workers require and their consequent training will vary widely throughout the world. But whatever their level of skill, it is important that they understand the real health needs of the communities they serve and they gain the active confidence and backing of the people." Professor V. Ramalingaswami, while receiving the Leon Bernard

Foundation Award stressed that this system of community-based health services employing auxiliaries must not be understood by the people as "providing inferior medicine to the rural poor." He went on—"An Auxiliary is a health educator, a rudimentary physician, a social worker and a preventive person, all in one. . . .The education and training of auxiliaries is the most challenging task that medicine faces today. Auxiliaries served to bridge the catastrophic separation between hospital-based, fragmented, episodic medicine and mass public health. The principles of educational science and technology must diffuse into their training programmes. It is on our willingness and ability to experiment with auxiliary training programmes that the chances of success will depend. The moment modern medicine penetrates the social veil in developing countries, that is the moment of triumph of modern medicine. Here is medicine in the raw, medicine rooted in the reality of rural life."[18]

3. The Closer links with General Development

Community health actions cannot be effective in isolation. These must be linked with the effort of total community development. These should be supported by a community-based organisation. As WHO has stated "since Primary Health Care is an integral part both of the community's health system and of overall economic and social development without which it is bound to fail, it has to be coordinated on a national basis with the other sectors that contribute to a country's total development strategy."[19]

4. National Resources and Political Will to Support Primary Health Care

National resources are needed to support primary health care. We have to find resources partly from the community and partly from the national exchequer. We have to change priorities of investment in the interest of the poor. The responsibility of the state must be there to provide continuous support in terms of technical knowledge, guidance and supervision, training, supplies and maintenance, the solving of specific problems, and the care of patients referred to other levels of the health system. The presence of a supportive health service infrastructure is essential for primary health care. Political leadership must also understand and appreciate the needs and aspirations of the rural poor. We are sure to provide an acceptable level of health to all the people by the year 2010 if each government has the political initiative, courage, boldness, innovation to reorient for the population, its health priorities according to their socio-economic conditions.

A Sivathanu Pillai, Distinguished Scientists, Chief Controller, Research and Development, Defence Research and Development Organisation, GOI New Delhi in his convocation address on 29th June 2005 observed that seventy per cent of our population resides in villages and they are deprived from modern medical facilities. Therefore health care needs to be improved in a big way in rural areas. The advent of communication technology and IT have made telemedicine a popular means of treatment. By using telemedicine it is possible to connect remote villages to major hospitals wherein a patient's condition is diagnosed by a doctor in the hospital and his views communicated through the link. Such systems have been installed by ISRO connecting super specialty hospitals to remote areas like Andaman and Nicobar Islands, Lakshadweep, etc.

Health care can be improved in rural areas by Providing Urban Amenities in Rural Areas (PURA) by providing proper health infrastructure, physical and electronic connectivity's. The PURA model is an annular ring shaped town connecting 10 to 15 villages resulting in the decrease in transportation time, and having access to facilities like schools, hospitals, internet kiosks, etc. Besides public health centers, mobile clinics can be deployed in such areas.

5. Role of WHO

Mohamed Abdelmoumene in his article, "To Support the poorest of the Poor", in the *World Health,* March 1990 clearly gave his remarks that the poorest countries often have great difficulty in accurately analyzing situations, putting integrated strategies into effect and managing their meager resources rationally.

Moreover, the work of the international organisations and even that of the different programmes of WHO is often insufficiently coordinated at the national level. This can lead to situations where certain activities are duplicated while others—which may well be the most essential—are sadly lacking. WHO as well as its member-countries are ready to re-think the direction of their efforts and to re-cast the firmly held notions of the past, so as to create a new approach which will truly permit ideas to be transformed into concrete realities.

The countries have committed themselves to taking a long hard look at their priorities in the light of the resources at their disposal, even if this might oblige them to start from scratch.

For its part, WHO commits itself to re-examine the way its own resources are allocated, to show more flexibility in the use of funds within the countries, and to ensure a better integration of its activities.[20]

Over and above all this, the Organisation will further reinforce the offices of the WHO representatives in the countries concerned, since they will have a crucial role to play in the new initiative. The WHO representatives will assist the countries to improve their capacity for planning, programming and management in the health sector, so as to arrive at better-integrated, well-coordinated and more realistic national health plans. They will thus seek to harmonise international health activities in such a way as to ensure that the health services use resources to the best possible advantage, serving all the possible advantage, serving all the population without exception. WHO hopes in this way to succeed in anchoring its activities in the very heart of each country, and bringing about a truly effective partnership.

C. EXPERIMENTS OF PHC IN DIFFERENT PARTS OF THE WORLD

In this section we would review (on the basis of case studies conducted by the health experts in different parts of the world) the progress of the implementation of primary health care. After this we shall discuss the analysis of primary health care in India.

Experiment of Old Soviet Union (Kazakhstan)[21]

Before the Russian Revolution of 1917, Soviet Kazakhstan was one of the most backward and neglected provinces of Tsarist Russia. Not more than two per cent of the total population could read and write. In the field of health, there was not a single medical institution and the number of medical personnel was negligible. Today, this region enjoys all the health facilities. Five medical schools and 26 junior medical colleges have helped to train some 40,000 doctors and more than 130,000 intermediate level medical workers. The bed-population ratio is 12:4.

After the revolution, primary health care formed the basis of the health system. It provided service through out-patient and posts staffed by midwives and fieldscher (medical auxiliaries). Each post is staffed by a nurse as well as a fieldscher and a midwife and covers about five hundred people. Those posts enlist the support of the population to carry out health activities. These also train assistants voluntary health workers from the Red Cross Society. The posts are also helped in their work by members of the rural workers' councils, by school teachers, by students, by rural youth groups, and by the managements of collective and state farms. The function of each post is to organise and carry out primary preventive health measures, i.e., immunization, home visiting of patients and new born babies, sanitary inspection of land and installations, primary epidemic, central measures, health education, etc. In addition, the post carries out primary curative measures including treating patients, carrying out instruction to the rural or district physician, or referring patients to the physician for medical advice/treatment. There is a medical store attached to every post.

Primary Health Care in Kazakhstan as in all the erstwhile Republics of the Soviet Union is closely integrated with socio-economic plans of the rural districts and also with the overall medical care system.

Soviet Kazakhstan had 60 years experience in the organisation and successful development of a national public health system and of primary health care. The conditions under which the people of the Republic were able, virtually from scratch, to build up a public health service closely resemble conditions in developing countries that are still experiencing the aftermath of colonial oppression. The study of Kazakhstan public health experience should therefore prove useful for all public health administrators particularly for representatives of the developing countries.

Experiments of Columbia[22]

The problems of health in Columbia is typical of the situation in most developing countries. In tact, mortality rate was very high, 45 per cent of the rural population have no access to safe drinking water. The former health system has not been meeting existing demands of the population. Thirty-six per cent of the population in rural and urban slums never or rarely use doctors or hospitals. They are organising a new mode, called M.A.C. system (Modulo de Amplication de Cobertura). Dr. Norberto Martinez explained the thinking behind it. We were aiming at people who had been inaccessible, culturally, economically and geographically to formal health provision. There were rural people and rural migrate living in belts of misery around the cities, not participating in modern economic and social life. These people were not using the health services, so we needed to build a bridge between them and the services by using auxiliaries drawn from their own communities. High technology was not appropriate because it cost much and our resources were limited. Moreover, most people were dying of a few basic diseases that could be cured or prevented by using a fairly simple technology without the need for highly qualified personnel.

The key to the new system is Columbias own brand of the barefoot doctor selected from the area to be served. These workers are trained for four months and receive an allowance of US $ 850 a month. They serve 3,000 people in the fringe urban areas or 1,000 in the more scattered rural areas. Each group of 6 workers is backed by a MAC health centre to which they can refer difficult cases.

"It is perhaps too soon to judge just how effective the MAC system will be. But even in its two years, it seems to have reached out to a section of the population previously untouched by the health services. It has made a start on the crucial vaccinations and environmental health campaigns that will prevent so much disease. Above all, it has begun to get people out of their traditional fatalistic attitudes which lead them to suffer patiently, believing that basically nothing could or should be done about it unless they were at deaths door. The marginal millions of Columbians are becoming actively interested in doing something individually and collectively to improve their own health."

Experiments in Thailand[23]

More than half of Thailand's approximately 7500 graduate physicians live and practice in Bangkok. The doctor-population ratio was 1:22,070 for the provinces and 1:84,000 for the countryside. The people in the countryside do not have any access to medical care. WHO (UNICEF assisted) provincial health care project was formulated whereby it is planned to train 22,400 village health volunteers, about 200,000 village health communicators, 2800 tambon doctors and 8400 granny midwives during the next five years. Although Thailand still has a long way to go before health care reaches all its citizens, the adoption of Primary Health

Care programmes will do much to alleviate the feeling of hopelessness that many villagers had thought was their inevitable fate.

Experiments of Costa Rica and Mexico[24]

There were no organised health services available in these countries. The shortage of health workers hampered the development of health services. In 1972 WHO and other agencies began collaborating in a local development effort (PRODESCH) to identify and stimulate the type of activities that could be meaningfully undertaken by the community itself. The progress is going on. They are both examples of how communities with outside support can resolve their own problems and thus can generate enough confidence in themselves to go ahead with other socio-economic efforts.

Most of the countries in Asia, Africa and Latin America have either introduced or are planning to introduce Primary Health Care system to provide health care to the unprivileged section of their countries. This is a challenging task which requires constant, continuous and persistent efforts of their governments and especially the health departments. All these countries may learn from each other's experiences and improve the mechanism of primary health care programmes. If such programmes are successful, it is sure that the health care would be available to all the people in the world by 2000 A.D. without exception.

Primary Health Care in India

The provision of adequate health care to 1 billion people is a challenging task. The Government has been trying to provide health care through primary health centres, dispensaries and mobile units. The quality and quantity of medical care available is extremely variable-ranging from organised, sophisticated and advanced in urban areas to the most primitive in rural areas. The Fifth Five Year Plan emphasized that the correction of the regional disparities and heavy concentration of health infrastructure and manpower in the urban areas is the imperative need of the social justice in the health sector. With this objective a re-orientation of the health programmes and policies was planned as envisaged in the Master Plan considered by the health and Family Planning Conference held in Delhi in December 1970. The consensus was that a minimum infrastructure for the entire country particularly in the rural areas should be set-up with the resources available. Many expert committees were appointed from time to time to look into these glaring contradictions during the last three decades. These committees have made some concrete and some general suggestions but because of the implementation crisis in the developing countries, nothing much substantial has been achieved. We are much concerned about these 70 per cent of the people living in rural areas. It is a stupendous task.

Village Health Guide Scheme

The Village Health Guide Scheme was initially started as Community Health Workers' Scheme on 2nd October. 1977 in all the States except

Arunachal Pradesh, J&K. Kerala and Tamil Nadu. The Scheme was renamed as Village Health Guide Scheme in 1981, when it was made 100% centrally sponsored scheme under Family Welfare Programme. According to the scheme, the village community selects a volunteer as Village Health Guide, who after training acts as a link between the community and the governmental health system. He/She mainly provides health education and creates awareness on MCH and Family Welfare Services. He/She has to keep track of communicable diseases, treat minor ailments and provide first aid to the patients.

At present, about 3.23 lakh VHGs are reported to be working. Each VHG is paid an honorarium of Rs. 50 per month. The Scheme has recently been reviewed by a committee of experts, which has looked into various aspects of the scheme such as the usefulness of the scheme, the work done by VHGs, capability of VHGs in the context of institutional arrangements available in the country, enhancement of honorarium and other facilities available to VHGs, etc. The committee obtained feedback from the states and visited some of the states to get first hand information and it has submitted its final report/recommendations and the same is being examined in the Ministry.

D. CRITICAL APPRAISAL OF THE PRIMARY HEALTH CARE IN INDIA

Primary Health Care in India has not made much impact so far. It was initiated to provide health care for the people and by the people. A seed can flourish and develop into a full-fledged plant only in a congenial soil and environment. Similarly Primary Health Care Scheme can be successful if a sound organisation set-up is provided for its growth. Let us analyse the reasons which are responsible for its failure in the areas where the scheme was introduced. If we want to put the scheme on a sound footing. we may keep the following facts and suggestions in mind.

Health Experts Lack Commitment

There persists widespread negative and unhelpful attitude among health personnel towards the health care of the poorest strata in the rural and urban population. They are not aware of the social responsibility to the society. If the doctors at the primary level are not mentally convinced of the scheme, changes at the grassroots are unimaginable and impracticable. Most of the doctors and health experts contacted by the writer pointed out that, "Such schemes are unworkable as the community health workers cannot learn much during such a brief training. Instead of being an asset to the health care system, they may reverse the trends and they may create more problems than solutions." Others remarked that, "They are already overworked. They do not find any time to have intimate contacts with the community." A few remarked that, "the present health care system cannot meet the needs of the society. The new system may be given a trial but the care may be taken to plan the scheme effectively before the introduction."

The Medical Association has been vocal enough and described this scheme as a "cruel joke." The major hurdle is the opposition to change, established health associations, institutions and organisations find it difficult to come out from their ivory towers and adjust to change and accept new challenges and responsibilities. Their resistance may be an attempt to defend their false prestige or traditions. Thus, there is a need to convince and train the health experts and their organisations before launching such schemes. We may cultivate a change in their attitudes in the interest of the programme.

At the Golden Jubilee Celebrations of the Indian Medical Association, its President, Dr. J.V.R. Sarma, said that the IMA had not been consulted by Planning Commission in the matter of evolving an effective pattern of rural health care and a national policy on health. He complained that various Governments had instead devised schemes arbitrarily to "suit the fancies and philosophies of changing personalities." If the entire medical manpower could be involved through their professional organisations he was confident that it would be possible to achieve the objective of the scheme. There is an element of truth in this criticism. The Government should not only consult experts before formulating any scheme but should also be able to energize, enthuse and develop a rapport with the professional organisations and, through them, their individual members to take an active part in the community health programmes.[25]

Dr. N.S. Deodhar in the 50th Anniversary of India Independence, Vol. I, p. 43 by gave his remarks that the major cause of failure was apathy and poor management. Evaluation of MPW and CHW schemes revealed that many programme managers lacked full knowledge and understanding of the schemes. The health system failed to perceive the high potential of these schemes towards Health For All by 2000 A.D. Major revamping of the health system is expedient. Premature up-scaling and hasty expansion of CHW scheme to cover the entire country was disastrous. Trainers were poorly trained and equipped. Training has to be effective and quality cannot be compromised. Tools and supplies to serve the people were not provided in time or were inadequate or not proper.

Opposition from Local Practitioners

The scheme is being opposed by the established personnel of traditional system of medicine and local allopathic practitioners. They view this scheme as an encroachment on their authority and prestige. Most of the community health workers interviewed by the writer remarked, practitioners of all the systems of medicine are making a lot of money by exploiting the illiterate poor in the villages. They think that if the scheme becomes successful, their future existence is uncertain. Besides, they have a strong hold on their clients and through them they spread propaganda against the utility of this scheme. One of the workers went on to the extent, "These practitioners would warn community that those people who would consult the community health workers would be in trouble as they knew nothing." Thus, there is a need to educate these practitioners properly and associate them in the planning and implementation of the scheme.

Insufficient Training to Community Health Workers

The training imparted to the community health workers is quite inadequate. He has a very weak educational base. Dr. C. Parkash, the then Senior Medical Superintendent, Medical College, Rohtak, remarked about this scheme to *The Tribune*. "The scheme is conceptually sound since the success of the scheme will largely depend on the quality of personnel chosen for the job. . . . A bare three months training to a person who had schooling up to sixth standard is not likely to adequately equip him for the job."[26] The same opinion was expressed by Prof. S.P. Gupta, Professor of Medicine in Medical College, Rohtak,[27] The Indian Medical Association suggested that the qualification for a CHW should be matriculation and that he must undergo at least 15 months' training to acquire the fundamental knowledge needed for his work. He is to be trained in medicine, art of communication, leadership, etc. The people pointed out that the community health workers do not have much education and training to discharge the responsibilities entrusted to them. The success of the scheme would depend upon the confidence of the community in these workers. There is need for screening these workers so that we retain only those workers who can really be effective. Besides, it has also become apparent that the process of retraining is essential in order to fill the gaps in the initial training or to refresh the health and medical knowledge imparted on a poor educational base.

Medical Education is Urban-oriented

There is national commitment to reorient medical education profession and health services, so as to serve the needs of rural people. All the expert bodies have agreed to modify the syllabus of under-graduate medical education so as to produce a basic doctor who would have the ability to cater to the needs of the rural area. It is necessary to make the medical colleges act not as ivory temples in majestic isolation but take on the responsibility for providing total health care for specified segment of the rural population.[28] The aim of medical education should be to promote happiness through better health of most of the deprived hundreds of millions of human beings. With the contemplated changes in the contents of the under-graduate course, the students would be in a position to appreciate the problems of rural people and would develop proper motivation to help them.

Village Community not Educated

Rural people lack functional literacy which is *sine qua non* for any endeavour towards community development. This requires a great effort on the part of the State governments; voluntary institutions and the health administrators should properly educate and enlighten the people. Properly planned programmes of health education would go a long way in propagating the ideals of a primary health care. It was observed by the writer that no regular efforts are being made to educate the public either by the health department or by the CHW. CHW devotes most of his time in providing curative care rather than laying much emphasis on educational approach. We must provide elementary and simple health education to the community. It should be based on indigenous technology. According to Dr. Mahler, the required new type of health education should be, "neither over sophisticated nor condescending but rather gains the confidence of the individuals and communities by explaining health technology in a language they can understand so that they can participate genuinely in taking decisions concerning their health. In short, a replacement of passive health education by active health learning." Besides, the beneficiaries should be asked to contribute to the cost of Primary Health Care. Everyone should realise his responsibility towards the health coverage of the community. When the rural people would be contributing, they would like to participate and take interest in its functioning. Some nominal contributions may be taken from the people themselves depending upon their income.

No Mechanism for Community Participation

Community participation is the way to development but how to go about it? In the field of primary health care, it was pointed out by the workers that, "It is impossible to educate all the people by them. They have to carry out their own work, and this is only their part time duty. At present, there is no system to involve the community." It is suggested that we may involve teachers, Panchayat members and other influential men and women to diffuse the health education in the community. The constitution of Youth Clubs, Mother Clubs, etc., as has been done in DRK, may be set-up to promote functional literacy and health education among the community.

Exploitation by Community Health Workers

Community health worker is the pivot of the whole scheme. The success or failure of the scheme would depend to a great extent upon the attitudes, perception and ethos of the workers. It has been mentioned that "These workers are not being selected properly. The selection of Community Health Worker has become a political patronage." Such a scheme would have no chance to grow and ultimately survive if we do not find workers who are committed to bring about a social change in the villages. They must have missionary zeal. Their enthusiasm should not be dampened by unfavourable local conditions. They must have zeal and perseverance to reorient the attitudes of the people, otherwise the whole scheme would be a failure. Some people went to remark, "These community health workers have become the agents of the political parties. They are making a lot of money. They want to pose as doctors. They are not easily accessible. They are exploiting the poor people." A section of medical practitioners apprehends that, "half-baked and semi-literate persons masquerading as barefoot doctors will play havoc with the health of the masses." What is the difference then between the private practitioners and CHW workers. It is high time that we select, train and develop our community health workers properly. We must get a system by which we must be able to assess the work of these workers. *The Tribune* editorial, dated 17 July 1975 had rightly commented that, '"If picking good men is the most important of them all, dumping the bad one is the next most important." We know that even poorly devised machinery may be made to work if manned with well trained, intelligent, imaginative and devoted staff. On the other hand, the best planned organisation may produce unsatisfactory results if it is operated by mediocre or disgruntled people. So, we must find out workers who are committed, willing to accept hardships and prepared to work in a spirit of dedication.

Absence of Political Support to Solve Problems of Rural Areas

The political elite in the country are not sensitive and responsive to their duties. They are busy with manipulation of politics and find hardly any time to look into the problems of the people. Because of instability in politics, there is no continuous, concerted and consistent effort to weed out the obstacles in the path of development. What is required is a strong political will and determination to make these schemes successful. Political elite at all levels must support the cause of the rural poor and help them to enjoy the good standards of life which were promised to them at the inception of independence. Political powers and wisdoms are constantly required in a democratic set-up to resolve any problem arising out of the policies and implementation of the scheme. The political elite may have to take bold and unpleasant steps to reallocate the resources between urban and rural sectors.

No Sound Administrative set-up to Implement the Policies of Community Health

A revolutionary scheme of this type can be successful only if there is proper administrative set-up to implement it. Most of the health experts are of the view that the scheme has been rushed through without examining its requirements. It is suggested that some experts in Public Administration may examine the organisation and procedures which are being used to implement the scheme. They may also examine the problems of coordination. control, supervision and headquarters-field relationships. In the light of the suggestions, the existing scheme may be modified to suit the requirements and the scheme in new areas may be set-up according to new recommendations. One of the very important problems is the poor quality of supervision of the scheme. Multipurpose health workers who are supposed to be their immediate supervisors lack proper orientation and training themselves. It is suggested that the multipurpose workers may be given refresher courses to discharge their duties efficiently.

Dr. N.S. Deodhar again remarks in 50th Anniversary of India Independence that decentralization is essential, but we are very slow and half-hearted on his vital question. Panchayati Raj system has been introduced, but it lacks adequate authority and resource. Although, health is the state subject, excessive centralization has resulted in failure of the state Government to take initiative. States have become passive partners in health development. Central health administrative set-up fails to differentiate the federal functions from those for administration of the Union Territories. This has resulted in considerable neglect of federal duties. The officers in Central Health Services have no experience of the state health issues or administration. There is no lateral entry for the state Government officers to the top level posts in Central Health Services. Unfortunately, the state Governments are no better and have failed to decentralize authority and resources.

Absence of Proper Evaluation

Evaluation is one of the most important components of any scheme. The good evaluation is to measure the impact of this scheme on health, the process of operations and scheme replicability. When the writer contacted the health experts, they pointed out many difficulties. Most of them observed, "No evaluation machinery has been designed, No methodology has been designed to measure the output. There is no simple information system by which the assessment of the scheme implemented so far can be made." This situation leads to failure in taking timely decisions and lack of feedback. Without an appropriate feedback, the health workers of the PHC level feel frustrated and their function as agents for information becomes meaningless to them. This lack of feedback is probably one of the most important problems in the development of primary health care which need solution. It is suggested that a simple information system may be designed to suit the conditions prevailing in a particular area.

Insufficient Supply of Drugs

The drugs are very costly. Most of the workers mentioned that "The amount of Rs. 600 per year for drugs is too small to meet the demands of the people." It is suggested that:

(a) The Government must strengthen the drug industries in the public sector and manufacture essential drugs at cheaper prices.

(b) The indigenous medicine may be standardised and used to provide cheaper services.

(c) Beneficiaries may be asked to contribute two to five rupees per head per year to make the scheme viable and effective. This would also encourage more participation.

(d) Researches to exploit local flora and fauna as medicine may be encouraged.

(e) More treatment may be suggested through the control of diet and naturopathy which would lead to better health.

(f) The supply of drugs may be made in time to keep the morale of the workers high and win confidence of the people.

CONCLUSION

The experiment of Community Health Workers Scheme in India has not gone on long enough to reveal all the problems inherent in it. Besides, it has not acquired the sophistication and expertise that one associates with already existing health programmes. There has been great opposition from many quarters. They consider this system as inferior and primitive. But their opposition is based on superficial thinking. There is no substitute for a poor country like India where the people cannot afford the costly medical care system. It may be noted here that even highly industrialized societies are depending upon such schemes to provide effective health care to the community. There is no denying the fact that this is theoretically sound and can help the unprivileged people and deprived communities to take care of their health problems which otherwise would remain unattended to because of financial and professional constraints. The scheme is a vital link in the country's health schemes. The weakness of the scheme is because of the poor design of the implementation machinery which may be streamlined to provide the health facilities for all.

NOTES AND REFERENCES

1. Alastair Anderson, "Strengthening of Health Services: Adapt-Don't Adopt", in *World Health,* July 1976, p. 4.
2. Fifty Year of WHO in South-East Asia, 1948-58, New Delhi, p. 59.
3. Alastair Anderson, *op. cit.,* p. 4.
4. WHO, *World Health,* May, 1978, p. 26.
5. WHO, SEARO: Annual Report of the Regional Director (1966-77), p. 5, (SEA/RC3/30/2).
6. WHO, "The Role of Frontier Workers", *WHO Chronicle,* Vol. 29, No. I. (January 1975).
7. WHO: *World Health,* "Primary Health Care", May 1979, p. 6.
8. WHO: SEARO: SEA/RC. 30/Sept. 1977, p. 38.
9. Dr. Hiroshi Nakajima, *World Health,* No. 2, March-April, 1995, p. 6.
10. SEARO: Declaration on Health Development in the South-East Asia Region in the 21st Century, New Delhi, 1997, pp. 22-23.
11. *Ibid.,* pp. 38-41.
12. Giovanni, Sartori, "Concept Misformation in Comparative Politics", The *American Political Science Review,* Vol. LXIV, No. 4, December 1970, pp. 1050-52 (Pluralism. integrating, participation, mobilisation).
13. M. Soyasal, "Public Relations in Administration: The influence of the Public on the Operation of Public Administration, Excluding Electoral Rights", General Report to the XIII International Congress of Administrative Services, Paris, 1965 (Brussels II AS, 1966, p. 47.
14. P. Yadav Ram: "People's Participation: Focus on Mobilisation of the Rural Poor", UN Asian and Pacific Institute, *op. cit.,* p. 6.
15. H. Mahler, "Further Thoughts of WHO Mission", *WHO Chronicle,* 29, 253-56, 1975.
16. Lucan Pye, Aspects of Political Development, p. 64.
17. Ramalingaswami, *op. cit.,* p. 12.

18. WHO, *World Health,* July, 1976, p. 12.
19. For details refer to Chapter V.
20. See Chart 2.1 to understand the intricacies of Health Information System in relation to Primary Health Care System.
21. Based on the article, "A land transformed" written by Prof. T.S. Sharmonov, Minister Health of the Kazakh Soviet Socialist Republic, and corresponding member of the Soviet Academy of Medical Science, in *World Health,* May 1978, pp. 4-6.
22. Based on the article, "Building a Bridge" by Paul Harrison, British Journalist and Photographer in *World Health,* May, 1978, pp. 7-11.
23. Based on the article "Medicine Man" by Johan Loftus, A Journalist, *World Health,* Oct. 1976, pp. 17-19.
24. Based on the article, "Generating Self-Confidence" by Manual Carballo, a member of the unit of maternal and child health division of Family Health, WHO Headquarters in Geneva, *World Health,* May 1978, pp. 26-29.
25. *Sunday Standard,* Oct. 1, 1978.
26. *The Tribune,* Oct. 25, 1978, Chandigarh.
27. *Ibid.*
28. India: National Plan for Health Care Services in the Rural Area.

2

CHAPTER

National Rural Health Mission (NRHM)

Health Care is one of the seven thrust areas under the National Common Minimum Programme (NCMP). There is an increasing recognition that despite significant improvements in health parameters like life expectancy at birth of and the reduction of infant and maternal mortality there are large parts of the country where people continue to have very poor access to health care services and their health status continues to be abysmal. A high proportion of the population continues to suffer from and die of preventable conditions like maternal deaths, malaria and tuberculosis. Persistent malnutrition and high levels of anemia amongst children and women is widespread. Due to the poor status of public health systems people are also facing poverty and indebtedness from the costs incurred in seeking health care. Public spending on health in India, especially on preventive and promotive health is also very low in India. On the other hand the private, out of pocket, expenditure on health is very high, about three times higher than the public expenditure. Thus, there is an urgency to deal with the multiple health related crisis that the rural poor in the country had to faced with. There is also the need to transform the health system into an efficient, transparent and responsible system delivering affordable and quality services.

The National Rural Health Mission has been conceptualized and is being implemented to bring about these fundamental changes in the way health care services are being delivered to the rural poor. The Goal of the Mission is to improve the availability of and access to quality health care by people, especially for those residing in rural areas, the poor, women and children.

Goals

- Reduction in Infant Mortality Rate (IMR) and Maternal Mortality Ratio (MMR).

- Universal access to public health services such as Women's health, child health, water, sanitation and hygiene, immunization, and Nutrition.
- Prevention and control of communicable and non-communicable diseases, including locally endemic diseases.
- Access to integrated comprehensive primary health care.
- Population stabilization, gender and demographic balance.
- Revitalize local health traditions and mainstream AYUSH.
- Promotion of healthy lifestyles.

The NCMP mandates an increase in expenditure in health sector, with main focus on Primary Health Care from the current level of 0.9% of GDP to 2-3% of GDP over the next five years. The National Rural Health Mission (NRHM), which is the main vehicle for giving effect to the above mandate was launched on 12.4.05 by Hon'ble Prime Minister of India. It is being operationalized throughout the country, with special focus on 18 states, which includes 8 empowerment Action Group States (Bihar, Jharkhand, Madhya Pradesh, Chhattisgarh, Uttar Pradesh, Uttaranchal, Orissa and Rajasthan), 8 NE States, Himachal Pradesh and Jammu and Kashmir.[1]

The thrust of the Mission was on establishing a fully functional, community owned, decentralized health delivery system with inter-sectoral convergence at all levels, to ensure simultaneous action on a wide range of determinants of health like water, sanitation, education, nutrition, social and gender equality. Institutional integration within the fragmented health sector was expected to provide a focus on outcomes, measured against Indian Public Health Standards for all health facilities. From narrowly defined schemes, the NRHM was shifting the focus to a functional health system at all levels, from the village to the district.[2]

The NRHM further aims to provide overarching umbrella to the existing programmes of Health and Family Welfare including RCH-II, Malaria, Blindness, Lodine deficiency, Filaria, Kata Azar, T.B., Leprosy and Integrated Diseases Surveillance. Further, it addresses the issue of health in the context of sector-wide approach addressing sanitation and hygiene, nutrition and safe drinking water as basic determinants of good health in order to have greater convergence among the related social sector Departments, i.e. AYUSH, Women and Child Development, Sanitation, Elementary Education, Panchayati Raj and Rural Development.

The Mission is an articulation of the commitment of the Government to achieve the goals and objectives of National Health Policy and Population Policy and increase the outlays for Health from the current 0.9% to 2-3% of GDP over the next five years, and to undertake systemic correction of the health system to effectively utilize such increased outlay for sustainable outcomes.[3]

Let us analyse the components of this programme.

1. ASHA

The Accredited Social Health Activist (ASHA) is envisaged to be a trained female voluntary Community Health Worker in the eight EAG states, Assam and Jammu and Kashmir. Other states also have the flexibility to adopt it under RCH-II. ASHAs would reinforce community action for universal immunization, safe/institutional delivery, other Reproductive and Health-related Services, newborn care, prevention of water-borne and other communicable diseases, nutrition and sanitation. ASHAs would be chosen by the Panchayat and be fully accountable to them. Though she would not be paid any salary she would be entitled for performance-linked incentives under different programmes. Fully anchored in the Anganwadi system, ASHAs would work in close coordination with the ANM and AWW. ASHAs would be provided with a basic drug kit including AYUSH drugs. She would also be a depot holder for contraceptives and IEC materials developed for villages. So far the selection of more than 1 lakh ASHAs has been completed and the training process is on.

2. Strengthening of Infrastructure

(i) Additional SC/PHC/CHCs are to be set-up to bring the number in line with the current population norm. Repair/renovation of the existing public health facilities is planned and norms are being developed for support to the states for construction of new buildings and maintenance to the existing buildings. Incentives are being devised to encourage the State Governments for filling up of vacant posts of ANMs/LHVs/MPWs. An annual support of Rs. 10,000 as untied fund to be spent in direct supervision of the Panchayats has been given to each Sub-Centre. Fifty percent of the PHCs are proposed to be made operational on 24 x 7 basis by including an AYUSH practitioner. All the CHCs are to be upgraded over the mission period to the Indian Public Health Standards (IPHS) with posting of additional specialists/up-gradation of infrastructure, etc. Indian Public Health Standard (IPHS) is a novel concept to fix benchmarks of infrastructure including building, manpower, equipments, drugs, quality assurance through introduction of treatment protocols. All CHCs are also to be made operational as First Referral Units (FRUs) providing emergency obstetric and newborn care. Accountability to public is to be enforced through a prominently displayed Citizens Charter (indicating the range of services and the rights of citizens) to be monitored through Hospital Management Society. The Rogi Kalyan Samitis are envisaged at all levels. At all levels, additional drugs are also being provided to improve their credibility.

CHART 2.1

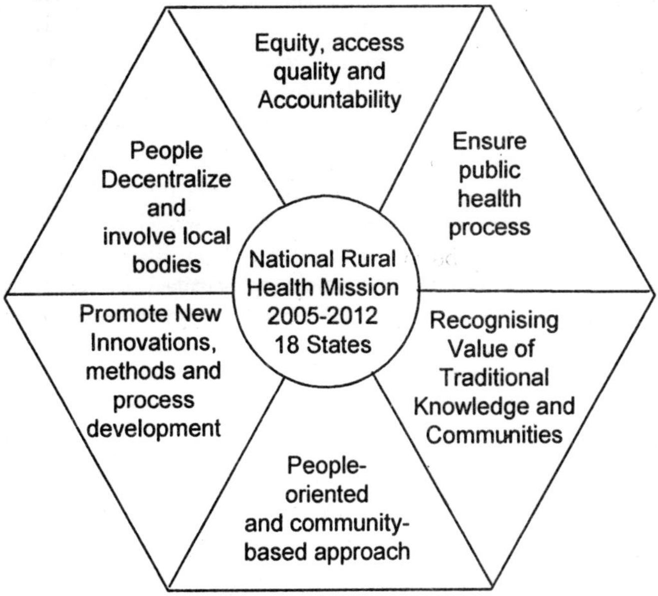
Equity, access
quality and
Accountability
Ensure
public
health
process
Recognising
Value of
Traditional
Knowledge and
Communities
People-
oriented
and community-
based approach
Promote New
Innovations,
methods and
process
development
People
Decentralize
and
involve local
bodies
National Rural
Health Mission
2005-2012
18 States

(ii) To meet the emergency type expenditures at Sub-Centre level, the untied fund of Rs. 10,000 per Sub-Centre per annum has been released which will be maintained by opening a joint account of the ANM and Sarpanch.

3. Decentralized Planning

Flexible, Decentralized Planning is the pivot on which the entire concept of the Mission revolves. The planning process under the guidance of the Village Health and Sanitation Committee is to start right from the village level. However, till such time that adequate capacity is built, the districts would be the starting points for this exercise. The district plans would thereafter converge into state plans. Planning would be taken up for the entire mission period as well as for each financial year. The district plans would be got appraised by the states, who thereafter would send the state plans to the Centre. These plans would be approved at the Central level before the beginning of the financial year.

4. Institutional Arrangements Under NRHM

The Mission Steering Group (MSG) has been set-up at the Centre chaired by the Union Minister of Health and Family Welfare with Deputy Chairman of the Planning Commission, Ministers of the Panchayati Raj, Rural Development, Human Resource Development, Secretary Expenditure and other senior officials from the Central as well as the State Governments and ten health professionals as members. The Empowered Programme Committee has also been set-up and is chaired by the Secretary (H&FW).

The Integration of the Departments of Health and Family Welfare at the national level has been replicated at the state levels. Advisory Group on Community health action has been set-up to guide the process of community participation. Most states have also set-up the State Health Mission to be chaired by the Chief Minister. The various societies at the state and the District level have been merged into an Integrated Society at the state level where it is the executive arm of the State Health Mission. The District Health Missions are being formed under the chairmanship of Zilla Parishad. The Integrated District Society is the executive arm of the District Health Mission. At CHC and PHC level Rogi Kalyan Samiti and the Hospital Management Society are being constituted to foster community participation in the management of Public Health Infrastructures. The Village Health and Sanitation Committee is the farthest link and guides the process at the village level.

5. Capacity Building under NRHM

The services of professional including MBAS, Chartered Accountants, etc. have been contracted in the EAG states to set-up the PMU. These professionals are assigned specific roles under the organogram of the State and District Health Society so as to bring them in the mainstream. Formation of the Mission teams both in terms of number as well as skills is one of the important preparatory activities. For ASHAs a minimum 23-day training is envisaged. Training Modules for this purpose have been developed and the training of trainers is currently on. ANMs and AWWs are also to be associated in the ASHA training process. A Mentoring Group comprising eminent health professionals has been set-up the guide the process. MNGOs are to be involved at the district level in planning process. Adequate provision to be made out of the Mission funds for training of the members of the Villages Health and Sanitation Committee, Zilla Parishad, Hospital Management Committee to equip them with the skills to take up planning, implementation and monitoring of the Mission activities.

6. Partnership with NGOs under NRHM

The Mission would forge suitable public-private partnership to meet the deficiencies in the public health delivery system. Guidelines are being developed for accreditation of private health providers. Pilots would be runs on different models in selected districts and based on the outcome they would be implemented on wider geographical area.

7. Monitoring and Evaluation under NRHM

A baseline survey is to be taken up at the district level incorporating Facility Survey (including private facilities) as well as survey of the Households. The baseline survey is to help the Mission in fixing decentralized monitorable goals and indicators. There would be community monitoring at the village level. The Panchayati Raj institutions, Rogi Kalyan Samitis, Quality Assurance Committees at the State and District level, State and District Health Missions, Mission Steering Group at the Central level, Planning Commission is to be the eventual monitor of the outcomes. External evaluation is also to be taken up at frequent interval.[4]

The first year of the Mission was the Preparatory phase during which the states were setting up the institutional framework of the Mission including the Merger of various departments in the health sector, constituting the State and District Health Missions, and notifying the State Health Societies formed by converging the several societies relating to the various national programmes. At the Government of India level, the detailing of the various strategies of NRHM was being firmed up during the year through a detailed process of stakeholder consultations with the state representatives, NGOs, public health experts and related departments. The guidelines for various activities under the Mission were disseminated to the states during the year and the same were then forwarded to the ground level functionaries for Operationalization.

The total outlay of the Department for the financial year 2006-07 is Rs. 11,505 crores, out of which the NRHM component is Rs. 9,065 crore. Working on the spending on health by the Central Government, it translates to 23.2% increase over the previous year. During the year 2005-06, an amount of Rs. 205.8 crore released to the states as United funds for Sub centers, Rs. 77 crore was released for ASHA selection, training and drug kits, Rs. 393.4 crore was released as seed funding for up-gradation of CHCs to IPHS standards. In addition to this additional funds were also released to the states under NRHM for improving the availability of essential drugs at all levels. Funds were also released to the states to accelerate the preparation of the Integrated District Health Acton Plans.

Community Link Worker

The original Cabinet note of the Mission envisaged the selection of a trained female community health worker called Accredited Social Health Activist (ASHA) in each village in the ratio of one per 1000 population in the 10 states. Under the detailed Framework of Implementation, the ASHA has been extended to all 18 High Focus states. For tribal, hilly, desert areas, the norm could be relaxed to one ASHA per habitation depending on the workload. ASHA is envisaged to be a primary resident of the village with formal education upto Class VIII and preferably in the age group 25-45. She would be selected by the Gram Sabha following an intense community mobilization process. She would be fully accountable to Panchayat.

The ASHA would reinforce community action for universal immunization, safe delivery, newborn care, prevention of water-borne and other communicable diseases, nutrition and sanitation. In order that ASHAs work in close coordination with the AWW, she would be fully anchored in the Anganwadi system. ASHAs would also provide immediate and easy access for the rural population to essential health supplies like ORS, contraceptives, a set of ten basic drugs and she would have a health communication kit and other IEC materials developed for villages.

Strengthening of Primary Health Infrastructure and Improving Service Delivery

There is a shortage of 21983 Sub-centres, 4436 PHCs and 3332 CHCs as per 2001 population norm. Further, almost 50% of the existing health infrastructure is in rented buildings, which coupled with poor upkeep and maintenance, is also a cause of high absenteeism of manpower in rural areas. The NRHM seeks to strengthen the Public Health delivery system at all levels. The Sub-centre and PHCs are proposed to be revitalized through better human resource development, clear quality standards, better community support and an untied fund to enable local planning and action and more Multi Purpose Workers (MPWs). The Indian Public Health Standards define structural, personnel, equipment and management standards and have already been finalized for the CHCs. Standards for the Sub-Centres, PHCs and District Hospitals are in the final stages of preparation and shall be communicated to the states shortly. All the states are undertaking facility surveys (regarding which detailed guidelines and formats were disseminated to the states) to identify the fund requirements for upgrading the facilities and provision of adequate funds has been made in this regard.

All the facilities are also being provided untied funds to enable the local management committee to carry out locally relevant initiatives for better service delivery. The Hospital Management Committees (Rogi Kalyan Samitis) at various levels are being set-up as registered societies with Panchayat Raj Institutions representation. These societies are also being given funding support under the NRHM to allow local action.

Community Ownership

The NRHM seeks to strengthen the service delivery by ensuring community ownership of the health facilities. The Sub centers are envisaged to be under the management of the local Panchayat. The Pradhan shall be operating the Joint account with the ANM for utilization of the Untied Funds. Similarly, the PHCs and CHCs are also proposed to be transferred to the local elected Panchayati Raj Institutions for management. The management committee of the health facilities, which would have the representation of the local SHGs and NGOs, elected representatives of the Panchayat Raj along with the MO of the facility shall be authorized to undertake local action for ensuring that the agreed service guarantees for the respective facility are fulfiled.[5]

Achievements till date

Under the NRHM, over the past 18 months, State Health Mission have been constituted in all States and District Health Mission have been constituted in all states. The merger of Departments of Health and Family Welfare has been completed in all states. Merger of State level societies has been completed in 28 states and is in progress in the remaining states. During 2005-06, 1.27 lakh ASHAs have been selected in the ten states as against the proposed one lakh and till date 2.39 lakh ASHAs have been selected out of which 1.84 lakh ASHAs have received the first module of training. Mentoring Group for ASHA has been set-up at the National level and detailed guidelines for ASHA support mechanisms have been communicated to the states. The training modules for ASHA training have also been finalized.

New Initiatives

New Initiatives like Integrated Management of Neonatal and Childhood Illness (IMNCI) have been started this year in 16 states namely, MP, WB, Jharkhand, UP, Haryana, Maharashtra, Delhi, Mizoram, J&K, Uttaranchal, Bihar, A&N Islands, Assam, Andhra Pradesh, and Chhattisgarh and Karnataka. Training on Newborn Care has been completed in 140 districts in the country. Integrated Disease Surveillance Project has been operationalized. Legal changes have been brought about to allow the ANMs to dispense medication and MBBS doctors to administer anesthesia. To strengthen Routine Immunization, accelerated Routine Immunization has been taken up in all EAG states. In addition, catch up rounds have been taken up in Bihar, Jharkhand, Orissa and Assam and other states. To prevent outbreak of Japanese Encephalitis (JE), vaccination for JE has been started. Groundwork for expansion of Hepatitis-B vaccine to 11 states has been finalized. To strengthen partnership with non-governmental stakeholders, 225 Mother NGOs have been appointed for 331 districts in 2005-06. Janani Suraksha Yojana has been launched all over the country to promote safe delivery and incentives are being provided to BPL families for institutional delivery. A Committee on Intersectoral convergence has been set-up and ground work for convergence with ICDS/Drinking Water/Sanitation/AYUSH/NACO has been completed. Monthly Health days are being organized at the Anganwadi Centres and many states have initiated school health programmes.

Progress Under National Rural Health Mission (NRHM)

1. Institutional Arrangements

- State Health Missions constituted in all states/UTs.
- State launch along with orientation of DMs/CMOs completed in all focus states.
- Merger of Departments of Health and Family Welfare completed in all states.
- Merger of State level Societies in 29 states. Rest in process.

2. ASHA

- Number selected as on 31.03.2006: 1,27,749.
- Number selected during 2006-07, till date: 1,11,396.

- ASHA trained: 1,49,855.
- Mentoring Group for ASHA set-up and meetings held.
- Detailed guidelines for the mentoring of ASHAs in the states and the associated generic funding have been disseminated to the states.
- ASHA Training modules finalized.
- State/District/Block level trainers completed.

3. *Infrastructure*

- Facility Survey has been completed in 1452 CHCs across the country.
- Untied funds of Rs. 10,000 released to all sub-centres in the country, Total amount released: Rs. 205.87 crore in 2005-06 and Rs. 55.03 crore during 2006-07.
- Joint account of ANM and Pradhan opened in 31580 sub-centres.
- Indian Public Health Standards finalized for Sub-Centres, PHCs and CHCs. Similar standards are in final stages of preparation for District Hospitals.
- 2045 CHCs have been identified for upgradation to IPHS. Total amount of Rs. 370.00 crores released during 2005-06 for starting the upgradation process and Rs. 326.40 crores during Financial Year 2006-07 till date for this purpose.
- 8080 Rogi Kalyan Samitis set-up at various levels.
- Mobility support being given for outreach programmes in the underserved areas. A total of Rs. 153.10 crores has been released for Mobile Medical Units to various states during 2006-07.
- 129 Integrated District Health Action Plans have been prepared in various states. These plans are sector wide in import and address all aspects of health including the collateral health determinants like nutrition, sanitation, drinking water, etc.

4. *Human Resource Development*

- Recommendations of the Task Group on Medical Education has been finalized and are under consideration by the Ministry.
- The Task Group on Identification, training and accreditation of RMPs in the final stages of deliberations.
- Positioning of accounts personnel at PHCs to strengthen the accounting of funds in view of the substantially larger number of transactions at that level has been approved by EPC/MSG.
- 22655 Doctors, ANMs and other paramedics have been appointed on contract by States to fill in critical gaps.
- Block pooling of doctors has been started in states so s to ensure that there is at least one functional health facility in each of the

block. The other health facilities in the territorial jurisdiction are being serviced through outreach visits.

- Over 700 professionals (CA/MBA) appointed in Program Manager Units (PMU) to support NRHM. Similar management support is being planned at the level fo the Block also.

5. *Training*

- National Health Resource Centre at Central level finalized.
- State level Health System Resource Centre for North East States set-up at Guwahait.
- Additional training initiatives undertaken including:
  - o Upgradation of State Training Institutes/ANMs Colleges.
  - o Integrated Skill Development Training ANMs/LHV/MOs.
  - o Skilled Birth Attendants Training MO/ANMs.
  - o Training on Emergency Obstetrics care for MOs.
  - o Training on No Scalpel Vasectomy (NSV) for MOs.
  - o Professional Development Programme for CMOs.
  - o Specialized skill development programme for MOs.
  - o Training program for Consultants of Program Management Units.

6. *New Programmes and Innovations*

- RCH-II launched and under implementation.
- Sterilization compensation scheme launched by GOI.
- Integrated Management of Neonatal and Childhood Illnesses (IMNCI) started this year in 27 States.
- With the help of Neonatology Forum initiated training on Newborn Care in 63 districts in the country.
- Integrated Disease Surveillance Project operationalized.
- Legal changes brought about to allow the ANMs to dispense medication and MBBS doctors to administer anesthesia.
- Short course for anesthesia being proposed.

7. *Immunization*

- Accelerated Routine Immunization (RI) taken up in all EAG states.
- Coverage expected to be around 80 per cent.
- Catch up rounds taken up in Bihar, Jharkhand, Orissa and Assam and other states.
- Organisation sessions in urban slums and under served areas by outsourcing the sessions where ever necessary (Hiring of vaccinator in service deficient areas or where ANM is not available).

- Mobilization of children by ASHA and Anganwadi Workers (AWW) to increase coverage and convergence of Nutrition with Immunization.
- JE vaccination initiated in 11 districts in 4 states—93 lakh children immunized.
- Groundwork for expansion of Hepatitis vaccine to 11 states finalized.
- AD Syringes introduced.
- Vaccine management addressed. BCG now in 10 dose vial.
- Development and implementation of a Routine Immunization Monitoring System Software.
- Neonatal Tetanus declared eliminated from 7 states.

8. Polio Eradication Programme

- Over 5 million children in transit administered polio drops (2005-06).
- During 2006, till date 583 cases have been reported.

9. Operational Guidelines Disseminated

- IMNCI.
- Skilled Birth Attendants.
- Emergency Obstetric Care.
- First referral Unit and Blood Storage Units.

10. Partnership with Non Government Stakeholders

- 297 Mother NGOs appointed for 404 districts till date.
- Providing services, RCH out reach services, Ambulance Services, Mobile Medical Units, Mentoring of ASHA, Management of Health facilities (as in Gujarat, Tamil Nadu, etc.), Involvement of Medical Colleges, Training programmes, ICCI, Partnership in polio/immunization programmes, etc.

11. IEC

- IEC Multi-media campaign on health issues including immunization, lodized Salt, Save the Girl Child.
- NRHM Newsletter.
- Health Melas organized in different states.
- Information booklets disseminated.
- Behaviour change workshops being organized for key stakeholders including state IEC representatives.

12. Supply of Drugs

- Empowered Procurement Wing set-up in the Ministry.
- Single Purchase Committee set-up under DGHS.
- Involvement of HLL for supply of drugs to EAG/North East States being finalized.

13. Janani Suraksha Yojana

- JSY launched all over the country to promote safe delivery.
- Incentive for BPL families of Rs. 1300 for safe delivery in EAG State, Assam and J & K and Rs. 1000 in all other states.
- Assistance also being given for Caesarian section.

14. Insectoral Convergence

- Insectoral Convergence Committee under Mission Director set-up.
- Convergence with ICDS/Drinking Water/Sanitation/AYUSH/ NACO ground work completed.
- School health programmes initiated by various states.
- Monthly Health day being organized at the Anganwadi Centres.

15. Monitoring

- New Monitoring format for NRHM developed.
- Household survey/facility survey introduced. NFHS proposed to be held every 2 years for half of the Districts.
- Scheme for appointment of Special Rapporteur finalized.
- Independent Monitoring by Population Research Centres/ Regional Research Centres.
- Mentoring Group/Advisory Group on Community Action.
- Internal monitoring by the Ministry.
- Internal monitoring by the Ministry through regular review meetings with State Secretaries, Directors of Family Welfare/ Mission Directors, etc. One-to-one meeting with High Focus States.
- Independent evaluation by Planning Commission.
- Community monitoring through Rogi Kalyan Samitis/PRIs.
- Monitoring by the community through Rogi Kalyan Samitis/ PRIs.
- Mentoring by Empowered Programme Committee, Mission Steering Group.

16. Financing of NRHM

- Out of Rs. 6731.16 crore allocated, an amount of Rs. 5702 crore has been released for all Program under NRHM in 2005-06. In 2006-07 Rs. 9065.00 crore has been allocated for NRHM out of which Rs. 3668.00 crore has been released.
- Risk Pooling and Health Insurance models being prepared.

17. Signing of MOUs by State Governments.

- Received from 33 States out of 35 States.

18. Moding and e-Banking

- E Banking fully operationalized in the states of Kerala and Gujarat and started in all other states. Funds are being transferred to the states through the e-Banking mode.

19. Status of Disease Control Programmes: RNTCP

- New adult out patients registered for TB diagnosis (target 2-3%): 2%.
- New Smear Positive case detection rate: 44%.
- Annualized Total case detection rate (per 1 lakh population): 115
- Success rate of new smear positive patients: 86%.

NAMP:

- Annual Blood Examination Rate for Malaria (per 100 population): 7.32.
- Annual Parasitic Incidence of Malaria (per 1000 population): 1.15.

KALA-AZAR

- Cases of Kala-azar: 18824.
- Death due to Kala-azar: 104.

NLEP

- Prevalence Rate/10,000 population: 0.86.[6]

CRITICAL APPRAISAL

Jeffrey D. Sachs, Professor of Economics Columbia University in his Articles, "The healthier poor" in Economic Times dated 3rd September, 2007 observes.

"Indeed, India is doing much more with its remarkable National Rural Health Mission (NRHM), which is the single largest mobilization of public health measures in the world. An astounding half-million young women have recently been hired as health workers to link impoverished households and public clinics and hospitals, which are being improved, and to increase women's access to emergency obstetrical care in order to avoid tragic and unnecessary deaths in children.

Another remarkable success in India is the safe home-care of newborn infants in the first few days of life. Currently, an alarming number of newborns die because of infection, mothers' failure to breastfeed during the first days, or other preventable causes. By training community health workers, the NRHM has achieved a marked reduction in newborn deaths in Indian villages.

All these programmes refute three widely held myths. The first is that the burden of disease among the poor is somehow inevitable and unavoidable, as if the poor are bound to get sick and die prematurely. In fact, the poor die of known and identifiable causes that are largely preventable and treatable at very low cost. There is no excuse for millions of deaths from malaria, AIDS, TB, Polio, Measles, Diarrhoea, or Respiratory infections, or for so may women and infants to dies in or after childbirth.

The second myth is that aid from rich countries is inevitably wasted. This fallacy is repeated so often by ignorant leaders in rich countries that it has become a major barrier to progress. The rich like to blame the poor, partly because it lets them off the hook, and partly because it gives them a feeling of moral superiority. But poor countries are capable of establishing effective public health programmes rapidly when they are helped. Recent success stories have been made possible through a combination of increased spending from poor countries' budgets, supplemented by aid from rich-country donors.

The third myth is that saving the poor will worsen the population explosion. But households in the least developed countries have many children—an average of five per woman—partly because fear of high childhood death rates leads them to overcompensate with large families. When childhood death rates come down, fertility rates tend to decline even more, since families are now confident that their children will survive. The result is lower population growth.

It is time to make good on a basic global commitment—that everybody, poor and rich alike—should have access to basic health services. If just 0.1% of rich-world income were devoted to life-saving health care for the poor, it would be possible to raise life expectancy, decrease child mortality, save mothers in childbirth, slow population growth, and spur economic development throughout the poor world.

The success stories in public health for the poor are multiplying. Given the low cost and the huge benefits of supporting such efforts, there is no excuse for inaction.[7]

Sweden's also formulated

A policy of "good health and health care on equal terms for the entire populatin" underlies HS 90—a special project, which foresees the shape of the health services in the 1990s.

The HS 90 plan represents a very serious effort to change the structure of the Swedish health care system inot a shape that is more consistent with the new goals as indicated by WHO, and as expressed in the Swedish Health and Medical Services Act. Decentralization means that the actual development of care will be to a large extent controlled by the regional authorities-the county councils. But these bodies have already shown a firm determination to pursue the agreed national policy. These changes are already getting under way, and their effect will be to ensure that health care in Sweden will indeed result in "good health and health care on equal terms for the entire population" in 14 years' time.[8]

Singapore Scheme

The government wants to provide a good health service of the highest quality, which is not only available and accessible to the population, but is also affordable and has to be paid for. So prior savings have had to be enforced to meet the expected rising costs of health care.

These considerations form the underlying basis for the National Health Plan formulated by the Ministry of Health in 1983. Its key proposal, the Medisave Scheme, attempts to impose compulsory savings and restructure the present system of health care financing.

The principal objectives of the National Health Plan are to secure a healthy, fit and productive population through active prevention and promotion of healthy lifestyles, and to improve cost-efficiency in the health services. In addition to promoting individual responsibility for maintaining it aims to build up financial resources so as to provide the y for medical care during illness.

gh Medisave is a uniquely Singaporean solution to local vertheless some useful lessons can be universally applied. The of "charity begins at home" and "saving for a rainy day" can kbone for viable long-term financing of increasingly expensive in any society. Such a compulsory family-centred savings have important implications for countries, which intend to heir welfare systems and wish to avoid potential social ing from a lack of financial planning for the future. This is gnificant in the light of competing claims on the scarce urces that are available to enable countries to pay for Health

ountries are still lacking a master plan that will husband ces between now and the new millennium. However such a nly way for countries to identify serious shortfalls, to find resources, to make better use of existing ones, and to span ıp between what must be provided and what reasonably can be financed from available sources. There is a need of drawing funds from all possible sources and combing them in an imaginative way, any given country can formulate the first essential key to equity in health.[10]

Democratic Republic of Korea

The Medical Assistance scheme is a programme for the needy, supported 80 per cent by the central government and 20 per cent by the local authorities, except in Seoul where the cost is shared equally. The Ministry of Health and Social Affairs sets the standards of eligibility for benefits, and the local government is responsible for assessing cases and for day-to-day management.

There are two categories of beneficiary, the indigent and the low income group. The indigent are those aged over 65, the disabled, children under 18 without parents or with parents over 60, and people residing at welfare facilities. These people receive yellow identity cards. The lower income group consists of those with an average income less than a certain amount and subsistence farmers. The level was set at 40,000 Won (about US $ 50) per person per month in 1985. People in this group are provided with green identity cards. The selection of eligible persons is made once a year.

The yellow cardholders receive medical care free of charge, whilst the green card holders have to pay 20 per cent of the in-patient fees (except in Seoul where they pay 50 per cent).[11]

Little can be said about the importance of health issues in terms of public political participation or expression, as this is an area in which evidence and analysis are largely absent. Public does not necessarily regard health as a key priority and hence it does not tend to become an issue of high politics. Perhaps because health reform has resulted in less drastic change than reform in many other areas of economic and social policy, it has been eclipsed as a critical political issue by other more immediate social needs such as employment, income housing and prices. It is appreciable that the Government of India has thought of reforms in health sector. It is too early to comment about its performance. However, it is sure that some health development would take place for the poor.

PREAMBLE

Recognizing the importance of Health in the process of economic and social development and improving the quality of life of our citizens, the Government of India has resolved to launch the National Rural Health Mission to carry out necessary architectural correction in the basic health care delivery system. The Mission adopts a synergistic approach by relating health to determinants of good health viz. segments of nutrition, sanitation, hygiene and safe drinking water. It also aims at mainstreaming the Indian systems of medicine to facilitate health care. The Plan of Action includes increasing public expenditure on health, reducing regional imbalance in health infrastructure, pooling resources, integration of organisational structures, optimization of health manpower, decentralization and district management of health programmes, community participation and ownership of assets, induction of management and financial personnel into district health system, and operationalizing community health centers into functional hospitals meeting Indian Public Health Standards in each Block of the Country.

The Goal of the Mission is to improve the availability of and access to quality health care by people, especially for those residing in rural areas, the poor, women and children.

Notes and References

1. NRHM, Health and Population Policies, Annual Report, 2006-07, GOI, Ministry of Health and Family Welfare, p. 17.
2. NRHM, The Progress So Far, p. 1.
3. Annual Report, 2005-06, Ministry of Health and Family Welfare, GOI, New Delhi, p. 23.
4. Annual Report, 2005-06, Ministry of Health and Family Welfare, GOI, pp. 23-25.
5. Annual Report, 2006-07, Ministry of Health and Family Welfare, Government of India, pp. 18-20.
6. GOI, Ministry of Health and Family Welfare, Annual Report, 2006-07, pp. 20-25.
7. Jeffrey D. Sachs, "The Healthier Poor", *Economics Times*, 3rd September 2007.
8. Marten Lagergren, Sweden's Plan for 2000, *World Health*, May 1986, pp. 7-8.
9. Kai Hong Phua, Singapore's Family Savings Scheme, *World Health*, May 1986, pp. 11-12.
10. A Budget for health for all, WHO, May 1986, p. 17.
11. Ok Ryun Moon, Towards equity in health care, WHO, May 1986, p. 20.

APPENDIX 2.1

(National Rural Health Mission 2005-12 Mission Document)

1. STATE OF PUBLIC HEALTH

- Public health expenditure in India has declined from 1.3% of GDP in 1990 to 0.9% of GDP in 1999. The Union Budgetary allocation for health is 1.3% while the State's budgetary allocation is 5.5%.
- Union Government contribution to public health expenditure is 15% while States contribution about 85%.
- Vertical Health and Family Welfare Programmes have limited synergisation at operational levels.
- Lack of community ownership of public health programmes impacts levels of efficiency, accountability and effectiveness.
- Lack of integration of sanitation, hygiene, nutrition and drinking water issues.
- There are striking regional inequalities.
- Population Stabilization is still a challenge, especially in States with weak demographic indicators.
- Curative services favour the non-poor: for every Re. 1 spent on the poorest 20% population, Rs. 3 is spent on the richest quintile.
- Only 10% Indians have some form of health insurance, mostly inadequate.
- Hospitalized Indians spend on an average 58% of their total annual expenditure.
- Over 40% of hospitalized Indians borrow heavily or sell assets to cover expenses.
- Over 25% of hospitalized Indians fall below poverty line because of hospital expenses.

2. NATIONAL RURAL HEALTH MISSION—THE VISION

- The National Rural Health Mission (2005-12) seeks to provide effective health care to rural population throughout the country with special focus on 18 states, which have weak public health indicators and/or weak infrastructure.
- These 18 States are Arunachal Pradesh, Assam, Bihar, Chhattisgarh, Himachal Pradesh, Jharkhand, Jammu & Kashmir, Manipur, Mizoram, Meghalaya, Madhya Pradesh, Nagaland, Orissa, Rajasthan, Sikkim, Tripura, Uttaranchal and Uttar Pradesh.
- The Mission is an articulation of the commitment of the Government to raise public spending on Health from 0.9% of GDP to 2-3% of GDP.

- It aims to undertake architectural correction of the health system to enable it to effectively handle increased allocations as promised under the National Common Minimum Programme and promote policies that strengthen public health management and service delivery in the country.
- It has as its key components provision of a female health activist in each village; a village health plan prepared through a local team headed by the Health and Sanitation Committee of the Panchayat; strengthening of the rural hospital for effective curative care and made measurable and accountable to the community through Indian Public Health Standards (IPHS); and integration of vertical Health and Family Welfare Programmes and Funds for optimal utilization of funds and infrastructure and strengthening delivery of primary health care.
- It seeks to revitalize local health traditions and mainstream AYUSH into the public health system.
- It aims at effective integration of health concerns with determinants of health like sanitation and hygiene, nutrition, and safe drinking water through a District Plan for Health.
- It seeks decentralization of programmes for district management of health.
- It seeks to address the inter-State and inter-district disparities, especially among the 18 high focus States, including unmet needs for public health infrastructure.
- It shall define time-bound goals and report publicly on their progress.
- It seeks to improve access of rural people, especially poor women and children, to equitable, affordable, accountable and effective primary health care.

3. GOALS

- Reduction in Infant Mortality Rate (IMR) and Maternal Mortality Ratio (MMR).
- Universal access to public health services such as Women's health, child health, water, sanitation and hygiene, immunization, and Nutrition.
- Prevention and control of communicable and non-communicable diseases, including locally endemic diseases.
- Access to integrated comprehensive primary health care.
- Population stabilization, gender and demographic balance.
- Revitalize local health traditions and mainstream AYUSH.
- Promotion of healthy lifestyles.

4. STRATEGIES

(a) Core Strategies:

- Train and enhance capacity of Panchayati Raj Institutions (PRIs) to own, control and manage public health services.
- Promote access to improved health care at household level through the female health activist (ASHA).
- Health Plan for each village through Village Health Committee of the Panchayat.
- Strengthening sub-centre through an untied fund to enable local planning and action and more Multi-Purpose Workers (MPWs).
- Strengthening existing PHCs and CHCs, and provision of 30-50 bedded CHC per lakh population for improved curative care to a normative standard (Indian Public Health Standards defining personnel, equipment and management standards).
- Preparation and Implementation of an inter-sectoral District Health Plan prepared by the District Health Mission, including drinking water, sanitation and hygiene and nutrition.
- Integrating vertical Health and Family Welfare programmes at National, State, Block, and District levels.
- Technical Support to National, State and District Health Missions, for Public Health Management.
- Strengthening capacities for data collection, assessment and review for evidence-based planning, monitoring and supervision.
- Formulation of transparent policies for deployment and career development of Human Resources for health.
- Developing capacities for preventive health care at all levels for promoting healthy lifestyles, reduction in consumption of tobacco and alcohol, etc.
- Promoting non-profit sector particularly in under served areas.

(b) Supplementary Strategies:

- Regulation of Private Sector including the informal rural practitioners to ensure availability of quality service to citizens at reasonable cost.
- Promotion of Public Private Partnerships for achieving public health goals.
- Mainstreaming AYUSH—revitalizing local health traditions.
- Reorienting medical education to support rural health issues including regulation of Medical care and Medical Ethics.
- Effective and viable risk pooling and social health insurance to provide health security to the poor by ensuring accessible, affordable, accountable and good quality hospital care.

5. PLAN OF ACTION

COMPONENT (A): ACCREDITED SOCIAL HEALTH ACTIVISTS

- Every village/large habitat will have a female Accredited Social Health Activist (ASHA)—chosen by and accountable to the panchayat—to act as the interface between the community and the public health system. States to choose State specific models.
- ASHA would act as a bridge between the ANM and the village and be accountable to the Panchayat.
- She will be an honorary volunteer, receiving performance-based compensation for promoting universal immunization, referral and escort services for RCH, construction of household toilets, and other health care delivery programmes.
- She will be trained on a pedagogy of public health developed and mentored through a Standing Mentoring Group at National level incorporating best practices and implemented through active involvement of community health resource organisations.
- She will facilitate preparation and implementation of the Village Health Plan along with Anganwadi worker, ANM, functionaries of other Departments, and Self Help Group members, under the leadership of the Village Health Committee of the Panchayat.
- She will be promoted all over the country, with special emphasis on the 18 high focus States. The Government of India will bear the cost of training, incentives and medical kits. The remaining components will be funded under Financial Envelope given to the States under the programme.
- She will be given a Drug Kit containing generic AYUSH and allopathic formulations for common ailments. The drug kit would be replenished from time to time.
- Induction training of ASHA to be of 23 days in all, spread over 12 months. On the job training would continue throughout the year.
- Prototype training material to be developed at National level subject to State level modifications.
- Cascade model of training proposed through Training of Trainers including contract plus distance learning model
- Training would require partnership with NGOs/ICDS Training Centres and State Health Institutes.

COMPONENT (B): STRENGTHENING SUB-CENTRES

- Each sub-centre will have an Untied Fund for local action @ Rs. 10,000 per annum. This Fund will be deposited in a joint Bank Account of the ANM and Sarpanch and operated by the ANM, in consultation with the Village Health Committee.

- Supply of essential drugs, both allopathic and AYUSH, to the Sub-centres.
- In case of additional Outlays, Multipurpose Workers (Male)/ Additional ANMs wherever needed, sanction of new Sub-centres as per 2001 population norm, and upgrading existing Sub-centres, including buildings for Sub-centres functioning in rented premises will be considered.

COMPONENT (C): STRENGTHENING PRIMARY HEALTH CENTRES

Mission aims at Strengthening PHC for quality preventive, promotive, curative, supervisory and Outreach services, through:

- Adequate and regular supply of essential quality drugs and equipment (including Supply of Auto Disabled Syringes for immunization) to PHCs.
- Provision of 24 hour service in 50% PHCs by addressing shortage of doctors, especially in high focus States, through mainstreaming AYUSH manpower.
- Observance of Standard treatment guidelines and protocols.
- In case of additional Outlays, intensification of ongoing communicable disease control programmes, new programmes for control of no communicable diseases, upgradation of 100% PHCs for 24 hours referral service, and provision of 2nd doctor at PHC level (I male, 1 female) would be undertaken on the basis of felt need.

COMPONENT (D): STRENGTHENING CHCs FOR FIRST REFERRAL CARE

A key strategy of the Mission is:

- Operationalizing 3222 existing Community Health Centres (30-50 beds) as 24 Hour First Referral Units, including posting of anaesthetists.
- Codification of new Indian Public Health Standards, setting norms for infrastructure, staff, equipment, management, etc. for CHCs.
- Promotion of Stakeholder Committees (Rogi Kalyan Samitis) for hospital management.
- Developing standards of services and costs in hospital care.
- Develop, display and ensure compliance to Citizen's Charter at CHC/PHC level.
- In case of additional Outlays, creation of new Community Health Centres (30-50 beds) to meet the population norm as per Census 2001, and bearing their recurring costs for the Mission period could be considered.

COMPONENT (E): DISTRICT HEALTH PLAN

- District Health Plan would be an amalgamation of field responses through Village Health Plans, State and National priorities for Health, Water Supply, Sanitation and Nutrition.
- Health Plans would form the core unit of action proposed in areas like water supply, sanitation, hygiene and nutrition. Implementing Departments would integrate into District Health Mission for monitoring.
- District becomes core unit of planning, budgeting and implementation.
- Centrally Sponsored Schemes could be rationalized/modified accordingly in consultation with States.
- Concept of "funneling" funds to district for effective integration of programmes
- All vertical Health and Family Welfare Programmes at District and state level merge into one common "District Health Mission" at the District level and the "State Health Mission" at the state level
- Provision of Project Management Unit for all districts, through contractual engagement of MBA, Inter Charter/Inter Cost and Data Entry Operator, for improved programme management.

COMPONENT (F): CONVERGING SANITATION AND HYGIENE UNDER NRHM

- Total Sanitation Campaign (TSC) is presently implemented in 350 districts, and is proposed to cover all districts in 10th Plan.
- Components of TSC include IEC activities, rural sanitary marts, individual household toilets, women sanitary complex, and School Sanitation Programme.
- Similar to the DHM, the TSC is also implemented through Panchayati Raj Institutions (PRIs).
- The District Health Mission would therefore guide activities of sanitation at district level, and promote joint IEC for public health, sanitation and hygiene, through Village Health and Sanitation Committee, and promote household toilets and School Sanitation Programme. ASHA would be incentivized for promoting household toilets by the Mission.

COMPONENT (G): STRENGTHENING DISEASE CONTROL PROGRAMMES

- National Disease Control Programmes for Malari a, TB, Kala Azar, Filaria, Blindness and Iodine Deficiency and Integrated Disease Surveillance Programme shall be integrated under the Mission, for improved programme delivery.
- New Initiatives would be launched for control of Non Communicable Diseases.

- Disease surveillance system at village level would be strengthened.
- Supply of generic drugs (both AYUSH and Allopathic) for common ailments at village, SC, PHC/CHC level.
- Provision of a mobile medical unit at District level for improved Outreach services.

COMPONENT (H): PUBLIC-PRIVATE PARTNERSHIP FOR PUBLIC HEALTH GOALS, INCLUDING REGULATION OF PRIVATE SECTOR

- Since almost 75% of health services are being currently provided by the private sector, there is a need to refine regulation.
- Regulation to be transparent and accountable.
- Reform of regulatory bodies/creation where necessary.
- District Institutional Mechanism for Mission must have representation of private sector.
- Need to develop guidelines for Public-Private Partnership (PPP) in health sector. Identifying areas of partnership, which are need based, thematic and geographic.
- Public sector to play the lead role in defining the framework and sustaining the partnership.
- Management plan for PPP initiatives: at District/State and National levels.

COMPONENT (I): NEW HEALTH FINANCING MECHANISMS

A Task Group to examine new health financing mechanisms, including Risk Pooling for Hospital Care as follows:

- Progressively the District Health Missions to move towards paying hospitals for services by way of reimbursement, on the principle of "money follows the patient."
- Standardization of services—outpatient, in-patient, laboratory, surgical interventions—and costs will be done periodically by a committee of experts in each state.
- A National Expert Group to monitor these standards and give suitable advice and guidance on protocols and cost comparisons.
- All existing CHCs to have wage component paid on monthly basis. Other recurrent costs may be reimbursed for services rendered from District Health Fund. Over the Mission period, the CHC may move towards all costs, including wages reimbursed for services rendered.
- A district health accounting system, and an ombudsman to be created to monitor the District Health Fund Management, and take corrective action.

- Adequate technical managerial and accounting support to be provided to DHM in managing risk-pooling and health security.
- Where credible Community Based Health Insurance Schemes (CBHI) exist/are launched, they will be encouraged as part of the Mission.
- The Central government will provide subsidies to cover a part of the premiums for the poor, and monitor the schemes.
- The IRDA will be approached to promote such CBHIs, which will be periodically evaluated for effective delivery.

COMPONENT (J): REORIENTING HEALTH/MEDICAL EDUCATION TO SUPPORT RURAL HEALTH ISSUES

- While district and tertiary hospitals are necessarily located in urban centres, they form an integral part of the referral care chain serving the needs of the rural people.
- Medical and para-medical education facilities need to be created in states, based on need assessment.
- Suggestion for Commission for Excellence in Health Care (Medical Grants Commission), National Institution for Public Health Management, etc.
- Task Group to improve guidelines/details.

6. INSTITUTIONAL MECHANISMS

- Village Health and Sanitation Samiti (at village level consisting of Panchayat Representative/s, ANM/MPW, Anganwadi worker, teacher, ASHA, community health volunteers.
- Rogi Kalyan Samiti (or equivalent) for community management of public hospitals.
- District Health Mission, under the leadership of Zila Parishad with District Health Head as Convener and all relevant departments, NGOs, private professionals, etc. represented on it.
- State Health Mission, Chaired by Chief Minister and co-chaired by Health Minister and with the State Health Secretary as Convener-representation of related departments, NGOs, private professionals, etc.
- Integration of Departments of Health and Family Welfare, at National and State level.
- National Mission Steering Group chaired by Union Minister for Health and Family Welfare with Deputy Chairman Planning Commission, Ministers of Panchayat Raj, Rural Development and Human Resource Development and public health professionals as members, to provide policy support and guidance to the Mission.

- Empowered Programme Committee chaired by Secretary HFW, to be the Executive Body of the Mission.
- Standing Mentoring Group shall guide and oversee the implementation of ASHA initiative.
- Task Groups for Selected Tasks (time-bound).

7. TECHNICAL SUPPORT

- To be effective the Mission needs a strong component of Technical Support.
- This would include reorientation into public health management.
- Reposition existing health resource institutions, like Population Research Centre (PRC), Regional Resource Centre (RRC), State Institute of Health and Family Welfare (SIHFW).
- Involve NGOs as resource organisations.
- Improved Health Information System.
- Support required at all levels: National, State, District and sub-district.
- Mission would require two distinct support mechanisms—Program Management Support Centre and Health Trust of India.

(A) PROGRAM MANAGEMENT SUPPORT CENTRE

- For Strengthening Management Systems-basic program management, financial systems, infrastructure maintenance, procurement and logistics systems, Monitoring and Information System (MIS), non-lapsable health pool, etc.
- For Developing Manpower Systems—recruitment (induction of MBAs/CAs/MCAs), training and curriculum development (revitalization of existing institutions and partnerships with NGO and private sector. Sector institutions), motivation and performance appraisal, etc.
- For Improved Governance—decentralization and empowerment of communities, induction of IT based systems like e-banking, social audit and right to information.

(B) HEALTH TRUST OF INDIA

- Proposed as a knowledge institution, to be the repository of innovation—research and documentation, health information system, planning, monitoring and evaluation, etc.
- For establishing Public Accountability Systems—external evaluations, community-based feedback mechanisms, participation of PRIs/NGOs, etc.

- For developing a Framework for pro-poor Innovations.
- For reviewing Health Legislations.
- A base for encouraging experimentation and action research.
- For inter and intra-Sector Networking with National and International Organisations.
- Think Tank for developing a long-term vision of the Sector and for building planning capacities of PRIs, Districts, etc.

8. ROLE OF STATE GOVERNMENTS UNDER NRHM

- The Mission covers the entire country. The 18 high focus States are Uttar Pradesh, Bihar, Rajasthan, Madhya Pradesh, Orissa, Uttaranchal, Jharkhand, Chhattisgarh, Assam, Sikkim, Arunachal Pradesh, Manipur, Meghalaya, Tripura, Nagaland, Mizoram, Himachal Pradesh and Jammu and Kashmir. GoI would provide funding for key components in these 18 high focus States. Other States would fund interventions like ASHA, Programme Management Unit (PMU), and upgradation of SC/PHC/CHC through Integrated Financial Envelope.
- NRHM provides broad conceptual framework. States would project operational modalities in their State Action Plans, to be decided in consultation with the Mission Steering Group.
- NRHM would prioritize funding for addressing inter-state and intradistrict disparities in terms of health infrastructure and indicators.
- States would sign Memorandum of Understanding with Government of India, indicating their commitment to increase contribution to Public Health Budget (preferably by 10% each year), increased devolution to Panchayati Raj Institutions as per 73rd Constitution (Amendment) Act, and performance benchmarks for release of funds.

9. FOCUS ON THE NORTH EASTERN STATES

- All 8 North East States, including Assam, Arunachal Pradesh, Manipur, Meghalaya, Mizoram, Nagaland, Sikkim and Tripura, are among the States selected under the Mission, for special focus.
- Empowerment to the Mission would mean greater flexibilities for the 10% committed Outlay of the Ministry of Health and Family Welfare, for North East States.
- States shall be supported for creation/upgradation of health infrastructure, increased mobility, contractual engagement, and technical support under the Mission.
- Regional Resource Centre is being supported under NRHM for the North Eastern States.

- Funding would be available to address local health issues in a comprehensive manner, through State specific schemes and initiatives.

10. ROLE OF PANCHAYATI RAJ INSTITUTIONS

The Mission envisages the following roles for PRIs:

- States to indicate in their MoUs the commitment for devolution of funds, functionaries and programmes for health, to PRIs.
- The District Health Mission to be led by the Zila Parishad. The DHM will control, guide and manage all public health institutions in the district, Sub-centres, PHCs and CHCs.
- ASHAs would be selected by and be accountable to the Village Panchayat.
- The Village Health Committee of the Panchayat would prepare the Village Health Plan, and promote intersectoral integration.
- Each sub-centre will have an Untied Fund for local action @ Rs. 10,000 per annum. This Fund will be deposited in a joint Bank Account of the ANM and Sarpanch and operated by the ANM, in consultation with the Village Health Committee.
- PRI involvement in Rogi Kalyan Samitis for good hospital management.
- Provision of training to members of PRIs.
- Making available health related databases to all stakeholders, including Panchayats at all levels.

11. ROLE OF NGOs IN THE MISSION

- Included in institutional arrangement at National, State and District levels, including Standing Mentoring Group for ASHA.
- Member of Task Groups.
- Provision of Training, BCC and Technical Support for ASHAs/ DHM.
- Health Resource Organisations.
- Service delivery for identified population groups on select themes.
- For monitoring, evaluation and social audit.

12. MAINSTREAMING AYUSH

- The Mission seeks to revitalize local health traditions and mainstream AYUSH infrastructure, including manpower, and drugs, to strengthen the public health system at all levels.
- AYUSH medications shall be included in the Drug Kit provided at village levels to ASHA.

- The additional supply of generic drugs for common ailments at Subcentre/PHC/CHC levels under the Mission shall also include AYUSH formulations.
- At the CHC level, two rooms shall be provided for AYUSH practitioner and pharmacist under the Indian Public Health System (IPHS) model.
- Single doctor PHCs shall be upgraded to two doctor PHCs by mainstreaming AYUSH practitioner at that level.

13. FUNDING ARRANGEMENTS

- The Mission is conceived as an umbrella programme subsuming the existing programmes of health and family welfare, including the RCHII, National Disease Control Programmes for Malaria, TB, Kala Azar, Filaria, Blindness and Iodine Deficiency and Integrated Disease Surveillance Programme.
- The Budget Head For NRHM shall be created in B.E. 2006-07 at National and State levels. Initially, the vertical health and family welfare programmes shall retain their Sub-Budget Head under the NRHM.
- The Outlay of the NRHM for 2005-06 is in the range of Rs. 6700 crores.
- The Mission envisages an additionality of 30% over existing Annual Budgetary Outlays, every year, to fulfil the mandate of the National Common Minimum Programme to raise the Outlays for Public Health from 0.9% of GDP to 2-3% of GDP.
- The Outlay for NRHM shall accordingly be determined in the Annual Budgetary exercise.
- The States are expected to raise their contributions to Public Health Budget by minimum 10% p.a. to support the Mission activities.
- Funds shall be released to States through SCOVA, largely in the form of Financial Envelopes, with weightage to 18 high focus States.

14. TIMELINES (FOR MAJOR COMPONENTS)

Merger of Multiple Societies Constitution of District/State Mission	June 2005
Provision of additional generic drugs at SC/PHC/CHC level	December 2005
Operational Programme Management Units	2005-06
Preparation of Village Health Plans	2006
ASHA at village level (with Drug Kit)	2005-08
Upgrading of Rural Hospitals	2005-07
Operationalizing District Planning	2005-07
Mobile Medical Unit at district level	2005-08

15. OUTCOMES

(a) National Level:

- Infant Mortality Rate reduced to 30/1000 live births.
- Maternal Mortality Ratio reduced to 100/100,000.
- Total Fertility Rate reduced to 2.1.
- Malaria mortality reduction rate -50% upto 2010, additional 10% by 2012.
- Kala Azar mortality reduction rate: 100% by 2010 and sustaining elimination until 2012.
- Filaria/Microfilaria reduction rate: 70% by 2010, 80% by 2012 and elimination by 2015.
- Dengue mortality reduction rate: 50% by 2010 and sustaining at that level until 2012.
- Japanese Encephalitis mortality reduction rate: 50% by 2010 and sustaining at that level until 2012.
- Cataract Operation: increasing to 46 lakhs per year until 2012.
- Leprosy prevalence rate: reduce from 1.8/10,000 in 2005 to less than 1/10,000 thereafter.
- Tuberculosis DOTS services: Maintain 85% cure rate through entire Mission period.
- Upgrading Community Health Centers to Indian Public Health Standards.
- Increase utilization of First Referral Units from less than 20% to 75%.
- Engaging 250,000 female Accredited Social Health Activists (ASHAs) in 10 States.

(b) Community Level:

- Availability of trained community level worker at village level, with a drug kit for generic ailments.
- Health Day at Anganwadi level on a fixed day/month for provision of immunization, ante/post-natal checkups and services related to mother and child health care, including nutrition.
- Availability of generic drugs for common ailments at Sub-centre and hospital level.
- Good hospital care through assured availability of doctors, drugs and quality services at PHC/CHC level.
- Improved access to Universal Immunization through induction of Auto Disabled Syringes, alternate vaccine delivery and improved mobilization services under the programme.
- Improved facilities for institutional delivery through provision of referral, transport, escort and improved hospital care subsidized

under the Janani Suraksha Yojana (JSY) for the Below Poverty Line families.

- Availability of assured health care at reduced financial risk through pilots of Community Health Insurance under the Mission.
- Provision of household toilets.
- Improved Outreach services through mobile medical unit at districtlevel.

16. MONITORING AND EVALUATION

- Health MIS to be developed upto CHC level, and web-enabled for citizen scrutiny.
- Sub-centres to report on performance to Panchayats, Hospitals to Rogi Kalyan Samitis and District Health Mission to Zila Parishad.
- The District Health Mission to monitor compliance to Citizen's Charter at CHC level.
- Annual District Reports on People's Health (to be prepared by Govt/NGO collaboration).
- State and National Reports on People's Health to be tabled in Assemblies, Parliament.
- External evaluation/social audit through professional bodies/ NGOs.
- Mid Course reviews and appropriate correction.

Some of the key areas that have been identified for concerned action within the NRHM framework of action are the following:

- Efficient functioning health facilities and services.
- Quality and accountability in the delivery of health services to the poor people.
- Prepare for health transformation with appropriate health financing and efficiency.
- Pro-people public private partnership to pool the resources.
- Convergence for effectiveness and efficiency to avoid duplication.
- Responsive health system meeting people's health needs.
- Special attention to aged, women and children.

Evaluation

National Rural Health Mission is an excellent scheme with excellent health infrastructure for planning, implementation and monitoring. However, the earlier health infrastructure to achieve health for all by 2000 AD created to fulfil the Alma Ata Declaration. That could not be achieved. The following suggestions are made to see that National Rural Health Mission achieves its goal and not become a routine programme like earlier ones.

It has become a fashion to set-up a new scheme without going into the causes of failures of earlier scheme. People were familiar with earlier scheme. What was needed was to improve upon that scheme and infect new inputs. The frequent changes in the schemes has poor impact and the period of 7 years for which National Rural Mission has been set-up would not be able to achieve much. The names of the schemes do not matter. What matters is the provision of health care to the rural people—

1. The success of the programme depends upon the human resources, therefore top most priority must be given to the development of human resource.
2. Health experts in secondary and tertiary health care are apathetic to such schemes. There persists widespread negative and unhelpful attitude among health personnel towards the health care of the poorest strata in the rural and urban population. They are not aware of the social responsibility to the society. If the doctors at the primary level are not mentally convinced of the scheme, changes at the grassroots are unimaginable and impracticable. The Government should not only consult experts before formulating any scheme but should also be able to energize, enthuse and develop a rapport with the professional organisations and, through them, their individual members to take an active part in the NRHM.
3. Absence of Rural Bias in Medical Education. There is national commitment to reorient medical education profession and health services, so as to serve the needs of rural people. All the expert bodies have agreed to modify the syllabus of undergraduate medical education so as to produce a basic doctor who would have the ability to cater to the needs of the rural area. It is necessary to make the medical colleges act not as ivory temples in majestic isolation but take on the responsibility for providing total health care for specified segments of the rural population.[1] The aim of medical education should be to promote happiness through better health of most of the deprived hundreds of millions of human beings. With the contemplated changes in the contents of the undergraduate course, the students would be in a position to appreciate the problems of rural people and would develop proper motivation to help them.
4. Lack of Proper Health Education of the Village Community. Rural people lack functional literacy, which is *sine qua non* for any endeavour towards community development. This requires a great effort on the part of the State governments; voluntary institutions and the health administrators should properly

1. India: National Plan for Health Care Services in the Rural Areas.

educate and enlighten the people. Properly planned programmes of health education would go a long way in propagating the ideals of a primary health care. According to Dr. Mahler, the required new type of health education should be, "neither oversopshisticated nor condescending but that gains the confidence of the individuals and communities by explaining health technology in a language they can understand so that they can participate genuinely in taking decisions concerning their health. In short, a replacement of passive health education by active health learning." Besides, the beneficiaries should be asked to contribute to the cost of Primary Health Care. Everyone should realize his responsibility towards the health coverage of the community. When the rural people would be contributing, they would like to participate and take interest in it's functioning. Some nominal contributions may be taken from the people themselves depending upon their income.

5. Absence of Political Support and Interest in the Problems of Rural Areas. The political elite in the country are not sensitive and responsive to their duties. They are busy with manipulation of politics and find hardly any time to look into the problems of the people. Because of instability in politics, there is no continuous, concerted and consistent effort to weed out the obstacles in the path of development. What is required is a strong political will and determination to make these scheme successful. Political elite at all levels must support the cause of the rural poor and help them to enjoy the good standards of life, which were promised to them at the inception of independence. Political powers and wisdoms are constantly required in a democratic set-up to resolve any problem arising out of the policies and implementation of the scheme. The political elite may have to take bold and unpleasant steps to re-allocate the resources between urban and rural sectors.

6. No sound Administrative set-up to Implement the Polities of Community Health. A revolutionary scheme of this type can be successful only if there is proper administrative set-up to implement it. Most of the health experts are of the view that the scheme has been rushed through without examining its requirements. It is suggested that some experts in Public Administration may examine the organisation and procedure, which are being used to implement the scheme. They may also examine the problems of coordination, control, supervision and headquarter-field relationships. In the light of the suggestions, the existing scheme may be modified to suit the requirements and the scheme in new areas may be set-up according to new recommendations. One of the very important problems is the poor quality of supervision of the scheme. Multipurpose health

workers who are supposed to be their immediate supervisors lack proper orientation and training themselves. It is suggested that the multipurpose workers may be given refresher courses to discharge their duties efficiently.

National Rural Health Mission

A seven year National Rural Health Mission (NRHM), which spans the duration of the 11th Plan, has been launched to address infirmities and problems across rural primary health care. Converging the public health approach with primary health care has been one of the primary objectives of this mission. Another objective is to genuinely empower and support Panchayati Raj Institutions to manage, administer and be accountable for health services at community levels. Supervision of health sub-centres by gram panchayats will improve attendance of staff, motivate appropriate quality of care and provide constant feedback on patient satisfaction. The NRHM will also converge the management of health delivery across all systems (including ISM) at primary health care levels—

- The National Rural Health Mission is expected to address the gaps in the provision of effective health care to rural population with special focus on 18 states, which have weak public health indicators and/or weak infrastructure.
- The Mission is a shift away from the vertical health and family welfare programmes to a new architecture of all inclusive health development in which societies under different programmes will be merged and resources pooled at the district level.
- It aims at effective integration of health concerns with determinants of health lie safe drinking water, sanitation and nutrition through integrated District Plans for Health. There is a provision for flexible funds so that the States can utilize them in the areas they feel are important.
- The Mission provides for appointment of Accredited Social Health Activist (ASHA) in each village and strengthening public health infrastructure, including outreach through mobile clinics. It emphasizes involvement of the non-profit sector, especially in the under served areas. It also aims at flexibility at the local level by providing for untied funds.
- The Mission, in its supplementary strategies, will aim at fostering public-private partnerships; regulating the private sector to improve equity and reduce out of pocket expenses; introducing effective risk pooling mechanisms and social health insurance; and taking advantage of local health traditions.[2]

2. Planning Commission, GOI, 17th November 2006, Towards Faster and More Inclusive Growth, An Approach to the 11th Five Year Plan, p. 71.

Conclusion

The experiment of National Rural Health Mission (NRHM) in India has not gone on long enough to reveal all the problems inherent in it. There is no denying the fact that this is theoretically sound and can help the unprivileged people and deprived communities to take care of their health problems which otherwise would remain unattended to because of financial and professional constraints. The scheme is a vital link in the country's health scheme.

3

CHAPTER

Inter-Sectoral Co-ordination for Health Promotion

Health Sector cannot achieve health for all on its own. Most of the determinants of health are outside the narrowly defined "health" sector. It is well known that education can play a significant role in the development of better health. The higher the level of education the better the health status. This is especially so with respect to female education. We can have health promoting schools. In all the developmental activities, health sector can (and should) provide technical expertise. Health sector can provide "added value." We should have partnership approach between the health sector and other sectors. Integrated approaches are needed. In the health sector itself, there is need for better partnership between the public, voluntary and private sectors, so as to provide better care, especially for the disadvantaged and improvement public health.

"Health profession has a key role to help ensure that the policies and strategies of various sectors and organisations contribute positively to health protection and promotion."

Inter-sectoral Action for Health, WHO, Geneva, 1997 calls for positive mutually supporting relationship between health sector and other sectors to achieve health outcomes, which are more efficient, effective, equitable and sustainable that could be achieved by the health sector alone. Whether within the Government or outside it, decisions affecting health should be taken collaboratively.

- The action taken should involve consideration of links between health and various factors in the physical, social and economic environment.
- The action must modify activities among the determinants of health so as to achieve better health.

CHART 3.1

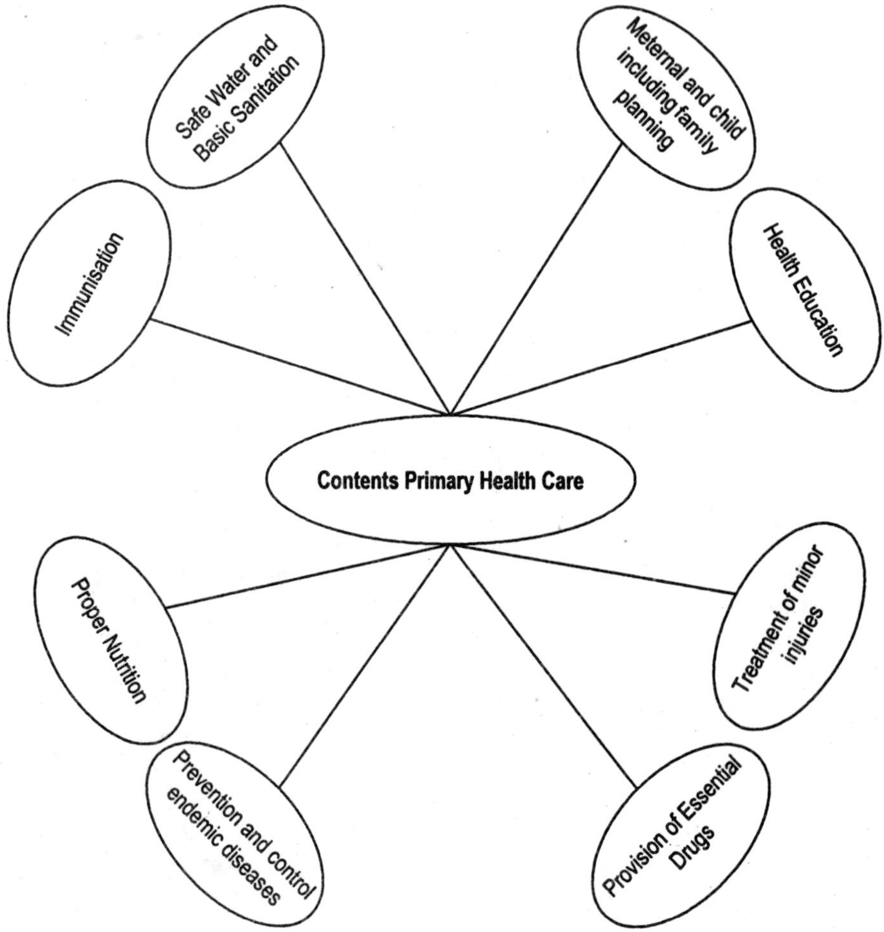

- The action should carry out the activities through widespread community participation.[1]

Closely allied to the concept of community participation is the fact that these programmes cannot be planned and implemented by the health sector alone. Only a multi-sectoral approach can set in motion the processes that lead to self-sustaining development. The benefits of visiting a health centre will be short-lived indeed if the person returns to the same environment that caused his ill-health in the first place. All conditions must improve—educational, economic, social, and of course health—if there is to be any real, lasting improvement.[2]

Alma-Ata-Declaration has desired multi-sectoral approach as one of the basic principles underlying Primary Health Care approach so as to enable the health organisations to attain 'Health For All'. The health status of the community is influenced by the various sectors such as Agriculture, Broadcasting and Information, Public Health Engineering, Education, Social Welfare and Rural Development. The programmes and schemes like Nutrition, Adult Education, Water and Sanitation, Integrated Child Development and Social Marketing need to be coordinated into an overall development effort.

National Institute of Health and Family Welfare in its document "Management Training Modules For District Health Officers" (New Delhi, 1990) states that the health and family welfare programme cannot function in isolation. The activities of other sectors directly as well as indirectly influence health development. Therefore, primary health care has to become a part of overall socio-economic development, including agriculture, irrigation, animal husbandry, education, social and women's welfare, housing and public works, communication, rural development, cooperatives, industries, panchayats and voluntary organisations. At present, extension workers and functionaries of these sectors/departments are operating in the field with few linkages of coordination. Mechanisms for coordination at the Central, state and district levels need to be developed so that the activities of the workers of all these sectors could be coordinated at the grassroot level. Arrangement should be made for working as a team, each member knowing who is doing what and for what purpose, so that programmes could be implemented in a more complimentary manner avoiding unnecessary duplication of efforts.

Coordinated planning at the community level will make it possible to link Primary Health Care closely with other sectors and with other agencies. The District Health Officer, therefore, needs to develop sound coordinating mechanisms at Community, Sector, Block and District levels. At present, extension workers of these sectors are operating in the field with few linkages. Mechanism for coordination at the Central, State and District levels also need to be developed so that the activities of the workers of all these sectors could be coordinated at the grass root level.

Arrangements should be made for working as a team, each member knowing who is doing what and for what purpose so that programmes could be implemented in a more complimentary manner, avoiding unnecessary duplication of efforts. Coordination means bringing about consistent and harmonious action of persons and programmes with each other towards a common goal. The coordination is lacking in the field of health care Administration resulting in poor delivery of health services. Professor Mofide (Iran) has rightly indicated the prevailing atmosphere when he states: "In the majority of countries with some or all of these problems (environmental) pollution, uncontrolled population growth; nutritional deficiencies; the high risk of disease: shortages and mal-distribution of trained staff; and insufficient financial, material and physical resources, there exists also a fragmentation of responsibilities for the delivery of health care, with overlapping, conflicting, and competing organisations within the health system and widely scattered funding mechanisms with the little control over costs. Health services authorities give only token recognition to those segments of the services that are not under their direct executive or financial control, and often plan only for that part of the national budget that is said to be their responsibility. The state of affairs is unjustified and harmful.[3]

Resources for the health care delivery are limited in the developing world. An effective health approach and strategy requires the coordinated efforts of sectors and agencies that can contribute directly or indirectly to the promotion of health care. Such coordinated efforts would promote health services that will be more efficient and effective from both the standpoint of the providers and that of the beneficiaries. The need of coordination is so great that according to Findlay, "It expresses the principles of organisation in toto; nothing less."[4]

The essential requisite to achieve coordination is to develop meaningful linkages with sectors of social and economic development, which can influence the promotion of health care, e.g., agriculture, public works, housing, communication, education, etc. The second step is to pool the efforts of all health agencies at all levels in a system to achieve maximum output—public and private; national and international; curative and promotive; peripheral, intermediate and central; western medicine and traditional medicine. This would avoid the dangers of dysfunctioal attitudes. Third, there is the need of welding different aspects of health services into a total health package, e.g., integration of maternal and child care, family planning, prevention of communicable diseases, health education, environmental sanitation.

Coordination and linkages on a systematic, rather than on adhoc, basis will definitely reduce costly duplications of effort and lead to increased health coverage of the needy population and neglected areas, while making the optimum use of the resources. Most of the countries in their reply to the WHO admitted that the lack of coordination in health care delivery system is a serious challenge. To quote WHO:

> "The consensus of opinion is that the most important managerial problems are foreseen in the continued reduction of the imbalance of the system and the lack of integration in the distribution of care with the existence of parallel systems with different objectives. Fragmentation and division of responsibility between the different levels of care have led to a lack of effective communication between the health and social welfare agencies. . . . As there are several agencies providing medical care there is overlapping and duplication of activities. . . . The major managerial problems. .....is to recognise the various components of this system in a way that reflects complementarily, eliminates duplication, and minimizes waste of resources."[5]

This problem becomes more acute in a federal country like India, where health is a State subject. It becomes important to coordinate the health programmes at the national level. The dilution of health standards in the State may affect adversely the whole country. There is a need, therefore, to give more powers to the central authority by making health a Concurrent subject. One of the health experts went on to say: "The present health situation in developing countries, especially India, is in a chaotic condition as non-scientific and realistic attempt is visible to coordinate the available inputs to produce maximum output. We can locate a large area without any health care facilities while in some areas, every third shop or house is providing medical care."[6]

How can we achieve effective coordination? According to Dr. White, its achievement may require. "The most delicate insights, the most mature wisdom, and perception of a truly artistic quality."[7]

It has to be achieved through formal as well as informal methods. The effective coordination and linkages would automatically result from effective planning, policy-making, and manpower planning.[8] After planning and policy-making, the effective instrument to achieve coordination is to design a sound organisation. Dr. White says:

> "An organisation characterised by clear lines of authority, adequate powers, well-understood allocation of functions, absence of overlapping and duplication of effort and proper delegation of work in itself reduce the necessities of coordination."[9]

Besides, if the organisational boundaries are properly demarcated. there would be little scope of confusion and misunderstanding and coordination would naturally flow from this inherent structure.

The coordination among different agencies. However, can be obtained through mutual consultation or information. This mutual consultation should be encouraged through setting up of inter-departmental agency/ committees for joint planning, joint decision-making and joint action in areas concerning more than one agency. While achieving coordination, we may keep the cost factor in mind. Such inter or intra-agencies can serve a useful purpose when the members come duly prepared with a sense of urgency and commitment. According to Key, "a session of an inter-departmental committee tends to be a place where departmental representatives come well prepared to defend their positions and level more convinced than before of the correctness of their attitudes."[10]

We are to take care that the benefits achieved through coordination should surpass the expenditure incurred to obtain coordination. Besides formal methods, we should adopt informal methods which are as effective as the formal ones, e.g., the Central Council of Health and the Central Council of Family Welfare (India) used the informal methods to achieve coordination among the different States and between the Union Government and the State Governments. "It is the most powerful cement in the whole executive structure."[11]

We must encourage such informal methods at all levels of Government. We must try to achieve coordination to obtain coherency in all the agencies dealing directly or indirectly with health care, all the systems of medicines, all the persons responsible for health care (team work) and at all the levels through well designed formal and informal channels with minimum costs to fulfil the goal-the betterment of the health of mankind irrespective of the status and location and to obtain optimum benefits from available and potential resources.

According to Dr. Halfdan Mahler,[12] there is one more illustration that health can only be attained through a combination of diverse measure in the health and other related sectors. These measures have to be applied within communities to deal with the full range of problems whose combined effects ravage the health of people. With the possible exception of smallpox eradication (which had unique features—the exception that proved the rule), attempts to deal with single communicable diseases in ways that were at best parallel and at worst divergent have proved to be ineffective. There is no escape from the need to deal in a concerted manner with those factors that in the final analysis are common to most of these diseases. This is the rationale for primary health care accessible to all in a spirit of social equity, and for health systems based on primary health care. The health and family welfare programmes cannot function in isolation. The activities of other sectors directly as well as indirectly influence health development. Therefore, primary health care has to become a part of overall socio-economic development, including agriculture, irrigation, animal husbandry, education, social and women's welfare, housing and public works, communication, rural development, cooperatives, industries, panchayats and voluntary organisations. At present, extension workers and functionaries of these sectors/departments are operating in the field with few linkages or coordination. Mechanisms for coordination at the Central, state and district levels need to be developed so that the activities of the workers/functionaries of all these sectors could be coordinated at the grass root level. Arrangements should be made for working as a team, each member knowing who is doing what and for what purpose, so that programmes could be implemented in a more complimentary manner avoiding unnecessary duplication of efforts.

Ale ya El Bindari Hammad[13] (*World Health*, March 1986, p. 3) in the Article, "Inter-sectoral cooperation in Primary Health Care" rightly mentions the need of forging alliances with other sectors of development to ensure good health. To quote him:

> Improvements in the health status of a population cannot be achieved simply by expanding and developing the health services. The prevention and control of disease and the promotion of health require a concerted effort for the improvement of human well-being as a whole. In this task, what has been defined as "health care" has to be supported by improvements in the social and economic infrastructure, and contributions from various sectors other than health.

Certainly there has been a broad understanding of the linkages between health development and development in other sectors. The health experience of the industrialized countries has contributed significantly to this understanding. We know that the major causes of sickness and death arising out of a large cluster of disease associated with poor sanitation, illiteracy and low levels of income were effectively controlled in these countries well before the discovery of antibiotics and other spectacular curative "break through." The control of diarrhoeal disease, tuberculosis and a wide range of communicable disease was primarily achieved through far reaching improvements in the urban infrastructure, housing and environmental sanitation, through the changes in health behaviour which accompanied higher levels of education and literacy, and through the improvement in nutritional status as income and living standards steadily rose. The positive outcome in health was therefore the result of an inter-sectoral effort.

In the initiative embodied in WHOs Health for all strategy, inter-sectoral action has been emphasized and articulated as part of the entire health strategy, mainly because of the basic re-ordering of health priorities. Today the major emphasis is on the prevention and control of disease and the promotion of health through primary health care. This shift in priorities has immediately highlighted the inter-sectoral character of health care. Agriculture and nutrition, housing, sanitation, water supply, literacy, health education and greater self-reliance in the health care all are integrated in the current primary health care strategies.[14]

Achievement of the Health for all goals will depend vitally on sound intersectoral action directed at specific health goals. And on the other, the broader aim of increasing well-being and resistance to disease as a whole while promoting and maintaining good health will require the combined efforts of many sectors not immediately related to health.

Neither the individual nor the household perceives well-being as fragmented into sectors—even if that well-being stems from a specific economic sector, or from education, or from health, or from employment. Well-being is a single unified condition. The same is equally true of the well-being of a community. It is with this perception in mind that health planners and health workers need to act when drawing up strategies or putting primary health care into practice. This will ensure that the health component is placed in the context of social development as a whole, and that other sectors are mobilized and motivated to lend their support towards achieving health goals.[15]

In the initiative embodied in WHO's Health for all strategy, inter-sectoral action has been emphasised and articulated as part of the entire health strategy, mainly because of the basic re-ordering of health priorities. Today the major emphasis is on the prevention and control of disease and the promotion of health through primary health care. This shift in priorities has immediately highlighted the inter-sectoral character of health care. Agriculture and nutrition, housing, sanitation, water supply, literacy, health education and greater self-reliance in health care are all integrated in the current primary health care strategies.

Achievement of the Health for all goals will depend vitally on sound inter-sectoral action directed at specific health goals. On the one hand, eliminating the major causes of prevalent sickness and preventing any specific cluster of diseases will require action in all those areas outside the health sector which currently contribute to the incidence of those diseases. And on the other, the broader aim of increasing well-being and resistance to disease as a whole while promoting and maintaining good health will require the combined efforts of many sectors not immediately related to health.

Neither the individual nor the household perceives well-being as fragmented into sectors even if that well-being stems from a specific economic sector, or from education, or from health, or from employment. Well-being is a single unified condition. The same is equally true of the well-being of a community. It is with this perception in mind that health planners and health workers need to act when drawing up strategies or putting primary health care into practice. This will ensure that the health component is placed in the context of social development as a whole, and that other sectors are mobilised and motivated to lend their support towards achieving health goals. World Health Organisation is also committed to this ideal.

More than ever before, the experts responsible for planning national economies are recognising that a country's health forms part of an integrated process of development. The experience of the world's industrialised countries showed that diseases associated with poor sanitation, illiteracy and poverty were eventually controlled, not by spectacular medical breakthrough, but by improvements in urban services, housing and the environment, higher levels of education and better diets. The moral for all the world today is that the health sector cannot do it alone! Many other ministries, services, institutions, official and unofficial bodies, and all levels of administration down to the community and the family must become involved in health. So the drive towards the goal of Health for all by the year 2000 can only be inspired and fuelled by concerted inter-sectoral action.

Our graphic model suggests only the eight elements included in WHOs definition of Primary Health Care: education about health, proper nutrition, safe water and basic sanitation, maternal and child care including family planning, immunization, prevention and control of locally endemic diseases, appropriate treatment of common diseases and injuries, and provision of essential drugs. (Chart 3.1)

But these symbolise a huge range of factors to which other sectors besides health must contribute if all people are indeed to attain a level of health that will permit them to lead a socially and economically productive life.

No sector engaged in socio-economic development can function properly in isolation. In the context of primary health care it is necessary to involve all the developmental departments in a coordinated effort. The inputs of one department have got to be synchronised with those of other departments-a total effort at the grassroot level. Success in the field of health and family welfare will largely depend on successful implementation of various programmes of social and economic development simultaneously. Particular mention may be made of education, social welfare, agriculture. animal husbandry, food, industry, works and housing, and communication with which health development programmes should be linked for the success of health and family welfare programmes.

ESSENTIALS OF INTER-SECTORAL CO-ORDINATION

(i) Clear-cut demarcation of the role of different sectors of development in the promotion of health.
(ii) Arranging meetings among collaborative Organisations to sort out duties and responsibilities.
(iii) Developing informal relationships.
(iv) Creating interest in other organisations.
(v) Joint monitoring of the programmes.
(vi) Developing good inter-personal relations.

In the new millennium, inter-sectoral coordination is going to be of vital concern. There has been lot of duplication, overlapping, and high expenditure in dealing with isolated problems of development. In 21st century, we have to integrate programmes to achieve multi-dimensional benefits. Area development through Inter-sectoral programmes is going to be the tool with the planners. In the 21st century, resources for health may not be unlimited. The solution to the problem of Primary Health care in new millennium lies in pooling resources from the sectors having impact on Primary Health Care directly or indirectly. Following are recommended to be pursued to ensure Primary Health Care:

(i) Health is an input into, as well as an outcome of socio-economic development.
(ii) The clear formulation of development policies, plans, actions and strategies keeping in view the focus on health. It also aims at defining of role and responsibilities of participating agencies and determining functional linkages.
(iii) The identification of area for inter-sectoral cooperation and the determination of the specific contribution of each sector to the attainment of the goals proposed in the normal process of planning for health.
(iv) Community participation to encourage an inter-sectoral approach at the local level through community empowerment.
(v) Locating the hurdles which stands in the way of inter-sectoral development.

(vi) Arranging informal meetings among agencies engaged in development tasks having bearing on health.

(vii) Conducting joint evaluations.

(viii) What does illiteracy mean to the illiterate? Let us note here that the map of illiteracy closely coincides with the maps of poverty, malnutrition, ill-health, infant mortality, etc. Hence, in the typical case, the illiterate is not only unable to read and write but he—or more usually she—is poor, hungry, vulnerable to illness, and uncertain that even his or her present miserable circumstances will not decline to the point where life itself becomes the issue. In these circumstances, does his or her literacy really matter? Would he or she even list illiteracy among life's major problems? While man does not live by bread alone, we can assume that the hunger of the body will normally take precedence over the hunger of the mind, particularly if the intellectual diet available to the new literate is as poor as is normally the case.

It follows that the best argument for doing something about illiteracy is not that it is part of the immense problem of inequality in our world, but that literacy can be part of the answer to remedying it.

Mark L. Schneider, in his article, "Rhetoric and Reality" in *World Health,* March 1986 observed that Inter-sectoral linkages which combine increased family income, education, and effective health services targeted to the most high-risk groups can yield positive improvements in health conditions. At the same time, there is a growing awareness that the failure to take account of the implications of macro-economic policies and projects on the environment and on health can have serious negative consequences for national health goals. What Latin America and the Caribbean have learnt from the economic and adjustment crisis is that understanding the nature of intersectoral linkages and promoting mutually productive intersectoral cooperation are not merely desirable; they are essential to the achievement of both Health for all and economic development objectives.

Experience with inter-sectoral support for primary health care is still in infancy and there is considerable doubt as to how such support can be harnessed. While the health sector must take a lead in promoting cooperation, effective action may require direction from outside the health sector, by a body with executive as well as coordinating powers. There is a need to set-up co-ordinating machinery at all levels.

CASE STUDIES

I. Urban Basic Services Scheme

Government of India, State Governments and UNICEF initiated urban basic services to make the life of slum-dwellers in the cities better and check degradation of cities.

J.S. Saksena and P.N. Govindarajuler in their Article "Health Care For Urban Slums with special reference to Bangalore City" have rightly sensed the problem. To quote them:

> "Slum-dwellers have the worst of both the worlds-urban and rural. On one side they suffer from economic hardships, lack of education and absence of health infrastructure like the rural population. On the other hand, they also suffer the ill-effects of overcrowding, pollution and rootlessness characteristics of large metropolitan cities."

They further add that "Most comforts and conveniences of the cities are sustained by the work done by slum-dwellers. As such, the affluent and the privileged have the moral responsibility to try to mitigate and alleviate their suffering. Rural population may be ignorant of the "goodies" they are missing but a slum-dweller is painfully aware of the privations suffered by him due to his constantly rubbing shoulders with urban affluence and conspicuous Consumption with resultant frustration and resentment."

The author conducted a research study in Una district of Himachal Pradesh to study the impact of the scheme. The Urban Basic services programmes in Una district was started in 1987-88, that it actually came up in May, 1988 when the first instalment of money was received. The programme is being implemented in all the five towns of the District, i.e. Una, Mehatpur, Santokhgarh, Gagret and Daulatpur. The Analysis of table indicates that out of a total slum population of 27,186 in all the five towns, 14,000 population is being covered under. UBS. The interesting feature of the population is that the Bastis are scattered being partly Hilly areas and these Bastis are not typical of Bastis in metropolitan cities in plains like Faridabad, Ludhiana, Delhi, etc. These Bastis do not pose problems to environmental sanitation except that the inhabitants, mostly belonging to scheduled castes, are poor and thus the women and children of these Bastis need special care to ensure their development and ultimately the total Development of the area.

There has been an effort to provide coverage of the basic services in all the Bastis. For improving the health services especially for women and children, there has been immunization (cent per cent) both for children and women, training of Dais, supplementary nutrition of children, medical checkup of children in Balwadis and primary schools. To ensure the education among children and women, the Balwadis and Adult Centres for Women have been set-up and to ensure economic independence for women, tailoring and knitting classes were started. There were also classes in food processing and soap-making. To maintain environmental sanitation, hand pumps have been installed, individual community and institutional latrines have been provided. Thus, women and children, especially of weaker sections of the society, have benefitted from the programme. For this, the Programme Officer has developed a liaison with District Information Officer to maintain Data Bank and information service.

The study found lack of inter-sectoral coordination to make sustained impact. Most of the components in these UBS programmes aim at providing fragments of services, while people need a total package. Most of the people narrated the same stories as given by Sister Agnestia in her article "Towards Health Care Directed For Social Transformation" (A Real Life Experience). To quote:

> "Can vitamin tablets satisfy their hunger and care their malnutrition? Can ORS eradicate the repeated attacks of diarrohea? What was I doing through my health education campaign? I was trying to conceal the real cause of the illness. The fact is that the poor are forced to lead unhealthy lives because of their poverty, which itself is a result of the exploitative and unjust practices of Society. Uncritical acceptance of health messages conveniently removes the responsibility for ill-health from those who exploit and instead place the blame on the very people who are victims of the exploitation."

It is evident that most of the functions carried out by UBS personnel relate to other sectors like Health, Education, Social Welfare, etc. In order to converge the benefits, we suggest the following to ensure effective linkages:

(a) Where services are already provided by other sectors the need is to make these services functional through the intervention of UBS staff rather than venturing their own services like Immunization, Training of Dais, etc.

(b) District Coordinator must see as to what can be provided by other departments without any consumption of resources. For example, all the places for conducting classes for women and children are hired while many such rooms are lying idle and thus can be provided free of cost. Similarly, this exercise need to be done at Municipal level. One is surprised to find that the Municipal Committee/Notified Area committees are charging rents of their unoccupied rooms from this project which is a sad reflection.

(c) Most of the Project staff is vied with the idea that whatever has been budgeted must be spent whether it is relevant or not, e.g. a community latrine was built in an area where most of the houses have household latrines.

(d) Linkage with the Community has not been developed, e.g. for the construction of community services, no community labour is used and thus the expenditure became high with the defeat of basic purpose.[16]

2. Women's Health

Government of India, Department of Women and Child Development,

Ministry of Human Resources Development presented country report to the Fourth World Conference on Women (Beijing 1995).[17] The report clearly mentions the need of inter-sectoral coordination to promote health of women.

Women's health covers mortality, morbidity, nutritional status and reproductive health. Linked to these are environmental degradation, violence and occupational hazards, all of which have implications for women's health.

The health status of a population is one of the crucial elements in the assessment of the quality of life. More precisely, indicators, namely, maternal mortality (MMR) and morbidity rates, infant mortality rates (IMR), life expectancy, fertility rates, studied along with statistics on female literacy rates, work participation rates, age at marriage, cases of recorded violence, malnutrition, etc., provide pointers to the physical status and well-being of women. The health of Indian women is intimately related to the socio-economic status of the households to which they belong and their age and kinship/marital status within the households. Given the predominantly patriarchal set-up, women and girls get a lesser share in the intra-household distribution of healthy goods and services, compared to men and boys. However, in the intra-household distribution of labour, women get the major share of economic, procreative and family responsibilities. Due to the competing demands on their time and energy, as well as their socialization, women tend to neglect their health. The lesser access to food coupled with neglect invariably leads to a poor nutritional status and a state of ill-health for most women.

Women's health plays an important role in determining the health of the future population, because women's health has an inter-generational effect. The cumulative impact of the low health situation of women is reflected in the high MMRs, the incidence of low-birth weight babies, high prenatal mortality and foetal wastage and consequent high fertility rates.

Asha Das in her article,[18] "Child Development and Empowering Women in India." Women in *IJPA*, July to Sept. 1997 rightly observes that: the major approach for the future will be to bring in holistic approach for women's development. This underscores harmonisation of various efforts in different fronts—social, economic, legal, political and cultural. This calls for consolidation of various programmes and efforts in different sectors of the Government. and their integration in a logical fashion to converge various services and facilities required by women. A sub-plan approach to package all relevant resources and benefits for women's development will be laid down to ensure their systematic focus on women.

3. Community Development Programme (CDP)

The programme of Community Development started after independence in India was a programme cutting across sectoral boundaries. It embraced education, health, drinking water, roads, agricultural production and cottage industries.

4. Integrated Child Development Services (ICDS)

ICDS, started in 1975-76, is an excellent example of Inter-sectoral coordination. The ICDS Scheme aims to improve the nutritional and health status of pre-school children, pregnant women and nursing mothers through providing a package of services, including supplementary nutrition, pre-school education, immunization, health checkup, referral services and nutrition and health education. In addition, the scheme focuses on effective convergence of inter-sectoral services in the Anganwadi Centres (AWC) which is the place for providing services to women and the children.

5. Integrated Rural Development Programme

In 1976, the Lok Sabha approved the new strategy of rural development, which is commonly known as Integrated Rural Development Programme. World Bank sector paper defines rural development as "Rural development is a strategy designed to improve the economic and social life of a group of people—the rural poor. It involves extending the benefits to the poorest among those who seek a livelihood in the rural areas. The group includes small farmers, tenants and the landless."

R.N. Azad defines it as "integrated development of the areas and the people through optimum development and utilization of local resources, physical, biological and human by bringing about necessary institutional, structural and attitudinal changes by delivering a package of services to encompass not only the economic field, that is, agriculture and rural industries but also the establishment of social infrastructure and services in the area of health and nutrition, sanitation, housing, drinking water, with the ultimate objective of improving the quality of life of the rural poor and rural weak. Integrated rural development implies functional, spatial, and temporal integration of all these parameters. Thus, Integral rural development is a multifacet framework involving a multi-disciplinary approach. In this process, self-help and community participation have a paramount role."[19]

The IRDP, launched in 1980, is a credit linked self-employment programme of assistance of the already identified rural poor families to augment their income and help them cross over the poverty line. The IRDP is implemented through the District Rural Development Agency (DRDA), which is a broad-based representative body that provides guidance and direction for programme implementation. At the grassroots level, Block Development Office is responsible for implementing IRDP. At the state and the Central Government levels, the Department of Rural Development and the Ministry of Rural, Areas and Employment respectively oversee the programme's implementation.

The ultimate thrust of IRDP need be on enhancing the quality of life of the rural people. The Public Accounts Committee (PAC) of parliament has recently given some suggestion about reshaping the Integrated Rural Development Programme (IRDP)."[20]

It lacks a comprehensive approach. A large number of poverty alleviation programmes pertaining to income, employment, quality of life, etc. of the poor are implemented simultaneously aiming at more or less the same group of people. This creates overlapping which results in confusion and weak planning. Secondly, these programmes, are implemented by a large number of ministries and departments of the central and state governments. This multiplicity of agencies, without any satisfactory level of co-ordination among them, adds to the confusion. And, thirdly, the IRDP approach aims at providing self-employment to the poor without giving due consideration to the, desirability and feasibility of self-employment for the poorest sections of the society. It has been observed that many times the poor and specially the poorest sections of the population, prefer wage employment. The committee therefore feels that the poor, who are not willing or are incapable of taking up self-employment should be given an option of wage employment. There is a need to integrate wage employment programmes with self-employment programmes.

The committee has recommended that a more comprehensive approach to rural development should be adopted which would aim at redesigning the whole rural economy and society, at elimination of the exploitation of the poor and at providing them with gainful employment, whether under the auspices of the public or private sector or under self-employment. IRDP can be effective only if there is integrated planning and coordinated implementation. The committee therefore suggests that as a first step in this direction, all allied programmes and activities, and the economic infrastructure required for effective implementation of these programmes are integrated and brought under one ministry to avoid overlapping and to enable the government to have an effective control over these programmes. All the programmes must be an integral part of a single development plan formulated by a single development authority and for whose effective implementation one single authority is responsible and accountable.

CONCLUSION (See Chart 3.2)

Health Policy 1983 suggests that all health and human development must ultimately constitute an integral component of the overall socio-economic developmental process in the country. It is thus of vital importance to ensure effective coordination between the health and its more intimately related sectors. It is, therefore, necessary to set-up standing mechanisms, at the Centre and in the States, for securing inter-sectoral coordination of the various efforts in the fields of health and family planning, medical education and research, drugs and pharmaceuticals, agriculture and food, water supply and drainage, housing, education and social welfare and rural development. The coordination and review committees, to be set-up, should review progress, resolve bottlenecks and bring about such shifts in the contents and priorities of program as may

CHART 3.2

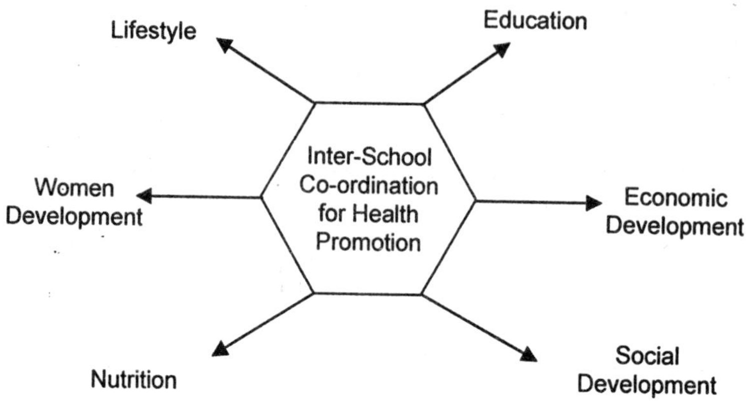

appear necessary, to achieve the overall objectives. At the community level, it would be desirable to devise arrangements for health and all other developmental activities being coordinated under an integrated programme of rural development.

Health policy 2002 recommends that It is well recognized that the overall well-being of the citizenry depends on the synergistic functioning of the various sectors in the socio economy. The health status of the citizenry would, *inter alia*, be dependent on adequate nutrition, safe drinking water, basic sanitation, a clear environment and primary education, especially for the girl child. The policies and the mode of functioning in these independent areas would necessarily overlap each other to contribute to the health status of the community. From the policy perspective, it is therefore imperative that the independent policies of each of these inter-connected sectors, be in tandem and that the interface between the policies of the two connected sectors, be smooth.

Sectoral policy documents are meant to serve as a guide to action for institutions and individual participants operating in that sector. Consistent with this role, NHP-2002 limits itself to making recommendations for the participants operating within the health sector. The policy aspects relating to inter-connected sectors, which, while crucial, fall outside the domain of the health sector, will not be covered by specific recommendations in this Policy document. Needless to say, the future attainment of the various goals set out in this policy assumes a reasonable complementary performance in these inter-connected sectors.

NOTES AND REFERENCES

1. Final Report, Karnataka towards Equity, Quality and Integrity in Health, Governmentof Karnataka, April, 2001, p. 304.
2. Dr. Hector R. Acuna, Community Participation, in *World Health*, Aug.-Sept. 1977, p. 6.

3. WHO, *World Health* Paper, 55, p. 83.
4. R.M. Findlay, Art of Administration. Edinburgh, Oliver, 1952, p. 48.
5. WHO, *Public Health Paper*, 55, p. 61.
6. Based on Personal discussion.
7. L.D. White, Introduction to the Study of Public Administration, Macmillan, pp. 213-14.
8. For details refer to the respective Chapters.
9. L.D. White, *op. cit.*, p. 214.
10. V.K. Key, Politics and Administration in White (Ed.), The Future of Government in the United States, p. 155.
11. S.E. Finer, Primer of Public Administration, London, 1950, p. 68.
12. Dr. Halfdan Mahler, "Defeat TB and Fore-ever", in *World Health*, January 1982. p. 3.
13. Ale ya EI Bindari Hammad. "Inter-sectoral Cooperation in Primary Health Care", in *World Health*, March 1986, p. 3.
14. WHO, *World Health*, March 9, 1986, p. 16.
15. S.L. Goel, "Planning and Administration of Urban Basic Services", in S. Bhatnagar and S.L. Goel, "Development Planning and Administrative" ed., New Delhi, Deep & Deep, 1992, pp. 167-206.
16. Aleya El Bindari Hammad, "Inter-sectoral Cooperation in Primary Health Care", *World Health*, March 1986, p. 5.
17. GOI, Department of Women and Child Development, Ministry of Human Resources Development, Fourth World Conference on Women, Beijing, 1995. (Country Report), p. 84.
18. Asha Das, "Child Development and Empowering Women in India", in *IJPA*, July-Sept., 1997, pp. 392-93.
19. R.N. Azad, Integrated Rural Development Dynamics of Development: An International Perspective, New Delhi, Concept, 1977, pp. 419-39.
20. A.K. Debey, "IRDP: The South Asian Experience" in *IJPA*, April-June, 1997, pp. 149-50.

4

CHAPTER

Community Participation and Health Development

Go in Search of People
Begin with what they know
Build on what they have

—*From a Chinese proverb*

According to Dennis E. Poplin (Communities- A survey of Theories and Methods of Research, McMillan, NY, 1972), A community is "a unit of social and territorial organisation in which people live, work, attend school, and carry on many other activities, which are a part of daily living. Indeed, communities are unique in that all of a person's needs can potentially be met within them."

Murray G. Ross defines community organisation as (Murray G. Ross and B.W. Lappin, Community Organisation, Theory, Principles and Practice, Harpa and Row, NY, Second Ed.) "a process by which a community identifies its needs or objectives, gives priority to them, develops the confidence and will to work at them, finds resources (internal and external) to deal with them, and in doing so, extends and develops cooperative and collaborative attitudes and practices within the community."

Kausar S. Khan, *et. al.* in their paper, "A Health Care Paradox" stress upon people's participation. To quote them: "Alma-Ata's challenge to view health as a human rights issue has not been adequately met by most Third World countries. Barring a few examples, health services continue to be either sub-standard, inaccessible, unaffordable and underutilised, or to suffer from varying combinations of these factors.

While governments of many countries, have spent millions on building physical infrastructures at district levels, the overall health status, especially of the urban and rural poor, remains deplorable. It is not more than evident that constructing a hierarchy of health centres, and even staffing them with doctors and paramedics, does not resolve the deeper issue of developing a health system that can achieve the goal of equity in health: universal coverage and care according to need.

This challenge is faced not only by governments but also by the non-governmental sector concerned with the health of the people. There is a pressing need to develop primary health care (PHC) systems which are technically sound and predicated on these principles of universal coverage and care according to need, but which at the same time involve communities so as to ensure that their own perceptions of their needs are fully recognised and that they are fully involved in the effort to address those needs."

Even the document "Action Plan for an Effective and Responsive government stressed that time has come for a strong message to be conveyed that administration is for the people and not the public servants themselves. There has to be a change of attitude, and public servants purport to offer, but in terms of public satisfaction. Simultaneously, there has also to be a cleansing of the services and codification of the ethics, value systems and the interface with the politicians.

The National Health Policy-2002 suggests that NHP-2002 recognizes the significant contribution made by NGOs and other institutions of the civil society in making available health service to the community. In order to utilize their high motivational skills on an increasing scale, this policy envisages that the disease control programmes should earmark not less than 10% of the budget in respect of identified programme components, to be exclusively implemented through these institutions. The policy also emphasizes the need to simplify procedures for government-civil society interfacing in order to enhance the involvement of civil society in public health programme. In principle, the state would encourage the handing over of public health service, outlets at any level for management by NGOs and other institutions of civil society, on as 'as-is-where-is' basis, along with the normative funds earmarked for such institutions.

MEANING OF COMMUNITY PARTICIPATION

What exactly we mean by community participation becomes rather enigmatic because every one interprets this term in his own way. The interpretation ranges from taking passive interest in local affairs as by reading newspapers, listening to radio, viewing TV and discussing matters with others, taking part in political activities like attending meetings, conferences, etc. and participating in processions and demonstrations. It may even include protest actions like strikes.

It is through participation that citizens at large are associated with the decisions taken by government. Participation can be at various levels and by different sets of people on different issues, in each case drawing different segments of community. It may be manifest in different degrees of intensity.[1]

People who share common interests and have the feeling that they belong together form a community. In a community people usually share common values, a common history (or background), and accept certain forms of behaviour as normal for all community members. People belonging to a certain religion or having the same political beliefs could also be called a community.

A community, then, is not the same thing as an area of land. Community is people, not land—but community members will often be able to point out the boundaries of land that belongs to the community.

Broadly speaking, the word participation is used to refer to the role of members of general public, as distinguished from that of appointed officials including civil servants, in influencing the activities of Government or in providing directly for community needs. It may occur at any level from the village to the country as a whole. It may involve decision-making, as in the case of governing bodies of local authorities and it may extend to actual implementation, as occurs when villagers/town-dwellers decide to carry out a community self-help project. The participation may be direct, as in community projects and in the work of private welfare organisations or it may be indirect, through elected officials or representative bodies responsive to public opinion. Individuals may participate through non-governmental or statutory bodies.

The extent of participation—whether direct or indirect—will ultimately depend upon citizens access to information and opportunity of presenting their views to elected representatives.

Lowell S. Levin in his article, "Listen to the Community" in the *World Health*, May-June 1992 observed that there is no mystery about community participation in health. The health care of ordinary people, for example, is mostly provided by self-care, or through family and friends, or through religious and voluntary groups. Only a small proportion of health care is provided by health professionals. Communities therefore have considerable responsibility for promoting good health through their investments in education, economic growth, social resources like recreation, and environmental protection. No professional service system could effectively or economically replace this "natural" social resource for health.

Professional planning and services should now be brought into clearer alignment with the community's priorities and preferences. This is not easily accomplished. It involves many stresses and strains on health professionals who, in the past, have not taken into account the community resources, priorities and views on how to proceed.

When the community is fully involved in all aspects of health development, new ideas and practices are widely and rapidly diffused through health education. Social networks are activated. People with similar values and experience trust and accept advice from each other more readily than they do from "authority figures", whose motives and social credentials may differ from those of the population they serve. Perhaps in the final analysis, reaching the hard-to-reach on their own terms may be the most valunale contribution of community participation.

May be we could conclude by saying that communities are concerned about their own health, and that there is already much collaboration with the health services. But governments should increases the possibilities for local communities to influence and participate in action for health. Health workers should be trained to understand their community and be taught how to work with people.

Yes, it is essential that everyone, clearly understands that communities should not only provide money, land and labour, but should contribute to health both intellectually and in decision-making. This is essential especially with regard to rural and poor urban communities.

Community participation is the process, of socio-economic development in which individuals and families assume responsibility and develop their capacity to contribute to development. This enables them to become agents for their own development instead of being passive beneficiaries of development aid. They are not obliged to accept conventional solutions that are unsuitable. They can improvise and innovate to find solutions that are suitable and sustainable. They have to acquire the capacity to appraise a situation, weigh the various possibilities and estimate what their own contribution can be. They are supposed to take active interest while the community must be willing to learn, the health system is responsible for explaining and advising, and for providing clear information about the favourable and adverse consequences of the interventions being proposed, as well as their relative costs.

Health personnel form an integral part of the community in which they live and work. A continuing dialogue between them and the rest of the community is necessary to harmonize views and activities relating to primary health care. Such a dialogue enables health personnel to acquire a better understanding of the community's feelings, the reasons for its views, the level of its aspirations and the pattern of its organisation and communication. For their part, the people will learn to identify real health needs, to understand the national strategy of primary health care and to become involved in and promote community action for health. Thus, society will come to realize that health is not only the right of all but also the responsibility of all, and the members of the health professions, too, will find their proper role.[2]

The management and monitoring of the basic health services that a community is entitled to by the community itself would go a long way to ensuring availability, accessibility and quality. It should be a tenet of policy to empower the people to do so or, in other words, to ensure that people's health is in people's hands. The community should be capable of determining their basic health needs, evaluating the local health situation and the services that exist and improving upon them. Mechanisms to create such awareness and to enable the local community to prepare Village Health Action Plans would need to be developed. These would include health campaigns, imaginative adoption of participatory techniques such as PRA, PLAINTIFF and micro-planning exercises. The involvement of youth and women's association, in conjunction with the panchayat institutions would be essential.

In the report on Primary Health Care presented at Alma-Ata by WHO and UNICEF, community participation has been mentioned as the essence of primary health care approach. It has been rightly pointed out that "self-reliance and. social awareness are the key factors in human development."

Development is a multi-dimensional phenomenon which cannot .be achieved unless the community itself is involved. Resources available with any Government are limited especially in the developing countries like India. Communities, according to their capacity, need to mobilise human, financial and material resources to supplement the resources provided by the national Government and other extra-community sources in order to effectively carry out local health improvement efforts. A community input for health care into the overall strategies, policies and work plan of the programme, which may range from unsystematic efforts by well intentioned health administrators to understanding varying community situations, to a systematic arrangement for the participation of people in health policy-making and for regular feedback of primary health care programme information from communities into the decision-making processes at different levels. Substantial financial and human resources can be mobilised from the community for health some of which may otherwise remain unused, such as the enthusiasm and energy of youth and women for community action. Communities with institutional structures such as local Government, a cooperative society, or a commune, which have a degree of control over the community productive assets, can mobilise resources for community health development programmes more easily than those relying on voluntary and individual contribution. Thus, the community participation is most widely seen as a way to mobilize resources for health that would otherwise not be available. A Government promoting health to meet the diverse needs of the people may be faced with expenditure it could not meet if the entire effort had to be financed out of the public purse. So, in order to cut costs, the intended beneficiaries themselves contribute to the extension of Primary Health Care coverage.

Community participation involves members of communities in planning, implementing and monitoring of health activities. Thus, community is wholly involved in the programme rather than being asked to either contribute or to take advantage of the services offered under it. Community participation is the process in which individual families assume responsibility for their own health. They come to know their own situation better and are motivated to solve their common problems. This enables them to become agents of their own development instead of passive beneficiaries of development aid. They, therefore need to realize that they are not obliged to accept conventional solutions that are not suitable. They have to acquire the capacity to appraise a situation, weigh the various possibilities and estimate what their own contribution can be.

Community participation is an educational and empowering process in which the people, in partnership with those who are able to assist them, seek to instil a sense of belongingness, self-reliance, confidence and competence to diagnose the problems, priorities the needs and assume critical responsibilities to manage, control and assess activities that affect them most and take collective actions that are proved necessary. It is a democracy in action. Community participation is of intrinsic value to the population group and ensures the involvement of local population in the decision-making process concerning development planning and implementation through their own efforts with the available local resources. The primary health care strategy is based upon effective community participation.

In Community participation, we have to safeguard the interests of the poor and the disadvantaged section of the society. Participation has objectives which the community commonly share. This common sharing makes the members of the community come together to take collective action to achieve the common goal. The goal gets the parameters and defines, in different situations, who the participants are. The roles different participants perform depend upon their capacity and capability like skills, technical knowledge, formal position, education, control over funds, connection with those in power, etc. The hierarchy makes the powerful participants active and others passive. This affects participation in favour of those who have the power to make decisions for and over others.

The poorer groups, who are generally the most affected by the development process, are the least endowed and least powerful. The poor are automatically excluded from the participation process. Decision-making is the first step in the development process. Therefore, a key objective of participation is to find out ways to include the hitherto neglected groups, who are directly affected by the negative impacts of development in the decision-making process.

Participation is a process of giving weightages to the poorer groups in the development process so that they may have a say and control over decisions which affect their lives; participation is a process of empowering the poorest. The indicator of genuine participation is the extent the poorer groups have power over decision-making and over resource management. Achieving sustainable development depends upon the extent of the participation.

Let us now discuss the essentials of participation:

- Full involvement at all levels, i.e. policy-making and planning.
- Framing/Developing programme.
- Implementation of programme.
- Evaluation of programme.
- Empowerment of powerless through giving weightage to them.
- Control over process and monitoring to ensure benefits. Keeping people well informed at all stages.

- According due recognition to people's contribution. Sincerity of government functionaries in enlisting people's support.
- Harnessing physical/economic/social resources of individual.
- Designing innovative plans for people's involvement in community.
- Empowered relationships.
- Voluntary contribution to programmes.
- Inculcating responsibility among the people for all development activities in the community.
- Ensuring that the people benefit from all development activities of the community.
- Selfless desire to work for the community.
- Respect faith in people's capacity and value the opinions and experience of the people.
- Develop on the basis of equal partnership.

P.K. Bajpai in his article, "People's Participation in Government" in *IJPA*, Oct.-Dec., 1998, rightly mentions that meaningful participation is concerned with achieving power, i.e., the power to influence the decision that affects one's livelihood. So power is the key variable to influence decision-making and lack of it not only causes but also perpetuates the well-being of the poor. Thus, participation, power and well-being are interlinked. Indian experience has been altogether different as policies and programmes meant for development of poor have rendered only intoxicating impact and have genuinely not been concerned with sharing power.

Government must understand that consciensation of the people and their active participation in the development process, on the one hand, and asserting their rights, on the other, does not weaken the authority of the State but is the symptom of true and mature democracy.

To encourage participation, you should try to:

- Keep people informed about activities that are being planned.
- Encourage suggestions to be made, directly or through a representative, to the planning committee.
- Set out specific tasks and jobs for everyone. You will need to explain the tasks and may provide some training. People should also understand how important their own job is to the success of the whole project.
- Find out on what date most people will be able to participate.
- Give praise and show appreciation to all who help. For example, you could take a photograph of everyone who helped with a project and display it where it can be seen by members of the community.

PURPOSES

Based upon our earlier observations, let us mention the important purposes that can be served by encouraging people's participation. (See Chart 4.1)

(i) Creating will and determination among the members of the community for improvement in their present and future life.
(ii) Identification and development of the local resources, thereby generating self-reliance among the community.
(iii) Achieving integrated area coordination among various agencies interested in primary health care.
(iv) Mobilising the available manpower for productive and useful activities.
(v) Keeping the members of the community constantly informed about the developments in the area.
(vi) Arranging functional literacy programmes which can help them in understanding new technology.
(vii) Organising various clubs of youth, women, to serve as centres of discussion and development.
(viii) Providing an open forum for the community to discuss its problems and find indigenous solutions which may be efficient and economical.
(ix) To develop local leaders who can further educate and mobilise the people in the area.
(x) Encouraging the people to adopt modern changes which can accelerate their socio-economic development.
(xi) Arranging extra curricular activities to generate social awareness through well designed publicity.
(xii) Encouraging the people to develop themselves rather than depend upon the Government for all activities and thus become self-reliant which is the key to development.
(xiii) Resource mobilisations from within the community to supplement organised health care services and keeping social control in the way resources are utilised.
(xiv) Encouraging non-governmental and voluntary organisations to become active partners in health care delivery.
(xv) Encouraging village health committees, panchayats, mahila mandals and youth clubs involvement in health care.
(xvi) The health care service providers and voluntary agencies should not behave as providers rather they should consciously make efforts to be viewed as agents of change enabling the community to use its own resources, improve skills to improve its own health.
(xvii) Recognizing the need to develop inter-sectoral coordination and multiple support linkage with health and health-related sectors of development to provide for the interest of varied sections of the community to avoid segmentation.

CHART 4.1

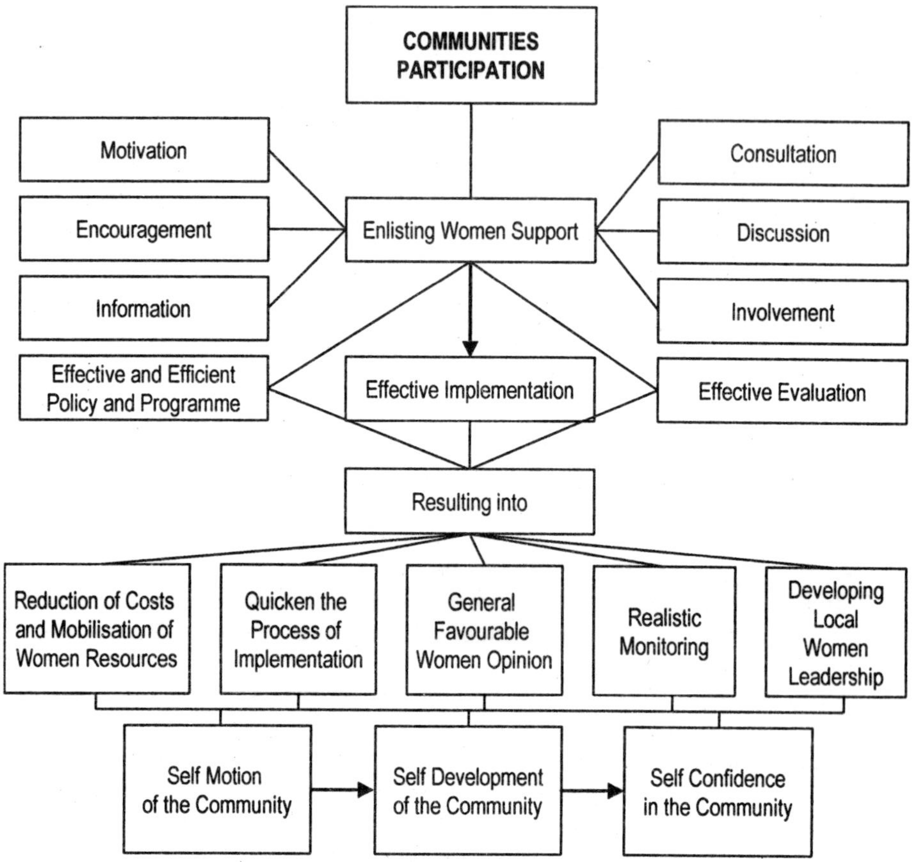

(xviii) Motivate and strengthen the skill of grass root level workers to improve their credibility in the community.
(xix) Catalyst for further development.
(xx) Generate kinetic energy for health development.
(xxi) Making people aware of their health needs.
(xxii) Higher achievement at a lower cost.

Mr. Etienne Berthet, Honorary Director General of the International Children's Centre, Paris has rightly said that all human behaviour aims at satisfying a need or an aspiration, and people will only agree to change their habits when they are convinced that it will be to their advantage. So it is through informing, motivating and encouraging the people that we can best hope to improve their living conditions.[3]

The Fifth Five Year Plan has also recognised this need. The Fifth Plan says, "The involvement of the people and their elected representatives is a prerequisite for effective planning. A plan which does not take into account their aspirations and preferences can have no operational validity, especially since its successful implementation can be ensured only if the majority of citizens functioning as entrepreneurs and decision-makers in relation to consumption, savings, investment, etc., endorse the envisaged policies and programmes by their whole hearted participation."

WHO and UNICEF, fully aware that the vast masses of humanity live in a state of abject poverty and, as a result, carry a great burden of ill-health, place a high priority on alleviating this burden. The strategy recently adopted for accomplishing this is that of providing primary health care. to all under-served populations, through the integration at the community level of all resources, both human and material, needed to make an impact upon the health status of the people. The approach emphasizes the need for community involvement in the general development process—a process of which better health can and should be both an ingredient and a derivative (WHO/UNICEF, 1977a: 3).

Primary health care addresses the main health problems in the community providing promotive, preventive, curative and rehabilitative services accordingly. In order to make primary health care universally accessible in the community as quickly as possible, maximum community and individual self-reliance requires full community participation in the planning, organisation and management of primary health care. Such participation is best mobilized through appropriate education which enables communities to deal with their real health problems in the most suitable ways.

Dr. Hiroshi Nakajima, former Director General of World Health Organisation stresses the need of exploiting people's potentialities. To quote him:[4]

> "People are the true measure of the success of policies and programmes. At the same time, people are the determinants of success. Experience teaches us that, whether in the most sophisticated cities or in the most remote villages, when people act with determination and understanding in pursuit of goals they deem essential, they achieve success. Previously insoluble problems are solved and resources are mobilized. Miracles happen, "We must learn to harness the energy, wisdom and will of the people we serve."

Health functionaries should have firm conviction in the ability of the people to participate. Judith long-staff Mackays[5] in his Article, "Profile of a Health Advocate" rightly says: Health advocates are crusaders for health-people with a strong sense of mission.

Dr. H. Mahler, Director General of World Health Organisation in his Article "Health for All—Everyone's Concern", stresses the need of people's participation. To quote him:[6]

Its primary responsibility is to promote individual and social awareness leading to people's involvement and self-reliance. If the individual, the family, the community do not fully realise the value of health, nor the potential consequences of the health hazards to which they are exposed or to which they voluntarily expose themselves, our goal of health for all will not be achieved. Nor will it be achieved if the people do not fully become involved in efforts to control disease and promote health.

The focus placed by the PHC approach on community involvement means that decision-makers, in developing new policies for health education, must understand and accept the need to make provision for communities to define and pursue their own goals, to mobilise their own resources, and to control and evaluate their own efforts.

It also means that mechanisms must be developed or strengthened to ensure that individuals and communities can express their views on their country health policy and take an active part in the planning and delivery of health programmes, including health education. We have to find ways of building up this process of community involvement to a point of providing continuous guidance from the grass root to national policy-makers. Eventually, national priorities should evolve from the synthesis of local priorities.

PROCESS OF COMMUNITY PARTICIPATION IN HEALTH PROGRAMMES

1. Analysis of the Needs and Requirements of the People in the Community

The understanding of the community is the first ingredient of the process of participative management, since the community consists of many heterogeneous groups. Such understanding would help us in assessing the positive as well as negative factors that will influence the success of the participation process. This analysis must be done on scientific lines and efforts should be made to locate the informal leaders through the process of sociometry, who can be helpful in changing heterogeneity into homogeneity to avoid the wastage that would result from the friction among the different groups.

2. Designing the Health Programmes to Meet the Needs of the People with the Involvement of the People

The Health workers in the areas must design the PHC programmes which meet the priority needs of the community. It would be desirable to involve the opinion leaders—both formal and informal, so that they can give information which one has not come across during the survey already made. This will also kindle interest in them.

3. Educating the People through Formal and Informal Channels to make them Aware of the Programme and Utilising the Resources Available with them

After designing the programme and getting it approved from their headquarters, it becomes the duty of Health workers to educate the people through formal and informal channels so that they become aware of the potentialities of the programmes. Here the health workers can also assess the resources which can be tapped locally with no cost or very little cost so that the people can manage the health programmes later on themselves.

4. Kindling and Generating Interest among the People to keep up the Momentum through the Provision of Resources not Available locally

The most important step in the process of participative management is the leadership role of the health workers, that is why we insist on giving adequate training to health workers in the art and science of participative management. The success or failure of participative management would thus depend to a great extent upon the administrative capability, leadership and motivation of health workers. Administrative capability is an important means of converting programme inputs into outputs with economy and efficiency. It has been mentioned by Y.L. Gabriel that, "what makes the leadership variable so crucial in the implementation process is its dynamic, not passive quality, i.e., its capability to act and react on these critical inputs. It is this administrative and transferring quality of leadership that could significantly determine the administrative capability of implementing organisation."[7]

Administrative capability is the capacity to obtain intended results through organisation. Katz says, "Administrative capability for development involves the ability to mobilise, allocate and combine the actions that are technically needed to achieve development objectives."[8]

Health workers must be the persons with vision, initiative and desire to achieve the operational goals with dedication and perseverance. In the words of Shri Jawaharlal Nehru: "No administrator, I suppose, or anyone else for the matter of that, can really do first class work without a sense of function, without some measures of a crusading spirit. I am doing this, I have to achieve this, as a part of great movement in a big cause. That gives a sense of function not the sense of individual, narrow approach of doing a job in an office for a salary or wage, something connected with your life's outlook or anything, perhaps being interested, as people inevitably are, on one's personal preferment in that particular work."[9]

5. Leaving the Programme to the Care of the People with Aided Guidance

It is also very important for health workers to encourage the people to run the programme without their help, i.e., the health workers must become intentionally passive and monitor the interest of the people. This will give the people a feeling of responsibility and confidence, which is *sine qua non* for the success of any health programme.

6. Providing Aided Guidance to Handover the Programme to the People

The health workers should occasionally see the running of the programmes to sort out any problem that the people may have experienced while implementing the programmes. Such problems can be in different areas—political, religious, social, economic, psychological or administrative. The health workers should provide their seasoned guidance to sort out such problems which may look petty in the beginning but can lead to disastrous results in the long-run. Therefore, he should work on the proverb 'A stitch in time saves the nine'.

In this way a programme of PHC would take deep roots in the soil of the community which would continue till there is a need of such programme by the community.

There are many ways in which the community can participate in primary health care. It must first be involved in the assessment of the situation, the definition of problems and the setting of priorities. Then the community helps to plan primary health care activities, and cooperates fully when these activities are carried out. Such cooperation includes the acceptance of a high degree of responsibility by individuals for their own health care, such as adoption of a healthy lifestyle, norms of good nutrition and hygiene, or use of immunization services. In addition, members of the community can contribute labour as well as financial and other resources towards promoting primary health care.

7. Occasional Follow-up to Sort Out any Problem

It is also a concern of the community to keep the implementation of primary health care under constant review. This community involvement will help identify and resolve difficulties.

Community participation also requires mutual support between government and community, reinforced by two-way communication. It is the government's responsibility to stimulate this kind of support, to set-up the necessary intersectional coordinating mechanisms at the different administrative levels, to pass legislation to support primary health care, and to provide sufficient human, material, technical and financial resources.

This will give birth of a permanent community managed primary health care programme and ultimately the birth of a healthy society.

METHODS TO ASCERTAIN COMMUNITY PARTICIPATION (See Chart 3.2)

Ana Filgueriras[10] in his Article, "Among the Street Children", in *World Health*, talks about these methods.

How can we find out to what extent there is community participation in health action, and how can it be stimulated and improved? A group could be created to evaluate the situation. It could consist of some health workers, representatives from local voluntary organisations, women's groups and youth groups, and may be a teacher or other specially interested individuals. The purpose of the evaluation is not to report to some higher authority, but to provide information to the local community so that community participation could be improved. This is why it is

CHART 4.2

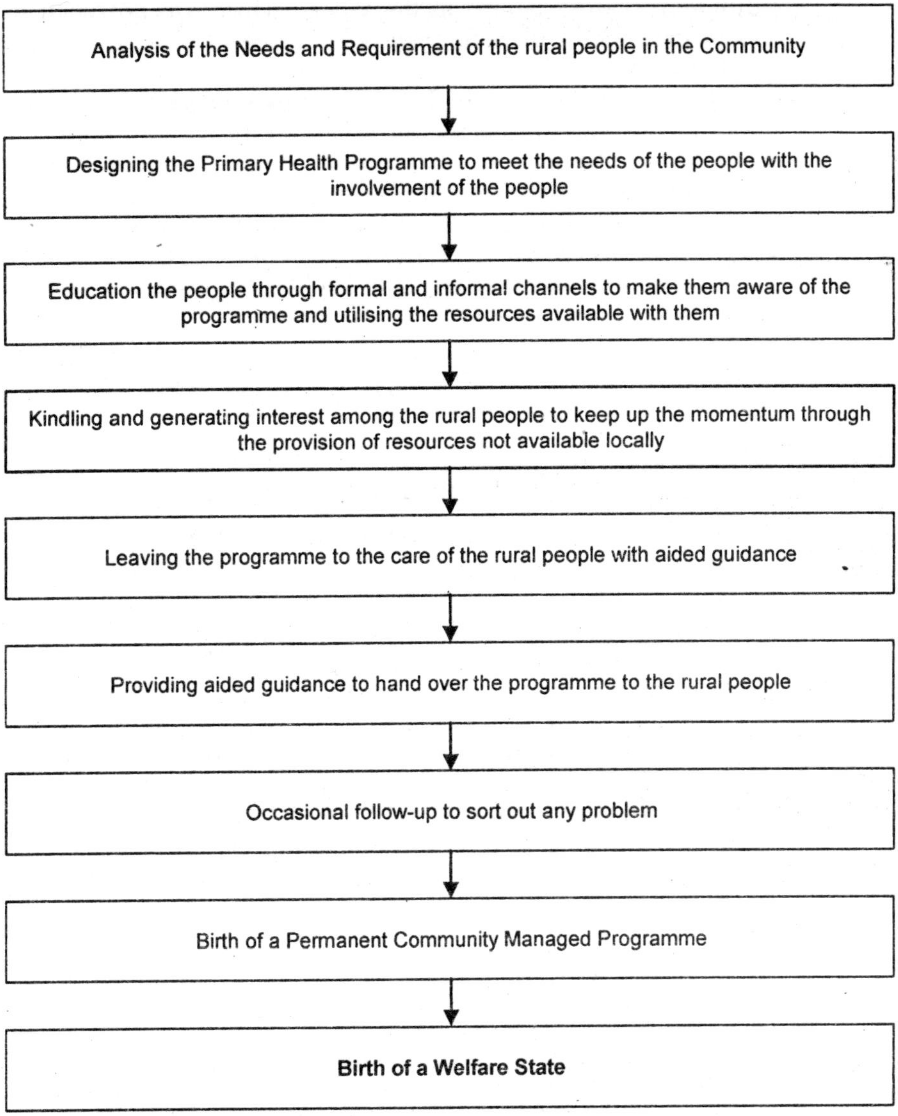

important for the local people themselves to be responsible. The evaluating group should look into the following aspects of participation:

- What are the relations between the community and the health workers? Do they meet regularly? Do they collaborate on specific projects?
- Do the health workers agree to let the community decide on local matters such as the working hours of the health post? Is there a health council or other group that meets regularly, and which has well-defined responsibilities?

- Are people willing to participate? If not, why not? Are there different interest groups in the village which 'do not want to work together? Is there no perceptible interest for health matters in the village? Why?
- In what activities does the community participate—in planning and evaluation, in decision-making, in providing funds or voluntary labour, in contacting higher political and administrative authorities to obtain support?
- What have been the results of community participation?
- Have people become more aware of the importance of health? Are they more satisfied with the health care provided? Has it improved? Is health improving?
- The findings should be written down and discussed. Hopefully, they will result in better collaboration between the health workers and the community. Things can always be improved!

Obstacles to Community Participation

There are quite a few obstacles to participation. Some are structural and need special attention while some others can be eliminated with committed effort. These are:

- Absence of confidence and ability of people in the machinery of health administration.
- Unequal domination of power relations in favour of rich and to the disadvantage of the poorer sections of the society. Inaccessible services in right quantity and quality. Rigid bureaucratic set-up impeding the people to participate.
- Legal hurdles as the courts delay the issues.
- Inadequate understanding of local talent, abilities and resources: professional experts underestimates people's knowledge and ability to handle local problems.
- Absence of identity with the community among people.
- People's dependence on Government and not in their own self.
- Heterogeneity of Interests.
- Resistance to empower people.
- Health system not oriented to Primary Health Care approach.
- Resistance on the part of certain segments of population to participate.
- Health workers indifferent attitude.
- Sustained efforts missing or luke warm attitude.

People's participation can improve through well designed and functional NGO's.[11]

> "The NGO sector has the potential to be a much greater force than it is at present. . . A working partnership between government agencies and NGOs can make tremendous progress in the next fifteen years."

Health development pre-supposes a creative teamwork involving self-help and self-care by the people themselves, supplemented by adequate health care services based on an appropriate health technology. It demands fulfilment of conditions beyond the narrow confines of medical concerns of disease, its diagnosis, cure or even prevention, and embraces the very quality of life of the people and their essential needs. The primary health care concept, which is the key to the achievement of Health for all by the year 2000 objectives, engenders all this and more. In its quintessence it is an interface between the extension of essential services, including health as an integral part of the role and responsibility of the government, and the vibrant, dynamic, upward struggle of the people in the community for the betterment of their own quality of life.

Action for this vital interface, where both these development streams meet, is crucial for the well-being of the community. It is here that the voluntary groups, societies and organisations called by the unsatisfactory term "non-governmental organisations"—NGOs for short—have their greatest strength. They are the bridges between people and the government. They are the pace-setters, innovators and reformers. Their contribution to the Health for all movement could make all the difference!

Guiding Principles

Certain guiding principles can be laid down to help resolve the kind of problems already mentioned:

1. Channelising the NGO's to Promote Health Plans

A country's health care strategy should be consistent with its socio-economic development plans. NGOs, when planning PHC programmes with the community, must like-wise take into account the socio-economic development plans for the area and the cultural characteristics as well as the existing health care facilities, so as to provide for coordination of services as well as allowing for expansion.

NGO-supported and organized health care services must be an integral part of the total health care system of a country, including the referral system.

NGOs should coordinate their health care activities among themselves and with the governmental health plan, and their PHC projects, including supportive services should not be financed in isolation from the overall development of health and related activities.

The mobilisation and allocation of both national and external resources for the development of NGO-supported or NGO-organized PHC programmes must be in harmony with the national health care strategy, and must be run in such a way as to ensure continuity of financing. In addition, external resources are a contribution to in international solidarity. For more effective participation in policy formulation and planning with the government, NGOs should actively pursue the monitoring and evaluation of their own work as well as carrying out or supporting relevant operational research.

2. *Strengthening of NGO's/Voluntary Agencies and Ensuring their Accountability*

Voluntary agencies have a long history of active involvement in the promotion of human welfare and well-being. Lord Beveridge called them "a private enterprise for social progress." Voluntary agencies come into existence spontaneously, voluntarily and without any compulsion or control to fulfil the particular needs of some groups of people. These agencies are flexible and possess the virtues of human services with dedication. Voluntary action is the soul of democracy as this medium secures the active involvement of the people from policy-making to implementation. It is the life and blood of democracy.

A voluntary agency may be defined as: "An organisation that is administered by an autonomous board which holds meeting, collects funds for the support, chiefly from private sources, and expends money, whether with or without paid workers, in conducting a programme."

According to Dharma Vira: "Work of voluntary organisations and citizen participation are two sides of the same coin. Citizens work in organisations but on their work depends the quality of the service the organisations render. Voluntary Organisations provide a frame for citizen participation. Without effective citizen participation, the organisation would only be empty forums."[12]

It is very difficult to provide all the services to the people through the Government, as it is very costly. The voluntary agency can exploit the unused energies of the people for the development of the country. Energy of the people, if unused, cannot be preserved. This unused energy "like the unused vast water resources flowing down in Himalayas is not only wasted like those rivers, but also, like the river waters that take with them the top soil of the Himalayan region causing permanent losses in social erosion, cause permanent damage to the human spirit and will in a community through dependence and frustration born out of ever-increasing level of abject poverty over the generations.[13]

Voluntary agencies can help in the programme implementation, collaboration and co-ordination with other activities. They can contribute to social welfare development in many ways through programme implementation. They can:[14]

(1) Provide assistance to develop and/or strengthen local NGO capabilities and activities with particular attention to local community development groups.

(2) Conduct reviews and assessment of existing development programmes and assist communities in the exercise of their own role in such reviews. A greater emphasis on evaluative techniques will render all new programmes more accountable to real community needs.

(3) Develop innovative programmes in the context of comprehensive human development.

(4) Ensure that their existing programmes and new initiatives promote full participation by individuals and communities in the planning, implementation and control of these programmes.
(5) Expand their training efforts to respond to the needs of programmes, e.g., training of health workers, supervisors, administrators, planners and various agricultural and development workers.
(6) Extend their efforts to develop locally sustainable and appropriate technologies and use of resources, with particular attention to energy, water, agriculture, sanitation and medical care.
(7) Contribute to the creation of new and effective methods of education, which enable both individuals and communities to assume greater responsibility for their own health.
(8) Recognise the essential rôles of women in the promotion and in the full range of community development concerns.
(9) Further extend their capacity to work with poor, disadvantaged and remote populations enabling them to break the cycle of deprivation, and in this way contribute to the search for greater social justice.

N.V. Lalitha and Mathu Kohli have given the following points to enhance performance of voluntary sector:

(i) The government should spell out clearly the policy towards voluntary organisations indicating the relative role of the government and the voluntary sector, entitlement to funds, etc. This is very necessary in view of the fact that social welfare programme suffer from *ad-hocism* and uncertainty which come in the way of promoting voluntary efforts.
(ii) There is an urgent need to make a serious review of the working of voluntary organisations in terms of assets, financial soundness, service conditions of staff, quality of service, etc. Such a review would help identify the genuine agencies and give them all the support they need financial and technical because voluntary agencies can do excellent work and bring in better results. The government should also have certain controls in terms of audit, submission of accounts, work report, etc.
(iii) The Directorates of Social Welfare should equip themselves with facts and figures regarding voluntary organisations, their specialised areas of work, problems faced by them in their day-to-day functioning, etc. so that they can deal with them better. The inadequate and scanty information available at present create considerable difficulties both for the government and the voluntary organisations.

(iv) The government should insist on certain rules and procedures of recruitment, salary scales and working/service conditions so that voluntary organisations would get properly qualified persons to man their programmes.

(v) Grants should not be released as a matter of routine. The government should see that the organisations qualify for grants.[15]

These associations can perform the following functions:

(a) Provision of information and advice to the citizens in the making of applications and complaints.

(b) Educating the citizens in regard to their duties to the State and advising them about what should not be expected from administration.

(c) Lending support to the citizen's genuine demand and complaints.

(d) Bringing to bear influence on the Government departments and agencies for improvement of policies, programmes and procedures in the interest of the citizen's welfare and satisfaction.

(e) Promotion of high standards of public morality for good governance.

The women's voluntary organisation in the form of Mother's Club in the Republic of South Korea have been quite useful in raising the status of women. By mid-2005, nearly 90,000 such clubs had been organised. The clubs provide opportunities for village women to get-together to talk about health, education of children and improvement of environment. The club helps in family planning, vaccination and treatment of emergency cases. The mothers' clubs are a genuinely grass-root community network which owes little to outside administrators or planners. I.C. Abcede, in his article on "Women-Power in Korea" observes that mother's clubs are helping to change age-old social attitudes towards women. He says, "The growth of women's clubs in Korea has coincided with considerable changes in social attitudes towards women.

The trend is towards greater recognition of womens' contribution to the Community, better communication between husband and wife, and more open discussion of family planning matters. . . it seems clear that the enhanced status of women and the growth of mothers' clubs have gone hand-in-hand and are contributing significantly to the development of rural communities in Korea."[16]

Such clubs should be set-up in other countries as well. These would help mobilise voluntary resources lying idle and if not used can be a source of destruction. In the developing countries like India, voluntary organisations are urban-based and serve the urban area. These organisations must create a strong base by setting up such clubs in rural and uncovered areas and diffuse information to them to be passed among the members of the community. This would bring about a socio-economic revolution and contribute substantially to modernisation and development.

However, NGO's should aim at making people self-reliant and not dependent on them. Touching upon the critical role to be played by the NGOs, the former Prime Minister Shri P.V. Narasimha Rao, while addressing the NGOs on March 7, 1994 at Vigyan Bhavan said:

> In all this, we have to remember that the people must occupy the centre stage. At all times, they should be the focus of all that we aim to do. Therefore, when I talk of a participatory approach to development, I have in mind an approach where the people would be helped to help themselves. In other words, we should envisage a situation in our country, where people would deal with their problems on their own in the not too distant a future, without having to depend upon outside agencies. In the ultimate analysis, the people should not merely change their masters; people should be their own masters. That is what people-centred development is all about. Therefore, if a particular area is taken up by a NGO, it is not expected that it would function there for all times to come. A time should come when the people would have been fully mobilised and made aware of and empowered to deal with their own problems. In other words, the NGOs should withdraw after the task is done and shift to other areas, where their services are needed.

3. *Effective Training of Health Personnel in Appropriate Technology*

The training of health personnel should be oriented towards appropriate technology and appropriate methods. The training should be task-oriented and practical; it should include technical as well as managerial tasks. There should be provision for supervision and continuing education.

4. *Responsive Administration*

A good and responsive administration can prompt people's participation. Mr. M.G. Devashyam in his article, "Towards Good Administration" talks about the image of the Government functionary in the country, which he thinks though not uniformly bad, but is largely negative. In order to make the administration responsive, he suggests the following:[17]

1. Openness in the sense of having wide contact with the people.
2. A sense of justice, fair play, and impartiality in dealing with men and matters.
3. Sensitivity and responsiveness to the urges, feeling and aspirations of the common man. Securing the honour and dignity of the human being, however humble he or she might be.

Humility and simplicity in the persons manning the administrative machinery and their easy accessibility. Creating and sustaining an atmosphere conducive to development, growth and social change.

4. Honesty and integrity in thought and action. As early as 1959, The Secretary General of the United Nations Pointed out that "Any systematic effort towards economic development must be preceded by or coupled with efforts to make more effective, the functioning of the Government machinery."
5. Creating and sustaining an atmosphere conducive to development, growth and social change.
6. Honesty and integrity in thought and action.[17]

As early as 1959, the Secretary General of the United Nations Pointed out that "Any systematic effort towards economic development must be preceded by or coupled with efforts to make more effective, the functioning of the Government machinery.[18]

5. Effective Public Relations

A responsive administration has to attach a lot of importance to its Public relations, which comprises of:

(1) Spread of awareness about the health activities of the Government within the given constraints and feed the Government with the expectations and aspirations of the people. The local voluntary organisations imbued with a spirit of service and Civic sense could be extremely helpful in creating citizen's consciousness and also in giving a micro-level feedback about the lapses, loopholes and snags if any.
(2) Speedy redressal of public grievance through a systematic and well thought out mechanism.

The above measures would thus infuse confidence in the people about the relevance of development programmes and their participation therein.

In the new millennium, we have to devise new methods to ensure people's participation. Hiroshi Nakajima in his article, "The State of the World's Health" rightly says—[19]

> A fundamental principle in the health for all philosophy is that participation in planning and decision-making is an important process enabling individuals and families to contribute to their own development and to that of the communities in which they live, work and socialize. If, by the year 2000, all people must become active participants. They must be in charge, rather than being passive recipients of the consequences of other people's decisions and of their perceptions concerning the development of the health system infrastructure and the planning and delivery of primary health care.

6. Attitudinal Changes among Personnel Responsible for Services

A democratic reorientation of the attitudes of the officials towards the citizens has become very much necessary for both the prevention of the citizen's complaints and their prompt redress. Local Bodies should pay great attention to the opinions of the people. Reorientation of the attitudes of the officials towards the citizens is a very difficult task. It will require thinking on several fronts such as in-service training, recruitment from a wider social base, special assignments in rural areas and the like. The officials of local bodies of today should not only possess traditional service virtues like efficiency, integrity and loyalty but should also shake off all the feelings of exclusiveness and superiority. There should be a desire to establish contacts with the citizens to understand their problems. Unless the change in the attitudes of civil servants as a whole is brought about, all other measures to deal with the citizen's grievances will be of limited use.

C.N. Ray has rightly felt that the Government of India has been concerned about the frustration and dissatisfaction among the people, especially the vulnerable groups of the civil society regarding deterioration in the performance of agencies meant for delivery of public services. Despite recognition of the critical role of responsive State, public administration and civil services at all levels, in terms of eroded credibility and effectiveness of the civil services, public perception of an unholy nexus between politicians, civil servants and criminals (as illustrated in the Vohra Committee Report), has been growing with an increasing criticism of low levels of honesty, transparency and accessibility of the democratic elements in-charge of administration. In order to restore the faith of the people in the fairness and capacity of the administration, the Prime Minister had inaugurated a Conference of the Chief Secretaries in November 1996 on "an agenda for an effective and responsive administration." The objective of the conference was to make public service more efficient, clean, accountable and citizen-friendly by evolving a concrete action plan. The adoption and implementation of the proposed action plan would require strong political will and commitment from the Central and State Governments.[20]

It is of utmost national importance that the civil servants are honest and upright in the discharge of their public duties, particularly at a time when clouds of political uncertainty and instability are hovering over our national life. It is at this time that the civil servants should serve the nation honestly by giving a sense of continuity. If they fail, the future of the nation may be dark.[21]

Former Prime Minister, Atal Bihari Vajpayee, rightly stressed: "My greatest concern today is in the area of implementation. The National Agenda for governance has clearly spelt out our priorities. In the light of these priorities, a large number of good policies, programmes, and schemes have been worked out of course. We have also inherited a large number of good policies, programmes, and schemes from the previous governments. Where we fumble, however, is in implementing them in a manner that satisfies the people. I have said it before, and I say it again, that I cannot accept delays and slippages in implementation. I cannot, because the people cannot. The people want to see action, and not just hear words of promise repeated again and again.

I want to see the entire administrative machinery, from top to bottom, work with a sense of mission and result-oriented approach. I want to see them work with their hearts and minds fully in the administrative responsibility they hold. I want to see them work faster and work better. I want to see them work with a sense of mission and accountability. In doing so, I want to see them work without any fear or favour."[22]

7. Sound Health System

The health system should be consonant with each community's political, cultural and administrative traditions. Existing mechanisms may already be appropriate, or new ones may be created, so that people can express their views concerning what they see as priority health problems and make their own decision about the best ways of solving them.

8. Understanding Public Needs and Values of the Community

The first important step in public relations is to understand the community. Every community is different and there are differences between each local community in the same country in terms of their work culture and living standards, family life, social structure, population structure and attitudes. Besides, values, beliefs and customs, religious practices, etc. differ in different areas. There is a need to understand the need of the people based upon this diversity before launching any field operations. How to learn about the people and the community? Some of the important methods are:

(i) Discussion with People

Discussion can be both formal and informal. Discussion can be held with formal groups of the people. However, informal discussions with people in the markets and common places will throw light as to what concerns people most. In ascertaining the health needs of the people, CNA (Community Needs Assessment) surveys are carried out before introducing facilities in the area. Mahatma Gandhi had to tour the country to understand the problems of the country. Jawaharlal Nehru advised bureaucracy not to retire in their cells after work but should mix with all kinds of people, which would provide them with material that is not in their files

(ii) Study of Newspapers, Magazines and Other Published Literature

A public relations department needs to study the published material wherein people express their needs and mention their likes and dislikes. This is a rich source of information.

(iii) Complaint and Suggestion Boxes

Most of the departments have put complaint and suggestion boxes. The analysis of complaints and suggestions can help the organisation in understanding the needs of the people.

(iv) Surveys

A well designed survey, opinion poll, or census can help us to know the reactions of the people about organisations. Researchers generally use such surveys to understand the problems.

Thus, the understanding of the people is vital for public relations to be effective. Hiroshi Nakajima, Former Director-General of the World Health Organisation, has rightly stressed the need of understanding the people. To quote him:[23]

> "People are the true measure of the success of policies and programmes. At the same time, people are the determinants of success. Experience teaches us that, whether in the most sophisticated cities or in the most remote villages, when people act with determination and understanding in pursuit of goals they deem essential, they achieve success. Previously insoluble problems are solved and resources are mobilised. Miracles happen."

9. Informing People and the Community

Public relations departments/sections need to make the people aware about the people's benefit programmes they want to undertake for the people's benefit or the benefit of the country/area. This would aim at educating the people about the schemes in operation—their objectives, services, eligibility criteria, agencies and functionaries for the delivery of services. A good public relations exercise would provide the information in a way as to generate community's conviction about the efficacy and usefulness of the services. It would also lead to community's clear understanding of its participation and contribution.

10. Creating Satisfactory Climate

For any public relation campaign to be effective, it is important to create an environment of goodwill based on equity. People must be given their due status and must be taken into confidence based on trust.

11. Advising People

The government may advise the people to act in a way, which may be beneficial to them and to the government/agency concerned. Public relations through its various channels need to inject the desired changes to generate development, dynamism and modernization. Thus, the advice to be effective should be preceded by extensive planning of the public relations strategies to be followed.

Prem Kumar has rightly stressed the right to participate in the affairs of the country is meaningless unless the citizens are well informed on all sides of the issues, in respect of which they are called upon to express their views. One-sided information, disinformation, misinformation and non-information-all equally create an uninformed citizenry, which makes democracy a farce when medium of information is monopolised either by a partisan central authority or by a private individual. This is particularly so in a country like ours where about 48 per cent of the population is illiterate and hardly 6.5 per cent of the population has access to the print media, which is not subject to pre-censorship. When, therefore, the electronic media is controlled by one Central agency or a few private agencies of the rich, there is a need to have a Central agency, as stated earlier, representing all sections of the society. Hence, to have a representative central agency to ensure viewer's right to be informed adequately and truthfully is a part of the right of the viewers under Article 19(1)(a) of the Constitution of India.[24]

12. Creating Independent and Attractive Mass Media

The media of any society are among the most important institutions. Democracy without free media is a contradiction in terms. Mass media should be the watchdog of democracy, and not the poodle of the establishment. The media has a greater responsibility today than they ever had to guide the nation and make every citizen conscious of his fundamental duties enshrined in the Constitution.

(a) Press

Press is a very important channel of public relations, especially in metropolitan cities where literacy rate is very high. However, it has its limitations because of low literacy in developing countries like India. Besides, the press in developing countries does not co-operate with the Government in creating positive atmosphere, which is ideal for development. Rather, the press generally concentrates on negative aspects of the government resulting in alienation between the Government and the people. Besides press release, the Government publishes useful books to highlight Government programmes and projects. Besides, Directorate of Advertisement and Visual Publicity (DAVP) publicises the policies, programmes and performance of the Government of India through advertisements in the press, posters, brochures, folders, cinema slides, etc. These are not done regularly and on a continuous basis, but intermittently to deal with particular situations.

(b) Radio and Television

Radio and Television also play an effective role in public relations. Television has become very popular and its visual impact is high. However, the programmes aiming at development are not presented in a way as can influence the minds of the people, besides, the time devoted for development activities is very less.

(c) Films

Public relations departments make films in the areas of health, education, family planning, literacy, grow more food, agriculture, etc. which are quite useful. These films are screened with the films shown in theatres as well as screened in villages by mobile units. However, the contents of these films are not attractive to motivate the people to attend.

(d) Songs and Dramas

Public relations departments arrange folk, songs, drama, dances to make the people understand the problems. For example, songs and dramas are used for depicting population problems. Public relations in the Government of India at the Union and State levels have not been effective in meeting the needs of the country. Public relations is quite effective in the private sector but the government sector needs improvement. Let us discuss some of the problems and suggest remedies.

1. Wrong Presumptions about the Homogeneity of the Population

Population differs in different areas in terms of their knowledge, values and attitudes. It is, therefore, important for the Government to understand these variations and divide the population into homogeneous units through segmentation and direct its public relation activities accordingly to be productivity useful and usher an era of good governance.

2. Public Relations Directed to Promote Vested Interest

Public relations in government is done to promote the Interest of the ruling party as well as to project the personalities of key persons, which is nothing but propaganda. This type of public relations creates misgivings and misunderstandings among the masses in general and affected interests in particular. There is a need to adopt impartiality and scientific attitude in public relations to ensure its fruitful results. Morton R. Davies rightly mentions: "Politicians must resist the temptation to use the information services for party/political advantage; administrators must equally resist the tendency to acquiesce in the demands of their political master, and be constantly vigilant of the limitations that should be imposed on their role."[25]

3. Public Relations Mainly Directed to Urban Areas

Most of the formal public relations aim at influencing the public opinion of urban population as they are the vocal and influential segments of the society. It is quite discouraging that 70 per cent of the population living in villages and other backward areas is not covered through the desired programmes of public relations. According to F.C. Gera, "It is not enough for mass media to be blaring forth statement of Government's policies and programmes. There must be deliberate and organised attempts also to assess the needs of people, to listen to their grievances and to redress them. And the people, particularly the uneducated people, must be treated with courtesy instead of being shouted at and compelled to shell out bribes."[26]

4. Very Little Research in Public Relations

Most of the research in public relations are elementary and urban-based and have been adopted from foreign models. It is suggested that indigenous models may be developed which can serve a developing country like India. This is succinctly stated by Ross when he said, "As public relations field has grown in sophistication, this no longer means simply advertising as news report, nor even highly polished receptionist and telephone-answering service, but careful study (again often using social scientists) of employees, consumers, and the community at large, so that there is awareness within the organisation of the strength and weakness of its own position in the community."[27]

Public relations programmes need to be fair, honest, truthful, impartial, open, authoritative and responsive. They must be conducted in the public interest. It should attempt at lubricating Government and public relationship based on trust and confidence.

As media is both under Government controlled and in private sector, there is all the more need to formulate a comprehensive media policy. There has to be a close co-ordination with the concerned local body and other institutions responsible for programme implementation. The vast potential of the mass media has to be utilised for making different sections of the society conscious of their constitutional responsibilities and fundamental duties while integrating entertainment with socially relevant and useful message in the entertainment programmes themselves.[28]

13. Personnel Communication

The art of developing common understanding about people is vital to bring about change of attitudes and behaviour among bureaucracy. Sociologists have classified the diffusion process, which leads to a widespread acceptance of the programme into five stages:

1. Awareness (the individual's first introduction to a new idea or practices);
2. Interest (the stage at which he actually seeks further information and background data);
3. Evaluation (the stage of assessment on theoretical grounds);
4. Trial (a limited phase of experiment), and finally
5. Acceptance or adoption.

Naturally, the duration of the process depends upon personality factors. which differ with individuals. Mass media helps in creating awareness. in providing stimulation and motivation and in giving ready access to information. But at the specific stage of evaluation, trial and adoption. inter-personal. face to face, communication counts for much more and the inability of the mass media to maintain a two-way dialogue with regular feedback restricts their utility.[29] Therefore, no medium of communication is as effective as one human being talking to another. The UNESCO has rightly stated:

> "The process of social and economic development is a process of human development, for people are the targets as well as the essential variable in development. Communication being a two-way process. provides for participation at whatever stage of enlightenment of the individuals composing a society find themselves. Change agents are key factors in the communication development process since they are instruments for getting facts to the people upon which decisions can be based."[30]

There has been heavy, and perhaps unwarranted, reliance on mass media. be it printed, projected or broadcast. There is a need to re-examine the methods, materials and mass communication media currently in use and to determine what methods and materials are appropriate to achieve a proper mix between the individual, group and mass communication.

Thus, the impersonal methods are relatively simpler and even less time consuming. The radio, TV, newspapers, posters, and pamphlets can also help in improving public relations. Experience with personal and impersonal methods of public relations has revealed that if both the methods are used simultaneously, one can obtain better results than simply using one or the other method. Alastair Metheson, Deputy Director of UNICEF's division, remarks on the basis of his research that "to get people to act in ways that conform to new values almost always requires that mass communications be reinforced by personal influence."[31]

14. Empowerment of the Poor

Eric R. Ram[32] in his article "Information is power" stresses the need of empowering the people for ensuring participation. For most of the people in the world, the root cause of poor health is poverty, and the people's powerlessness to do anything about it. Primary Health Care (PHC), as described in the Declaration of Alma Ata, is a comprehensive process and in its fullest sense, has a liberating and empowering potential. By helping people to gain control over some aspects of their lives, it can bring about collective action for social change. People work together to improve the total situation of their community, and deal with the underlying causes of poor health and poverty. This requires organized action on the part of poor people themselves in developing their own strategies, selecting priorities, controlling interventions and carrying them out. Running village communities and using PHC as a strategy to achieve the target of health requires a strong commitment to social justice, human values and respect for life, by communities and governments alike.

Making people aware of their rights and responsibilities helps them to determine their own health priorities and take part in solving their own health problems, a step so essential in the process of empowerment of the people. We have to employ all credible channels of communication, including the traditional methods of story-telling and drama, in order to reach all people. Films, radio and television whenever available can be useful, but we have to recognise their limitations; they are useful in creating awareness among people in their communities, but to bring about a real change in health practices people have to decide for themselves and take responsibility for their own health.

15. Developing Social Networks

Lowell S. Levin's[33] in his article stresses the need of developing social networks. Such networks would develop bond of exchange.

Merle Fainsod remarks: "The most favourable setting for progress in development administration exists where a politically influential and dynamic modernizing elite strongly desires development and can successfully project this attitude into both the bureaucracy and the population at large."[34]

Many well-intentioned and technically sound programmes aimed at solving health problems have been frustrated by a lack of popular acceptance and community participation. "It has been observed that such programmes are either not actively associated or passively ignored because they do not 'belong' to the population they are designed to help; they are rather seen by the population as imposed external programmes that belong to the government and consequently deserve and require little, if any, of the population's attention, action, or other response. We must be clear that health cannot be imposed, it can only be acquired. This requires participation based on enlightenment of the beneficiaries."[35]

Dr. Madiou Toure, Director Hygiene and Health Protection, Ministry of Public Health, Republic of Senargal, in his article, "The Health Revolution", in *World Health* (November, 1979) has rightly said: "The medicine of tomorrow will be shapped by the people for the people, because the people themselves will determine their own condition, their own destiny."[36]

The greatest obstacle in achieving Health for all, the goal agreed by all of WHO's 191 member-states, is poor planning, organisation and management, particularly at the local level, where the most intensive action is supposed to be. This is why WHO launched the initiative which it calls "Strengthening district health systems."

Better health does not just mean going to the doctor for treatment-when one is sick. For one thing, millions of people particularly in the Third World—have no doctor to go to even if they wanted to. Instead, people need to know how to adopt more healthy lifestyles, and how to make changes in their home and community environments, which are effective, feasible and affordable. And they need support to obtain better nutrition, better sanitation, better education and better housing—all this in addition to better health care. So the people who staff health centres, clinics and local hospitals need to recruit positive support from people at all levels in the locality and by 'district'. WHO indicates merely a local area which is manageable in size. And they must encourage coordination between government bodies and private and non-governmental institutions.[37]

Primary health care at the district level offers the best possible opportunity for even the remotest of rural communities to reach out for health.

We may conclude in the words of Dr. H. Mahler, Ex-Director General of World Health Organisation, "Economic growth, without being specifically attuned to human needs and human realizations, is not worth very much. Once more you hear everywhere people speaking about nuclear energy, oil energy, solar energy, wind energy, and everybody seems to be overlooking the fact that without human energy, there would be no kind of progress either socially or economically."

For the success of health administration to function effectively and efficiently, the citizen has also to be equipped for being a good citizen. Citizen should be well enlightened. It has been rightly said by the Poet that it is not gold but only men of right quality who can make a nation great and strong. "The citizen fails to have confidence in himself—a confidence that comes out of being important and useful to society. Confidence in oneself is necessary for being self-reliant, disciplined and work-oriented, a condition that is a basic necessity for the success of a democracy."[38] In order to improve the citizenship, Prof. B.S. Khanna has suggested that the programmes of human and socio-economic development are necessary to bring about structural and behaviour changes on the following lines:

1. Lessening substantially the rigidities of social stratification and achieving increasing egalitarianism (Social and Economic).
2. Removing of poverty, social backwardness and social injustice.
3. Stimulating the organisation of more and more groups with Socio-political objectives to aggregate, articulate and safeguard the interest of the citizens.
4. Achieving a suitable equilibrium between consensus and dissent so as to avoid regimentation as well as social fragmentation.[39]

In addition to the administrative reforms and improvements, there should be immediate simplification of procedures. Most of the complaints of the citizens are the result of complicated procedures. Simplification of the procedures should take place in the matters like:

(a) Regard for public comfort and convenience.
(b) Speed in disposal of applications.
(c) Reduction in the number of levels required to examine cases.
(d) Minimum interdepartmental/office references.

(e) Reduction in the number of agencies with which the citizen has to deal with.

(f) Supply of detailed information to the citizen as to how is he to go about to receive a certain benefits or approval from administration.

Learning about your community

Women's groups, scouts, health volunteers, local organisations and health teams, should know their community, if they are to be effective in improving its health. You may already know many things about our community, especially if it is a small one. But do you know enough about it? You will learn more by talking in a systematic way with its leaders and other people. Do not ask too many questions tough; it is better to observe, listen and leant! Here are some of the things you should find out. How many people are there in the community, and how many of them are young, middle-aged, and old.

'How do people get food? How do they earn money'? Are they farm workers, fishermen, cattle-farmres, estate workers, factory workers? How do they sepnd their free time.

- Do they work at night?
- 'Do children work? How many of the children attend school'?
- Is the community poor? Is it becoming poorer or less poor? Is its standard of living higher or lower than the average for the country? Are there good markets. Good roads? Is there a clean water supply? Is there electricity. A telephone service, a bus service?
- 'How do families live? What are the houses like'? Do they have a system of Sanitation? 'Are the houses clean and free of pests'?
- 'Who makes decisions within the family'? How many children are there in the average family? 'How are the children fed and how are they taught'? What are the most common beliefs. values and traditions?
- What are the main health problems and what are their causes? Some causes of bad health are:
- Too many people living close together;
    - not enough water or the water is not safe;
    - not enough food of the right kind;
    - unclean houses in dirty surroundings;
    - no way to keep cool in the heat or to keep warm in the cold;
    - no latrines or the latrine are dirty;
    - no protection against insect that carry disease:
    - the health centre is difficult to reach;
    - people cannot read and thus do not learn about health and healthy habits.

Talk to various group and people: families or household (both rich and poor), those who make decisions for the community about the community and members of special groups. Try to find out:

- what part of their income do they spend on health?
- what community problems are they especially concerned about?
- What have they been doing about these problems?
- What do they think can be done?
- Who are the leaders, or those who make the decisions for the community? They may be tribal leaders, religious leaders or political leaders. They are the ones who are most likely to help in improving health. Other people whose opinions and support are valued may include the elders, landowners, money lenders or businessmen.

Find out how the community is organized and who runs its affairs. For example:

- 'Which group makes decisions for all the people'? Is it a development committee, a political body. Or some other group?
- 'Does this group deal with all the affairs of the community'? Or 'does it have subcommittees that look after different needs of the community, such as health, water supply and education'?
- 'Is there a health committee? Who are its members and how are they chosen'? What are their tasks?
- 'How often do they meet'! 'Are all sections or groups in the community represented'?
- 'What other groups are there'? For example, a women's group or a farmers' cooperative.

If you are a school teacher, 'why not ask your students to do a community survey based on questions like these'? Then you could call a meeting of parents and ask the students to present their findings. May be a movement to improve health could be started.

In the new millennium, we expect the people to be more dynamic, participative, self-reliant, as they will be well equipped with the info-technology. They would have all the means to know about the latest developments in the area of health and thus the community can be benefitted by this explosion of knowledge and new technology. In this way, they can be self-reliant.

For democracy to be successful at the national level, the grassroots organisations have to be strong. The local authorities have to respond to the felt needs of the people. The citizens have to have faith in the efficacy of the administrative system *so* that the distance between people and the government is reduced. The administration, for good governance has to be accessible. In developing countries, it is the government, which initiates and implements development programmes. It must gain support of the people in the discharge of these programmes, particularly at the cutting-edge. Such support would strengthen democracy as well as a positive response of the community to development programme which should be the ultimate goal of good governance."[40]

Late Dr. Y.C. James Yen has beautifully advised the Government functionaries through the following enunciation:

Go to the people;
Live among the people;
Learn from the people;
Plan with the people;
Work with the people;
Start with what the people know;
Build on what the people have;
Teach by showing, learn by doing;
Not a showcase, but a pattern;
Not odds and ends, but a system;
Out piecemeal, but an integrated approach;
Not to conform, but to transform;
Not relief, but release.

FOR
In every developing community there are
civic-minded leaders who want to help their
people, Give them a handle and they will
seize it and march like an armywith a banner.

CONCLUSION

The success of the Good Governance depends, to a great extent, upon the harmonious relationships between the citizens and administration. Local Government should not function as a machinery but in a humane and purposeful way. The people in Local Body should have a sense of dedication, responsibility, be responsive and alert to the aspirations of the citizens. Citizens, on the other hand, should also provide meaningful cooperation to Local Bodies. Under such an atmosphere, it would be very easy to implement the developmental tasks, to bring about social change and modernisation in the country. The strengthening of democracy in its social and economic aspect has to be attained through the participation on the part of the people. A similar shift is evident in international thinking.

If the citizens' grievances are allowed to mount up, the dissatisfaction with the administration may add to any existing social unrest and tensions.

The phenomenon of growing social discontent which erupts into frequent acts of violence finds substance in the citizen's frustration with the administration, it is, therefore, necessary that the citizen's faith in the Government of which the administration is the chief executive agency should not be allowed to deteriorate but should be reinforced adequately. This is important both for political stability and preservation of the social fabric. The dissatisfaction of the citizens with the administrative machinery has grown in recent years. There has been general agreement that the administration has not been able to provide efficient and timely service.

Notes and References

1. Roy, Darke and Ray, Walker, Local Government and the Public, London, Leonard Hill, 1977, p. 89.
2. NIHWF, Management Training Modules for Health Assistants, Male and Female, New Delhi, 1987.
3. Etinne Berthet, "The Fight Against Famine", in *World Health,* December 1980, p. 27.
4. Hiroshi Nakajima, *'Editorial, A Grand Alliance',* in *World Health,* May-June, 1992, p. 3.
5. Judith Long-staff Mackay, "Profile of a Health Advocate", in *World Health,* May-June, 1992, p. 3.
6. H. Mahler, *'Health For All, Everyone's Concern',* in *World Health,* April-May 1983, p. 3.
7. Gabriel V. Legisi as, College of Public Administration, University of Philippines, "Administrative Capability as a Neglected Dimension in the Implementation of Development Programme and Projects", Seventieth General Assembly and Conference of EROPA on "Implementations, the Problem of Achieving Results", October 24-31, 1973, Vol. III, p. 314.
8. Saul, M. Katz, "A Methodological Note on Appraising Administrative Capability for Development", in Appraising Administrative Capability for Development, U.N. Publication Sales No. E. 60. II, H. 2, p. 8.
9. Jawaharlal Nehru and Public Administration, IIPA, New Delhi, 1975, p. 88.
10. Ana Filguerias, "Among the Street Children", *World Health,* May-June 1992, p. 6.
11. Mechai Viravaidy, "Untapped Potential", *World Health,* March 1985, p. 45.
12. Dharam Vir, Citizen Participation in Encyclopaedia of Social Work, Vol. I, p. 102.
13. Malhotra, R.C., *op. cit.,* p. 11.
14. World Federation of Public Health Association, *op. cit.,* pp. 45-46.
15. N.V. Lalitha and Madhu Kohli, Satus of Voluntary Effort in Social Welfare, *Ibid.,* pp. 124-25.
16. WHO: *World Health,* May 1979, p. 19.
17. *The Daily Tribune,* 27th December, 1988.
18. U.N. Official Records of Economics and Social Council, E/1701, Agenda Item No. 10, p. 3.
19. Hiroshi Nakajima, "The State of the World's Health", *World Health,* No. 3, May-June 1993, p. 3.
20. C.N. Ray, Citizens' Charter in India: An Overview, in *IJPA,* Oct.-Dec. 1998, p. 236.

21. R.P. Dubhshi, Administrative Automony, in *IJPA*. Oct.-Dec. 1998. p. 102.
22. Atal Behari Vajpayee, Indian Administration Today, In *IJPA*. Jan. to March. 1999 p. 4.
23. WHO, *World Health*, May-June, 1992, p. 3.
24. Prem Kumar, Fundamental Duties and Media in *IJPA*, Oct.-Dec. 1999, pp. 698-730
25. Mortun, R Davies, 'Government and Administrative Responsiveness in Britain' in *IJPA*, Vol. XXXIII, No. 2 (April-June 1987), p. 209.
26. F.C Gera. 'Need for Public Relations in Administration' in *IJPA*, Vol. XXI, July-Sept. 1975, pp. 545-46.
27. Marray, G. Ross, Community Organisation, New York, Harper and Row, 1967, p. 25.
28. Prem Kumar, *op. cit.*, p. 718.
29. UNESCO, Communication in Media, Family Planning and Development, No. I, Paris, p. 1975.
30. UNESCO, Communication in Support of Population, Family Planning and Development, F/F/S/75, XIII, 5, p. 482.
31. UNICEF, UNICEF News, "Communication: A Tool for Development", Issue, 84/1975/2, p. 18.
32. Eric R. Ram, "Information is Power", *World Health*, January-Feb. 1989, p. 8.
33. Lowell S. Lewin, "Listen to the Community", in *World Health*, May-June 1992, p. 11.
34. Merle Fainsod, "The Structure of Development Administration", in Irving Swerdlow, (ed.) *Development Administration: Concepts and Problems*, Syracuse, N.Y., Syracuse University Press, 1963, p. 1.
35. For details, refer to the Chapter on "Primary Health Care Administration".
36. "Reach out for health. . . .", *World Health*, May 1989, p. 16.
37. Quoted in S.L. Goel, Public Health Administration, Sterling Publishers, 1998.
38. Ishwar Dayal, "Confident, Self-reliant and disciplined Citizen", in *Yojna*, xxii, 26 January, 1976, p. 41.
39. B.S. Khanna, Citizen and Administration, *IJPA*, Special Number, July-Sept. 1975.
40. A.P. Barnbas, Good Government at Local Level, in *IJPA*, July-Sept. 1998, p. 453, Special Number on Towards Good Governance.

5

CHAPTER

Financial Administration for Primary Health Care

Finance is the crux of the problem. Without adequate finances Primary Health Care cannot be achieved. However, in a developing country like India, finances are limited, therefore we have to find ways and means to obtain finances locally and make the best use of them.[1]

Brain Abel Smith in his article "Paying for Health For All" raises the pertinent issue of providing resources for Primary Health Care in national plans judiciously. To quote him:[2]

> "How is Health for all going to be paid for? Unless clear answers are found to this question, Health for all is at risk of remaining a dream. This means that it is vital in the first instance to work out the cost of national Health for all plans. A plan that does not take account of costs amounts to no more than window shopping."

Facing up to where the money will come from to pay for Health for all is now seen as a crucial step in health planning. Some early national plans proved to be far too ambitious. They started from the assumption that if an ideal plan was made, it was bound to attract funding. When it did not, it was attributed to the narrow outlook of the ministry of finance or the lack of sympathy of foreign donors. It is now increasingly accepted that detailed planning must start by looking at all possible sources of finance including money found from redeploying funds within existing services.

To be realistic, any national plan has to be tailored to fit the money likely to be made available. This does not mean abandoning Health for all. What it does mean is finding the most efficient way of providing the essential primary health care services to people currently without them, and ensuring greater efficiency in the way in which existing financial resources are used.

CHART 5.1

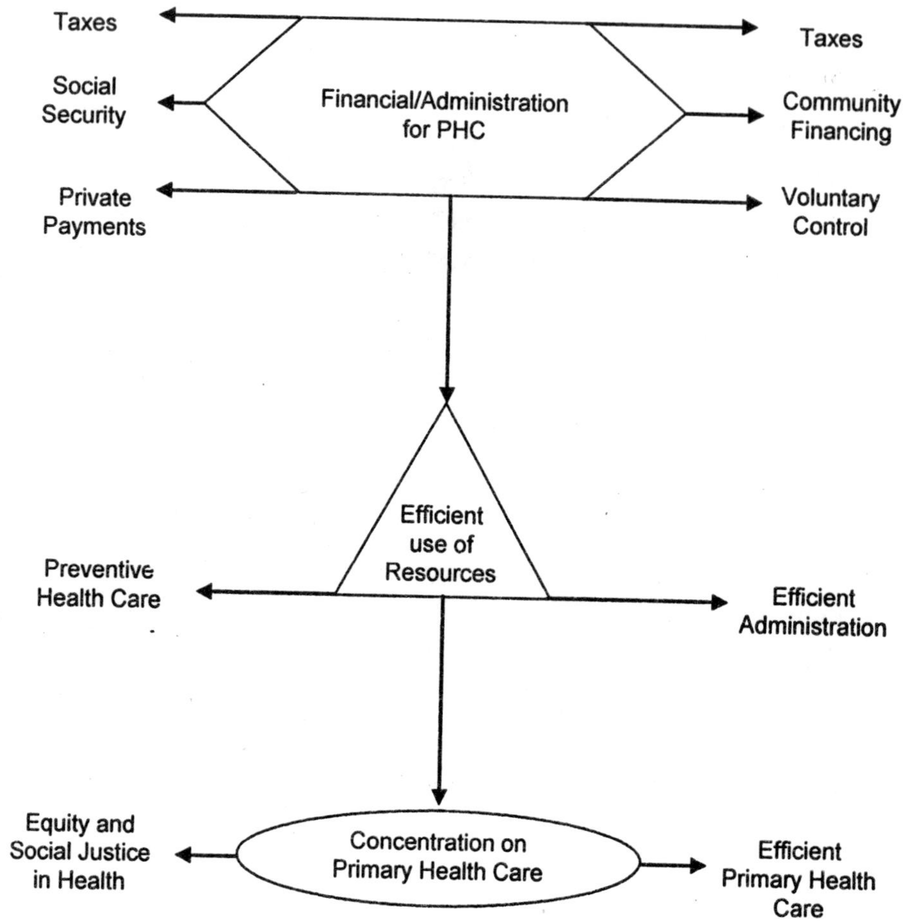

We must however be clear that we cannot apply the techniques of financial management like cost-benefit analysis in providing money for primary health care as the tools for these techniques in this area are still in infancy and not reliable. John S. Aken[3] in his article, "Equity for the Poor" rightly mentions the limitations of this technique. To quote him:

"The tradition of cost-benefit analysis in development planning means that there is perhaps greater pressure on the health sector in developing than in developed countries to justify its proposals in economic terms. Thus, there is considerable interest in the application of techniques of economic evaluation to the health sector. Unfortunately, the lack of economists with an interest in health, and the problems of obtaining adequate data on costs and consequences are considerable obstacles to good economic evaluation."

Moreover, the application of the techniques is still at an early stage and many studies aim to stretch the boundaries of the discipline rather than to provide practical guidance. The studies done under the umberalla of the WHO Expanded Programme on immunization provide a good example of the way in which early theoretical work can be developed into a methodology capable of application by health service managers. These studies further pointed the importance of choosing issues that are amenable to economic evaluation, where calculations or plausible assumptions can be made of the relationship between health, interventions and health consequences, and the need for collaborative work between economists, epidemiologists and other health researchers.

The results of economic evaluation are of assistance to decision-makers, but they do not dictate their course of action. While it is important to know the cost-effectiveness of different ways of organising primary health care activities, other consequences less easy to quantity, such as stimulating community participation and promoting the capacity to improve individual health, must not be neglected. Decision-makers will wish to take these also into account when they review the results of economic evaluation studies. We must husband resources from all and should not depend only on Government.[4]

No money, no Health for all. Yet in many countries health budgets are being drastically cut as a result of inflation and the world recession. Cutbacks present problems in the short-run, but they also provide opportunities to re-examine the deployment of resources so as to bring them in line with Health for all priorities.

Most countries are still lacking a master plan that will husband health resources between now and the new millennium. However, such a plan is the only way for countries to identity serious shortfalls, to find potential new resources, to make better use of existing ones, and to span the current gap between what must be provided and what reasonably can be financed from releasable sources. There is a need of drawing funds from all possible sources and combining them in an imaginative way, any given country can formulate the first essential key to equity in health: a budget for Health for all by the year 2000. These sources can be:

(a) Foreign Aid
(b) Community Financing
(c) Voluntary contribution
(d) Private payments
(e) Social security
(f) Taxes

W.A. Hassouna in his article, "A Strategy against poverty" also advocates the approach of using all resources. To quote him,[5] In most developing and some developed countries, governments have been the major providers of preventive and curative health care. These services used to be accessible to the poor since they were provided without charge. But the unprecedented escalation of the cost of health services in the last ten years and the adoption of economic reforms which usually resulted in sizeable reductions of allocations for health services have greatly reduced the access of the poor to government health services. Such reforms have affected curative more than preventive care since many governments provide the latter free or at minimal cost.

Several ways have been adopted in various countries to increase access to health services, all of which are aimed at reducing the patient's economic burden. Unfortunately, most of the approaches, such as health insurance and cost-sharing, are geared to helping middle income groups rather than the poor, who cannot afford to pay insurance premiums or even reduced fees, and in many cases will not have the cash to pay for health services when they are seriously sick.

It seems clear that what is needed is a system that ensures for the poor a reasonable access to health services with a minimal economic burden. This could be done by including specific health benefits within a compulsory social insurance system or making available interest-free loans from group savings to be used in case of sickness.

Certainly, increasing access to health services as a strategy for poverty alleviation should be dealt with in a comprehensive manner that takes into account physical, social, cultural and economic factors. The ultimate aim should be to put "reasonable quality of care" at an affordable cost within the reach of the poor, rather than offering low quality of care at cheaper prices.

Hakan Hellberg and Edward P. Mach[6] have rightly said that in many countries, the costs of PHC have not been fully worked out and sources of finance for health programmes in the future are left vague. Far more work needs to be done to ensure a realistic and sound estimation of costs.

One of the more essential requirements of primary health care is that it should be at a cost that people can afford right now. At the same time, it is vital to investigate and use all possible resources to support and finance PHC, since relying only on traditional sources of financing will not be enough. The very concept of PHC calls for changes in the traditional approaches to basic health services. People's involvement, inter-sectoral action for health and the need for appropriate technology all require new form of financing.

Health workers may be hammered again and again with the idea that they should depend more on community resources rather than Government. Experience has shown that people should not be merely on receiving ends but they should become partners in the development programmes. The realisation has come that any development programme designed for the users must involve the users' right from the planning stage. If development is meant for the people then it should be of the people and by the people. Health workers may be made aware of the successful projects being implemented and if possible some of them may be taken on visit to such project areas. Some of these may be mentioned as—The Ludheran World Service (India) Project in a slum of Calcutta. The Dharavi Slum Project by

L.T.M. Medical College, Bombay, RUSHA Project in North Arcot District, the Vishakapathan Slum Improvement Project, Hyderabad Slum Improvement Project.

The developing countries give low priority in the allocation of resources to the health care of their people. The health expenditure to the total .expenditure has been very low in South-East Asian countries, i.e. 1.6 per cent in Indonesia, 2.1 percent in India, 3.8 percent in Bangladesh. Mongolia has been spending 10 percent for the health care of its people. There is a need to raise the health allocations to improve the quality of life. Dr. White has rightly said that, "Nothing can be done without the expenditure of money. Available financial resources set a maximum limit on administrative activity as a whole and on each of its separate parts."[7]

A sound state of finance is of paramount importance to the political health of a nation. The soundness or public finance depends both upon the right policy and good organisation, but a great deal upon the latter. The scarcity of resources affects all aspects of the health delivery system. There is a need to step up the health allocations to the minimum of 10 per cent of the total budget.[8]

Secondly, there is mal-distribution of health resources. Most of the health budget (about 80 per cent) is being spent only on a few people (20 per cent). This deprives the people living in rural areas and urban slums. A WHO study group on the Financing of Health Services mentioned the following characteristics, which reflect the situation in the developing countries.[9]

(a) Disproportionate concentration of expenditure on health services in urban are compared with expenditure in rural areas.
(b) Heavy concentration of expenditure on secondary and tertiary care services compared with expenditure on primary care services.
(c) Heavy concentration of expenditure on curatives services compared with expenditure on preventive services.

We can correct this imbalance through the innovative health policies developed in tune with the needs of the country rather than based on any foreign model.[10]

The third serious problem in this area is of inefficient use of expenditure and non-utilisation of actual and potential resources judiciously and properly. In the developing countries, huge resources are being wasted because of the selection of inappropriate technology,[11] inefficient management,[12] and unsatisfactory control mechanisms.

> "It is necessary that public revenue should be raised in an equitable manner and spent economically so that the tax payers may get full value for his money."[13]

The objects of financial control are to ensure: (i) that no wastage of resources occurs; (ii) that public money is not misused, and (iii) that intended results are obtained with the money spent. We can exploit the potential resources through careful planning and management. The traditional system of medicine can be of immense value to provide health care at a very low cost provided this is properly tapped by the designers of health services. It was reported in a recent UN Survey (1976) that, these adverse trends are despite the higher percentage of government expenditure being devoted to health, compared with 1960s and the fact that ratio of population to the number of beds and of medical personnel have moved favourably. Essentially, the continuance of poor health standards is indicative, as opposed to preventive techniques embodied in the existing hospital systems, the inadequate development of indigenous medicine systems on which there is a continued reliance and the limited coverage of available medical facilities particularly in rural areas.[14]

In a paper presented by M. Siegel, Assistant Director-General, Department of Administration and Finance, WHO, Geneva, to the Advisory Group of Nursing Administration (16 December, 1977) it has been rightly stated:

> "If the resources for health work, in trained persons and in finances, were unlimited, the need for constant attention to those factors would not be so great. But the limitation in the number of trained personnel and the lack of adequate financial resources are major obstacles to greatly improved health in the world today. We must, therefore, husband our resources carefully to accomplish as much as possible with what we have available."

The fourth serious challenge in this field is the rising cost of health services beyond the reach of most of the people inhabiting the developing societies. It is very difficult to afford the costly urban-based hospitals using highly sophisticated technology. A huge amount is being spent on costly buildings and equipment which the developing countries cannot afford. The only services which can meet the health needs of the people are low-cost services which should be efficient and effective. This is possible if we use methods and equipment appropriate to the socio-economic environment existing in a country, e.g. the people can contribute voluntary labour to maintain health services. This would reduce the cost. We must take decisions and think of alternative solutions to provide health care to the people as financing and decision-making are complementary functions. The health administrator should encourage the low-cost service programmes beneficial to the larger section of the community.

The fifth problem in this connection is the lack of coordination among different agencies financing health care services. This may result in wasteful duplication of efforts. Besides, many health services may not get the desired financial allocation because of this wastage. The situation can be improved through proper coordination among such agencies.

In the new millennium, we have to give preference to primary health care. Aviva Ron[15] has rightly said in his article, 'Shifting Resources in Israel' that, if we analyse the budget of almost every health care system we will find that hospital care takes up the largest single proportion, usually accounting for more than half the total. Although it is clear that most medical care is given outside the hospital and does not require resources generally concentrated in hospitals, little has been done to divert manpower, equipment and capital away from these institutions. Today, changes in the economic situation and in the consensus view as to what constitutes good medical care provide us with the rational to shift resources to the community. We now accept that:

- A reduction in hospital services holds the greatest potential for cost containment;
- Patients should be kept within their homes and communities to the extent possible, to minimise the trauma of illness and maximise the support provided by their surroundings. When overnight care is necessary, it should be as short as possible, with the hospital stay forming a planned stage in the diagnosis and treatment within the referral chain;
- Primary health care can be most effective when it is provided in a facility which stimulates team work among health professionals at all levels, ensures continuity of care and encourages a concentration of both knowledge and equipment.

According to Sidney Ndeki,[16] Primary health care is gaining acceptance as a strategy for bringing basic health services to all the people. Such programmes can have a significant impact on health by focusing on a carefully selected number of health problems that are preventable by means of simple, and relatively low-cost interventions.

CRITICAL APPRAISAL

Finances for primary health care are not being allocated and spent prudently and rationally. We mention some of the facts and suggestions, which can improve the financial health of primary health care systems in the new millennium:

1. Undue Expansion leading to Dilution of Services

There has been undue expansion of health infrastructure, without proper facilities, because of financial constraints. For example, number of sub-centres has increased from 84376 to 144988 (from 1.4.85 to 31.3.2006). Similarly, primary health centres have increased from 9115 to 22669 during the same period. Concern Health Centres from 761 to 3910. It is time to consolidate and equip the already existing facilities fully. This would save the money for future expansion.

2. Low Time Utilization by Health Workers

The output of workers is very less in terms of health care delivery system. Strict disciplinary action may be initiated against those workers who are habitually late or are in the habit of wasting time. Besides, unessential activities may be withdrawn so that they can concentrate on essential services. It is no use paying salaries without any output. This may be strictly ascertained through supervision, performance appraisal, surprise checks, etc.

3. Less Emphasis on Curative Services

The main activity of primary health care is preventive care and not curative. The health workers should focus attention on ensuring provision of cheaper preventive services having lasting impact.

4. Improper Maintenance of Equipment

Equipment at health centres generally remains out of order, inspite of the fact that the equipment supplied is not old. Health workers do not take due care and also do not handle properly the equipment, resulting in the equipment going out of order. They should maintain equipment in good condition.

5. Intersectoral Coordination Missing

Many of the activities in the domain of primary health care can be better handled by some other agencies or Panchayati Raj System. There is a need to involve more and more other agencies like ICDS.

6. Performance Budgeting to make the best use of Resources

Performance budgeting is very useful in developing countries. It facilitates better programming, decision-making, review and control for a more intelligible presentation of governmental activities to the public and the legislature. Broadly speaking, the main purposes sought to be served by performance budgeting are:[17]

(a) to correlate the physical and financial aspects of every programme/activity;
(b) to improve budget formulation, review and decision-making at all levels of management in the government machinery;
(c) to facilitate better appreciation and review by the legislature;
(d) to make possible more effective performance audit;
(e) to measure progress towards long-term objectives as envisaged in the plan; and
(f) to bring annual budgets and development plans closely together through a common language.

7. Ineffective Utilisation of Resources

The most serious problem in India is not as much of Resource mobilisation as that of resource utilisation. The resources are not producing the desired impact.

K.N. Rao, in a paper on "Health in Developing Countries" pointed out: "It may be stated, however, that even funds allocated by WHO and UNICEF are not fully utilized in some developing countries including India due to administrative and procedural difficulties."[18]

Thus, a quantitatively inadequate or qualitatively deficient system of public administration will not merely retard the development process, but may defeat the entire development effort in an even more decisive manner than any temporary shortage of capital, or inadequate technical skills, or an unfavourable monsoon. Nigro has also remarked in this connection that "management experts from the highly developed countries find that these are serious obstacles to improvements." He adds that some developing countries in Latin America which have succeeded substantially in improving their respective administrative system, have been able to make better use of international assistance."[19]

Let us understand the nature of these problems. There have been a large number of administrative challenges and problems, which impede and bedevil the effective functioning of the governments in the developing countries. Let us mention some of them:

(a) Lack of effective policy-making, planning and decision-making to exploit the human and financial resources for the better health of the people.
(b) Lack of effective manpower planning resulting in the poor utilization of human resources.
(c) Lack of coordination among the allied agencies and within the various units of a department resulting in duplication and wastage of financial resources.
(d) Lack of reliable, timely and suitable information systems for the formulation, implementation and evaluation of financial policy.
(e) Widely scattered funding mechanism with little control over costs.
(f) Lack of effective mechanism to involve the employees and beneficiaries in the policy-making and implementation of the programmes of an organisation.
(g) Use of outdated methods and procedures in the operation of the financial administration.
(h) Lack of interest to improve financial administrative structures and procedures.
(i) Absence of innovative leadership, administrative capability and competence in general and financial administration in particular.
(j) Lack of equity of distribution and adequacy of coverage in relationship to need.

Resource mobilisation and utilisation can be improved to a great extent through improved administrative system, especially in the sphere of financial administration. Besides, all the resources must be utilised economically and efficiently and the expenditure on unproductive resources must be curbed.

CONCLUSION

We may conclude by saying that the policy-makers, planners and decision-makers may attend to the following carefully to husband all resources and to accomplish as much as possible with what is available:

(i) to identify who (action agents) needs how much money (cost) and for what (activities);
(ii) to define criteria for and priority in allocation of budgetary resources among different activities and different organisations responsible for performance of activities;
(iii) to provide flexibility in budgeting and financing, if necessary, beyond bureaucratic control;
(iv) to ensure the timely availability of funds to the programme activities of field level;
(v) to design Management Information System to get timely information on the utilisation of resources;
(vi) arrange statistical analysis to bring out what the performance data truly signify;
(vii) to explore and recommend possibilities of reducing costs with due regards to the maintenance of efficiency and quality;
(viii) to ensure the development of effective linkages among financial, personnel, materials and other resources; and
(ix) to ensure the full impact on the main objective: socio- economic development and modernisation.

Notes and References

1. Brian Abel Smith, "Paying for Health for All", in *World Health*, May 1986.
2. *Ibid.*
3. John S. Akin, "Equity for the Poor", in *World Health*, May 1986, p. 29.
4. *World Health*, May 1986, p. 17.
5. W.A. Hassouna, "A Strategy against Poverty", in *World Health*, Nov.-Dec. 1994, p. 6.
6. Hakan Hellberg and Edward P. Mach, "Financing Primary Health Care", in *World Health*, March 1985, p. 26.
7. L.D. White, Introduction to the Study of Public Administration, Macmillan, N.Y., p. 2101.
8. Gyan Chand, The Financial System of India, p. 1.
9. WHO: Technical Report Series, 925, p. 18.
10. Refer to Volume IV.

11. J.H. Bryant, Health and the Developing World, Ithaca, N.Y., Cornell University Press, 1969.
12. WHO, Modern Management Methods and the Organisation of Services, Geneva, WHO, 1974, (Public Health Paper, No. 55).
13. P.K. Wattal, Parliamentary Financial Control in India, Bombay, Minerva, 1979.
14. UN (ESCAP), Economic and Social Survey of Asia and the Pacific, 1976, Bangkok, April 1977, p. 18.
15. Aviva Ron, "Shifting Resources in Israel", in *World Health,* May 1986, p. 24.
16. Sidney, Ndeki, "Money of Health", in *World Health,* May 1989, p. 13.
17. ARC: Report of the Study Team, Financial Administration, May 1979, Chapter III.
18. Dr. K.N. Rao, "Health in Developing Countries", *Indian Journal of Public Health,* Vol. XIII, No. 2, April 1969, pp. 21-40.
19. Felix, A. Nigro, Chap. III: Administration and Culture, Modern Public Administration, (New York, 1966), p. 70.

6

CHAPTER

Personnel Administration for Primary Health Care

A task without a vision is a drudgery,
A vision without a task is revere,
A task with a vision is victory.

The success or failure of primary health care depends to a substantial extent upon the quantity and quality of health personnel, especially at the lower levels, where people have less opportunity of alternative health care because of poverty.

Primary Health care is a challenging and arduous task, which cannot be achieved without competent, dedicated, honest, hardworking and public spirited health functionaries, especially at the grassroot level. Since the policy of primary health care is to be formulated at the higher level, there is a need of intensive training to health professionals about the importance of primary health care and in behaviour sciences, so that they can act as agents of social change and development. The primary health care programme should rely more on action rather than paper work. It has been rightly said that words written or spoken are of no use unless put to action. The success and usefulness of other features of primary health care, e.g. community participation, intersectoral coordination, appropriate technology, health research, etc. would depend upon the sincerity, good intentions and urge of the persons responsible for delivery of primary health care.

Deepak Chopra, the new doyen of management in USA, draws inspiration from vedantic philosophy to redefine spiritual laws of success—Law of pure potentiality, Law of giving, Law of Karma or cause and effect, Law of least effort, Law of intention and desire, Law of detachment, Law of dharma and purpose of life. Out of these, two are being mentioned in some detail to be followed by primary health care personnel. (Quoted by

CHART 6.1

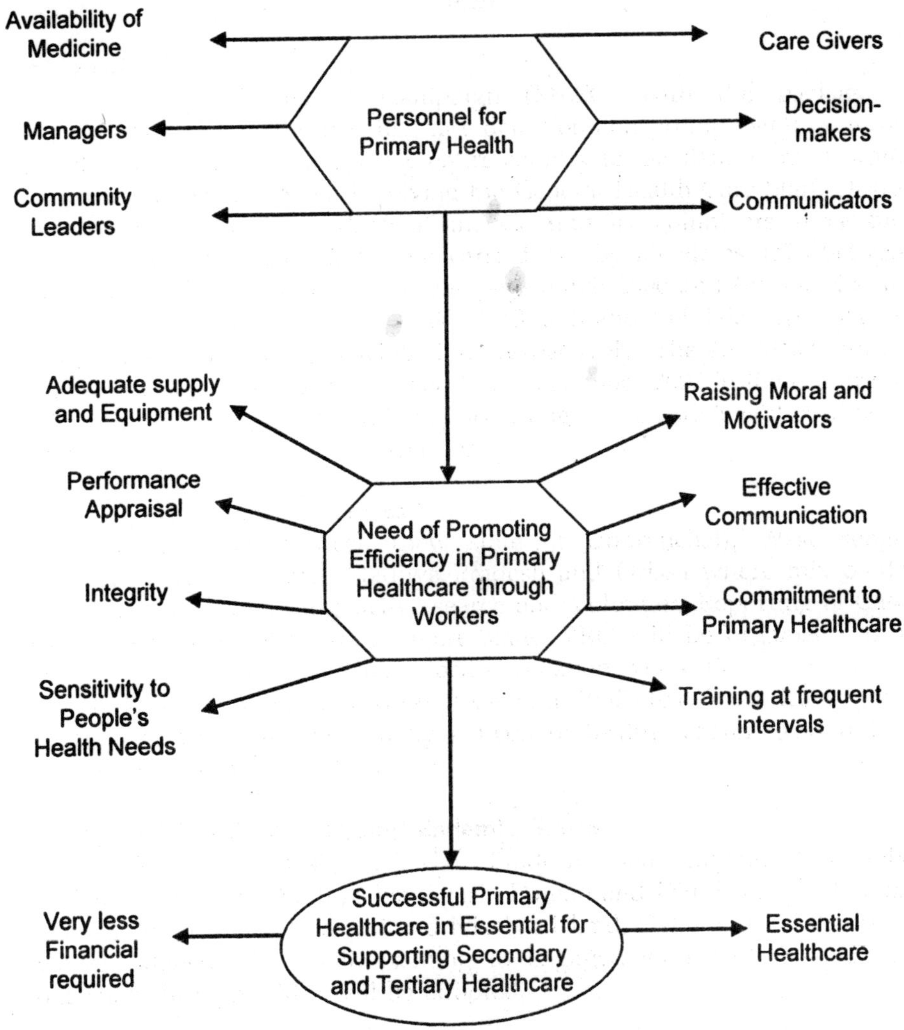

Krishan Mohan Mathur, in his article, "Vedantic Wisdom and Contemporary Management" in *IJPA*, January-March 1999).

The second spiritual law of success is the law of giving. The more you give, the more you receive, because you will keep the abundance of the universe circulating in your life. This law could be called the law of giving and receiving, because the universe operates through dynamic exchange. One's body is always in dynamic and constant exchange with the body of universe; the mind is dynamically interacting with the mind of the cosmos and one's energy is an expression of cosmic energy.

Karma is both action and consequence of that action. It is the cause and effect simultaneously, because every action generates force and energy that returns to us in like kind. We want happiness in our lives, we must return to sow the seeds of happiness. Obviously Karma implies action of conscious choice-making.

The author while giving a key note address to the participants of a training programme, held from March 17 to March 20, 1999, remarked that health personnel must follow the teachings of Guru Nanak Devji and share their health expertise with the suffering humanity and take this oath on the tricenitary celebrations of Khalsa Panth.

Peter Drucker regarded human resource as main organisational "input and equated it with capital resource and he considered that difference between success and failure in any organisation could be traced to the quality of people within the organisation. The initial step to optimise human resources is to attempt manpower planning. According to De. Ray, "A health manpower plan is meant to ensure that the right number and quality of manpower are available to staff the health facilities as the needs expand, so as to keep up with current and future demands of services from the people."[1]

According to Tamas Fulop, Director of the Health Manpower Development Division, WHO, the objective of a health manpower plan should be: "to concentrate all national efforts so as to satisfy the health services composed of balanced teams of health personnel; that is, to ensure that all health activities are undertaken at the most peripheral level of the health services as is practicable, bv workers most suitably trained to carry out these activities. Their emphasis should be put on the most 'suitably' trained as opposed to the most 'highly' trained since the latter term might entail confusing the most sophisticated and most costly with the optimal."[2] According to John Bland, information expert at Geneva, health manpower planning is: "a process of estimating the quality and type of knowledge skill and attitudes needed to introduce predetermined changes into the functioning of a health system. The object of the exercise is not merely to promote health in the widest sense, but to provide the appropriately trained staff who will, as far as possible, treat diseases, prevent their onset and meet the community's demand for services."[3]

COMPARATIVE COST OF TRAINING HEALTH WORKERS FOR PRIMARY HEALTH CARE

How to decide about the possible mixes of different sorts of health workers? We may decide on that mix which can train and retain the manpower to cover the whole of the country and be within the financial limits of the country. J. Bryant compared the cost of training of professional and auxiliary personnel. The comparison is indicated in the Table 6.1 given on next page.

These figures indicate that about 20 auxiliaries can be trained at the cost of training one doctor.

A substantial reduction in expenditure can be achieved as functions are transferred from high salary to low salary workers, because the main

TABLE 6.1

Example of Training Cost[4]

(In US Dollars)

Country	Doctors	Nurses	Auxiliaries
Thailand	6,600	1,200	350
Columbia	24.600	3,000	1,000
East Africa	26,000	9,800	1,000
United Republic of Tanzania	35,000	—	2,100

Source: WHO.

costs in the health industry are for services rather than goods. Improved health standards and the number of physicians don't definitely go together. However. there is evidence to show that the investment in para-medicals would give more dividends. Studies by Cunningham and Morrley[6] in Nigeria showed that either nurse or grade-2 midwives were effective in lowering under-five mortality rates.

The preparatory committee on medical education in India was of the view that doctors aren't the only important category of health personnel that the nation needed. There is a need of other categories of health personnel of right quantity and quality. The situation in regard to the members of the health team in the country is today the reverse of what it ought to be. To give only one example, Optimum utilization of health manpower required that there should be six nurses for one doctor, but in our case the doctors still outnumber nurses. It is only now that the annual out-turn of nurses has reached the same figures as that of the doctors., i.e. around 12,500 each. This applies to other categories of personnel as well.[7]

TABLE 6.2

Country	Number of nurses per doctor
Finland	3.7
Sweden	3.1
Japan	1.2
Turkey	.6
Sudan	.6
India	.4
Sri Lanka	2.49
Nepal	.19
Thailand	2.83
Bangladesh	.22

Source: Ibid.

The same phenomenon is visible in many developing countries. Table 6.2 shows the ratio of nurses to doctors in several countries.

There can be many reasons for this state of affairs. The most important is the low status and low salary scales accorded to paramedical staff. "Western consultants at collegiate schools of nursing in underdeveloped countries report that nursing shortages exist only because too few women wished to enter a downtrodden and unskilled career."[8]

Besides, physicians in developing countries often feel that nothing but physician care is the most important thing for their people. Baker emphasizes the potential of lower level health workers:

"Improvement of the training and utilisation of all members of the health team offers the greatest opportunities and challenges in the health field today. In most countries the greatest return will come from increased investment in lower-level health workers."[9]

TABLE 6.3

Comparative Costs of Services of One District Hospital and 15 Rural Centres in United Republic of Tanzania[10]

Population		*Input (in Thousand of Tanzanian Shillings (T.Sh.)) Capital*	*Recurrent*	*Output per cent: Outpatient*	*Inpatients Coverage*
200 bed Hospital	6,000	2,060.0	4000,000	9,000	10,000-30,000
15 rural health centres	6,000	2,225.0	1,000,000	15,000	300,000-500000

Source: Ibid.

Another study points out the comparative costs of services of the Urban and the Rural Health Centres.

The table indicates the far greater coverage of population that can be achieved through a network of smaller facilities as opposed to a hospital. There is a need of innovation in the concept of health manpower planning to make it relevant to present and future community health needs. The new innovations may take into consideration the following:

(a) Training and utilisation of more auxiliary and primary health workers and their supervisors.
(b) Training of health personnel should not be only hospital and disease-oriented but should be preventive and promotive. It

should help the health personnel to develop an effective link with the health of the community.

(c) Education of physicians may be made relevant to the needs of the society.

(d) Education must prepare health professionals for their leadership role in community development.

(e) The specialists must concentrate only on secondary and tertiary care and should not devote their time and waste the resources in promoting primary health care. More services can be made available if some of the health workers, trained for certain simple routine tasks, can release the professional personnel and enable them to concentrate on activities which require a higher level of competence.

Thus, the health manpower planners will have to decide about the proper mix between the different categories of health personnel to provide health care to the community.

"These changes should result in a sound health manpower system which will plan, develop, and manage/utilize efficiently the right 'mix' of health personnel within well-conceived health and other services, which will continuously monitor whether they all are functioning properly and which will adjust the planning and 'production' systems on the basis of such monitoring, so as to achieve a full health coverage for the entire population in the coming decades."[11]

Dr. Guillermo Soberon Acevedo rightly says: "The medicine that was practiced in the 19th century, i.e. liberal model as a personal undertaking has acquired such complexity in our own century that it has ad to give place to group forms of practice whether state run or private. A profession that is supposed to be self-regulating according to the law of supply and demand has, with the advent of new ways of organising the delivery of services and with the promises of the Welfare State that has been the ruling model since the Second World War, went out of control. As a result, it has created disparities between the health manpower that countries need, the manpower that they can employ, and the manpower that is actually trained."[12]

According to Oladipo O. Akinkugbem,[13] "If we are to relate health manpower to the attainment of Health for all by the year 2000 through Primary Health Care, we must first define the nature and structure of health services and the type of resources needed to sustain the best possible health care, having regard to the peculiar circumstances of the developing world."

Health manpower development is often taken to imply the training of doctors, nurses, dentists, pharmacists and so on, and hitherto little attention has been paid to a detailed characterisation of the skills to be provided in meeting adequate health care. The need to orient this traditional thinking towards a broader perspective has been made more urgent by the HFA credo, for it would be meaningless to undertake to provide adequate health care without clearly understanding just what personnel will be needed at all levels.

Zbigniew Bankowaski,[14] "rightly says: A glut of medical, graduates and an unprecededeted level of unemployment among medical and dental graduates is causing deep concern in many parts of the world today."

A conference on "Health Manpower Out of Balance: Conflicts and Prospects," held last autumn in Acapulco, Mexico, brought together about 120 health policy-makers, physicians, dentists, nurses, medical students and educators of health personnel from 40 countries. It was prepared in close collaboration with WHO, the Pan American Health Organisation, the World Federation for Medical Education and the Secretariat of Health of Mexico.

The conference recommended a number of preventive actions and other measures which would help to solve acute manpower imbalances. The aim should be to bring the supply of health professionals into line with the foreseeable demand of the population and the economic ability of a country to make adequate use of them. Urgent research is needed into this fast growing problem, and a regular exchange of information between countries. Among radical actions that might be taken to reduce the surplus doctors, the conference suggested the following:

- limiting the intake into medical schools or restricting the number of graduates; and
- postponing the opening of new medical schools or even closing existing ones; and imposing a compulsory retirement age for physicians.

Alastair Anderson[15] in his article, "Adapt-Dont Adopt" in *World Health*, rightly says that Primary health care integrates at the community level all the elements necessary to make an impact on the health status of the people. It calls for measures that are simple and effective in terms of costs, technique and organisation, that are easily accessible, and that improve living conditions. It should use available local resources including manpower material and funds generated within the community itself as well as strictly essential resources allocated by the government. It should be fully integrated with the national health system and with the other sectors involved in community development—agriculture, education, public works, housing, communications.

The most important functionary in Primary Health Care is front line worker or multipurpose worker. Charles Boelen'b in his article, "Frontline Doctors of Tomorrow" in *World Health*, rightly suggests the following functions for front-line workers:

Caregivers

Besides giving individual treatment, front line doctors must take into account the total (physical, mental, social) needs of the patient. They must ensure that a full range of treatment—curative, preventive or rehabilitative—will be dispensed in ways that are complementary, integrated and continuous. And they must ensure that the treatment is of the highest quality.

Decision-makers

In a climate of transparency the front line doctor will have to take decisions that can be justified in terms of efficacy and cost. From all the possible ways of treating a given health condition, the one that seems most appropriate in the given situation must be chosen. As regards expenditure, the limited resources available for health must be shared out fairly to the benefit of every individual in the community.

Communicators

Lifestyle aspects such as a balanced diet, safety measures at work, type of leisure pursuits, respect for the environment and so on all have a determining influence on health. The involvement of the individual in protecting and restoring his or her own health is therefore vital, since exposure to a health risk is largely determined by one's behaviour. The doctors of tomorrow must be excellent communicators in order to persuade individuals, families and the communities in their charge to adopt healthy lifestyles and become partners in the health effort.

Community leaders

The needs and problems of the whole community—in a suburb or a district must not be forgotten. By understanding the determinants of health inherent in the physical and social environment and by appreciating the breadth of each problem or health risk, the frontline doctor will not simply be treating individuals who seek help but will also take a positive interest in community health activities which will benefit large number of people.

Managers

To carry out all these functions, it will be essential for the frontline doctors to acquire managerial skills. This will enable them to initiate exchanges of information in order to make better decisions, and to work within a multidisciplinary team in close association with other partners for health and social development. Both old and new methods of dispensing care will have to be integrated with the totality of health and social services, whether destined for the individual or for the community.

The ideal frontline doctor of the future might be described as the five-star doctor someone who is equal in excellence to a five-star hotel or restaurant, but is accessible to everyone from the richest to the poorest. The skills of the doctors of tomorrow will serve the needs of all health system and services; these abilities will be desirable to a certain degree in health personnel at every level. Far from being a dream, these goals and skills must be seen as imperative for our doctors of tomorrow.

In the new millennium, we should overhaul our personnel system in favour of Primary Health Care. We suggest here some facts which may be taken into account for manpower planning and development:

(i) Eliminate haphazard growth of health personnel; there should be adequate manpower planning, so that there is logical forecasting of the manpower needs at least ten years in advance. It should be related to the health plans and health policy.

(ii) It is essential that the health organisations should have a declared and well-accepted personnel policy. It should reflect the total personnel system rather than attending, on piece-meal basis to the sub-systems. Manpower planning like health planning, is a continuous cyclical process with constant reviews and adjustments being made to ensure that the health service goals and manpower demands are matched by an appropriate supply of staff.

(iii) This declared personnel policy must be developed by a staffing section at headquarters or comparable level. It would be quite desirable if the academic guidance may be sought from the NIHFW and the universities.

(iv) The staffing section must be under the charge of a duly qualified and trained personnel officer. It is often forgotten that manpower planners, as well as health planners must acquire special skills, not only through experience but also by learning the principles and theories.

(v) Manpower planning should be based on a proper-mix of different categories of health workers. This proper-mix should be determined by the health policy and the socio-economic status of the country. They must have special aptitude and motivations if they're to be effective.

(vi) While formulating the personnel policy, internal as well as external sources may be explored. To supplement the internal data, the administration must collect information from external sources, e.g. associations/unions of employees.

(vii) There is a need of proper classification of health personnel so that their duties and responsibilities may be clearly demarcated. The ambiguity in this sphere result in confusion.

(viii) Manpower planning should ensure optimum utilisation of the capacity of the existing personnel.

(ix) There is a need to provide proper motivation which can help the employees for the maximum optimisation of goods and services. This would require judicious decentralisation, delegation, job enlargement and proper system of performance appraisal.

(x) Health manpower planning should be relevant to the existing disease pattern.

(xi) The personnel department must carry out research in various aspects of personnel administration in collaboration with training institutions and universities to identify future requirements and trends (futuristic approach).

(xii) A commission may be appointed to deal with all problems of personnel administration in the States of Indian Union. The members of the Commission may be taken from the top level health administration; legislature, training institutions and the universities. Based on the findings of this Commission, committees may be appointed by the various State governments to go into the applicability and efficacy of these recommendations in their respective States.

(xiii) Manpower planners must be involved in implementing their plans. The separation between planning and implementation must be broken down if plans are to be successfully converted into reality.

(xiv) Health manpower planning should not concentrate on the personnel and training resources of the public sector only but also take into account to private sector and voluntary sector.

(xv) The entire efforts in the field of health manpower development should be directed towards making the manpower relevant to the needs of the health services which should also be reoriented to provide wider coverage to the rural people and the under-served urban poor.

(xvi) Training programmes for health manpower should be formulated to make them need-based, task-oriented and relevant to specific situations where the trainees will work and apply their skills.

(xvii) More emphasis should be laid on the training and utilization of auxiliary and primary health workers rather than on the classical 'categories' of health workers (doctors, nurses, etc.)

An important operational objective for the 21st century is, therefore, to improve personnel systems, develop manpower planning in health services, and expand the opportunity for education and training of personnel to achieve developmental goals as it is the human capacities which transform the passive natural resources into active agents of production. Most developing countries confront the immense task of reforming their system of personnel administration so that they will assist rather than hinder development programmes. Thus, the most important task is the development of sound personnel planning and improvement of the policy-making and implementation capabilities of personnel units in health care administration. We should also encourage team work to provide support for workers directly engaged in Primary Health Care in the new millennium.

Most of the health workers are working in isolation, i.e., their activities are not coordinated properly, resulting in lower output of services.

The health workers should form part of health manpower planning system. According to Antonio Ordonez Plaja, "Team work requires, among other things, that the members have an image of their team-mates which coincides as precisely as possible with reality. In addition, each member must have a self-image which adjusts to reality as much as possible and thus coincides with the image the other members have of him."[16]

Team work would develop common practices and shared experiences. This would also raise the morale of the health personnel working at the grass-root level. Dr. Daniel Flahault, head of the team of Development Unit, WHO, has rightly said: "Backed up by health service officials working at a high level, conscious of belonging to a group and not being in isolation, the local health team will find its prestige and its credibility strengthened. It will find it easier to win the confidence of the local population, and that confidence in turn will facilitate the development of services that are better adapted to the needs."[17]

CASE STUDY

The author was engaged by Punjab Health System Corporation as a management consultant and course director to impart training to senior health functionaries in Punjab in 1998. The author visited some health institutions to find out the impact of training. A visit to one of the health centres in Ropar district in Punjab revealed that at 9.30 a.m., there was none in the health centre except a peon. There was stinking smell all around. All the rooms were unclean and the garbage was lying scattered. The examination room of the doctor had a tray of medicines, all the bottles were open and were not arranged. In one room, two broken iron folding beds were lying, making the room unfit for use!

The author contacted the people nearby and learnt that the doctor and other staff absent themselves without leave and are rarely punctual. Besides, they have no sense of cleanliness or improvement of the health of the people. They are keen to leave the health centre to reach their home in Chandigarh. How can we expect the success of primary health care from such personnel? Who have no interest in their job.

Dr. Naven Shah, in his article, "Doctors in India must be accountable" in *Economic Times* (30 December, 1999) rightly asserts that there is not enough accountability of doctors, few or no hospital records, a lack of quality care and responsibility. The author visited a number of sub-centres to find out the problems affecting primary health care, resulting into personnel apathy, indifference and slackness.

Based on discussion, observation and analysis of records, following problems in the area of health personnel responsible for the delivery of primary health care have been found:

1. Absence from duty without leave.
2. Lack of punctuality.

3. Apathy, indifference and insensitivity towards the health needs of the people.
4. Utilization time very less-ranging from 20 to 30 percent.
5. Lack of rapport with the people as most of them stay away from the place of work.
6. Lack of effective supervision and control.
7. Lack of professional competence.
8. Prevalence of corrupt practices.
9. No attention to main problems of primary health care.
10. Lack of faith and identity in primary health care.
11. Improper behaviour.

The personnel responsible for primary health care, on the other hand, blame the government for not providing them:

(a) Medicines
(b) Equipments
(c) Infrastructural facilities
(d) Incentives
(e) Transport
(f) Effective supervision and support from the health department.

We are of the opinion that in order to improve the performance of primary health care personnel, there is urgent necessity of focusing on the Human Resource Development (HRD) aspects. HRD, which in brief is change of potential human resources into kinetic human resources, that is optimisation of the potential capacity of employees.

Prof. Udai Pareek says, Human Resource Development in the organisational context is a process by which the employees of an organisation are helped in a continuous and planned way to:

1. Acquire or sharpen capabilities required to perform various functions associated with their present or expected future roles;
2. Development of their general capabilities as individuals and discover and exploit their own inner potential for their own and for organisational development purposes; and
3. Develop an organisational culture in which senior subordinate relationships, teamwork, and collaboration among sub-units are strong and contribute to the professional well-being, motivation and pride of employees.

According to Ishwar Dayal, three things are important in HRD:

(a) Ways to better adjust the individual to his job and the environment;
(b) The greatest involvement of the employee in various aspects of his work; and

(c) The greatest concern for enhancing the capabilities of the individual.

We may thus define HRD as a process of the development of employees through training, performance appraisals, potential development exercises, communication policies, job enrichment programmes, etc., and building of an organisational climate, which may encourage openness, risk-taking, role clarity, awareness of employee's responsibility, increased communication, improvement of personnel policies, management styles, etc., so that employees may be effective in translating their potential energy into kinetic energy and the organisation may be benefited in terms of better image, higher productivity, better utilisation of resources, etc. HRD in a way involves total management and for HRD to be effective, we have to introduce changes in management at all levels.

Although most of the factors are included in HRD, but still we mention only the headings which need attention to improve the working of primary health care functionaries:

1. Raising morale and motivation,
2. Effective communication,
3. Training at frequent intervals,
4. Adequate supply of medicine and equipment,
5. Performance appraisal,
6. Integrity,
7. Commitment to the Ideals of Primary Health Care, and
8. Sensitivity to People's Health needs.

CONCLUSION

Health Policy 1983 suggests that a dynamic process of change and innovation is required to be brought about in the entire approach to health manpower development, ensuring the emergence of fully integrated bands of workers functioning within the "Health Team" approach.

Health policy 2002 reiterates that Historically, it has been the practice to implement major national disease control programmes through the public health machinery of the State/Central Governments. It has become increasingly apparent that certain components of such programmes cannot be efficiently implemented merely through government functionaries. A considerable change in the mode of implementation has come about in the last two decades, with the increasing involvement of NGOs and other institutions of civil society. It is to be recognized that widespread debate on various public health issues has, in fact, been initiated and sustained by NGOs and other members of the civil society. Also, an increasing contribution is being made by such institutions in the delivery of different components of public health services. Certain disease control programmes require close inter-action with the beneficiaries for regular administration of drugs; periodic carrying out of pathological tests; dissemination of information regarding disease control and other general health information. NHP-2002 will address such issues and suggest policy instruments for the implementation of public health programmes through individuals and institutions of civil society.

Notes and References

1. Dev Ray, "Manpower Planning", in *World Health*, April 1979, p. 24.
2. Tamas, Fulop, "Who will care for Health", in *World Health*, April 1977, p. 4.
3. John Bland, "Basic Skills," in *World Health*, July 1976, p. 19.
4. J. Bryant, Health and the Developing World, Ithaca, Cornell University Press, 1969.
5. N. Cunningham (1969): An Evaluation of an auxiliary based on child health service in rural Nigeria", *Journal of the Society of Health of Nigeria*, 3, pp. 21-25.
6. D. Morlay (1963), "A Medical Service for Children under five years of Age in West Africa", Transactions of the Royal Society of Tropical Medicine and Hygiene, 57, p. 79.
7. *The Tribune*, Chandigarh, 26 August, 1979.
8. W.A. Glasser (1966), "Nursing Leadership and Policy: Some Cross-national Comparisons" in the Nursing Profession—Five Sociological Essays, (ed.) Davis, F., New York, John Wiley.
9. Baker D. Timothy (ed.), Paramedical Paradoxes-Challenges and Opportunity in Team Work for *World Health*, 8, London, J. II. A. Churchill, 1971, p. 137.
10. "Resource Allocation, Equality of Access and Health", *International Journal of Health Services*, Vol. 3, No. 3 (Summer 1973), New York, Baywood Publishing Company, Incl., 1973).
11. Tamas Fulop, *op. cit.*, p. 4.
12. Dr. Guillenno Sobcron Acevedo, "Health Manpower out of Balance", in *World Health*, April 1987, p. 16.
13. Oladipo, O. Akindkughe, "A Third World Perspective", in *World Health*, April 1987, p. 24.
14. Zbigniew Bankowski, "A Wasteful Mockery", in *World Health*, April 1987, p. 3.
15. Alastair Anderson, "Adapt-Don't Adopt" in *World Health*, July 1976, p. 6.
16. Antonio Ordonez-Plaja, "Teamwork at Ministry Level", in Team Work for *World Health* (ed.) *op. cit.*, p. 170.
17. Dr. Daniel Flahault, "Vital Team Work", in *World Health*, April 1977, p. 18.

7

CHAPTER

Appropriate Technology and Research for Primary Health Care

In this chapter, we are discussing two interconnected issues, i.e., (a) Appropriate Technology for Health, and (b) Research for Primary Health Care.

A. APPROPRIATE TECHNOLOGY

Technology stimulates science and science acts as a spur to new technology. Social progress depends on both technology and science, but both of these again depends on man's basic desire to live a life that is both physically and intellectually richer and fruitful. A piece of technology may be regarded as appropriate for a community if its design is related to the real needs of that community and its use fulfils these needs. Its use and promotion are based on that community's economic viability and technical competence to support, service, maintain and even improve upon it to suit local conditions. Appropriate technology is thus an approach in which technical innovation and adoption go hand in hand with social and cultural integration.

As stated in a WHO document, appropriate means: besides being scientifically sound, the technology is acceptable to those who apply it as well as those for whom it is used. This implies that the technology should be in keeping with the local culture. It must be capable of being adapted and further developed if necessary. As stated in a WHO document, health technology has been defined as an association of methods, techniques and equipment, together with the people using them. The use of appropriate technology is an important factor that will contribute to the success of health care. The following are some examples of these technologies:

CHART 7.1

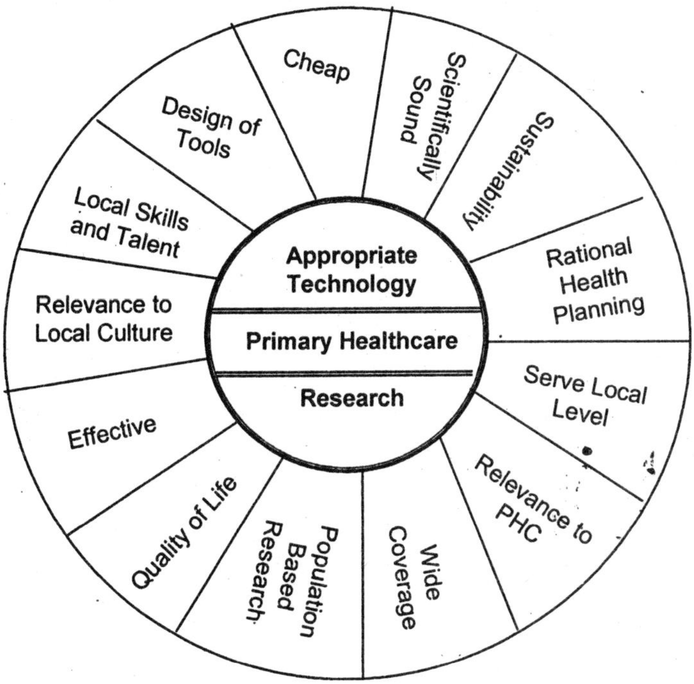

1. Biogas generation for cooking, lighting and refrigeration.
2. Use of plastic mouds for water-sealed latrines.
3. Indigenous cooling system using running water to help maintain the cold chain.
4. Use of bamboo to fortify concrete-based hand-pumps and community maintenance of these hand-pumps.
5. Organisation of community maintenance of hand-pumps.
6. Rain water storage tanks.

It is not defined in terms of the high level of technology used, but by the attention given to the local conditions and environment. Thus, appropriate technology, depends on the local skill, resources and talent. Appropriate technology is the only answer to promote primary health care. These are also reiterated by Alma Ata Declaration.

Ashok Khosla in his article, "Technology and Development" in *IJPA*, July to Sept. 1989, pp. 531-32 rightly defines appropriate Technology as: "Technology which serves the goals of development is defined as appropriate technology. Appropriate technology springs from creative, in response to local needs and possibilities. It is relevant and ready for use by the common people, and aims directly to improve the quality of their lives. It derives maximum leverage from the local cultural environment, by drawing upon the existing managerial and technical skills and providing the basis for extending them. It uses the physical potential of an area and maintains man's harmony with nature."

Claudine Brelet[1] in his article, "Appropriate Technology for Health" in *World Health*, June 1985, defines it as:

> Appropriate Technology for health is a concept that has launched thousands of projects and programmes all over our planet, initiated by governments, non-governmental organisations, small local voluntary groups and private individuals.

Generally abbreviated as A.T.H. or A.T. it has been defined by WHO as "technology that is scientifically sound, adaptable to local needs, and acceptable to those who apply it and those for whom it is used, and that can be-maintained by the people themselves in keeping with the principle of self-reliance with the resources the community and the country can afford." So from the start, the accent has been put on people's participation, and on their appropriation of the appropriate means to provide and use health care.

A.T. does not mean cheap, second-class technology, nor is it a fashionable label that can be used to sell cheap devices to developing countries. Although sometimes scornfully dismissed as "bamboo technology", this is to overlook the fact that, in some places, bamboo can indeed be a better adapted and more appropriate choice of material than, say, corrugated iron. One basic characteristic of A.T. is that it entails the choice of the cost locally available produce, irrespective of whether it stems from the indigenous culture or from the latest high-technology. Indeed, the pioneers of A.T. emphasized the need in today's world for "appropriate science and technology by and for the people."

It has become highly difficult to decide on the use of appropriate technology keeping in view the various factors—need, finances, nature of disease, etc. It has become a fashion to use complex technology for simple health problems thereby increasing costs and non-availability to majority of the people. Hukan Hellberg[2] in his article, "Technology for Health" suggests the basis of decision-making about the use of appropriate technology.

Sidney Nickhe in his article "Money for Health" in *World Health*, May 1989, "rites based on his experience in Kieto district hospital. The costs incurred in running a district hospital are often high because the technology used in providing health services is neither sustainable nor effective. An affordable technology could be helpful to district health managers especially in the areas of support services and energy use."

To cook for the 50 or so patients admitted each month to the Kiteto district hospital requires seven truckloads of firewood, each weighing seven tons. This does not only mean deforestation and destruction of the environment, but is also an expensive and inefficient use of resources.

Cooking is done on an open fire where three stones serve as a stove.

Money could be saved by using an improved energy-saving stove, which also bums firewood. Such stoves are produced at an appropriate technology centre in Arusha (CAMARTEC) and are sold to institutions which use firewood for cooking purposes. The stoves reduce fuel wood consumption by more than 50 percent compared to the three-stone fireplace. Where energy problems prevail, health services are inevitably adversely affected. For example, refrigerators for preserving vaccines use kerosene but practice shows that the unreliability of fuel supplies may result in spoiled vaccines. The use of kerosene for refrigerators, lighting and sterilising purposes is too expensive for most district hospitals. Alternative sources of energy are available but capital investments are forbidding. A biogas plant could be more efficiently and effectively used at a district hospital than wood-burning systems.

Biogas is produced when bacteria break down organic material under airless conditions. It is a simple technology and when carefully used in rural hospitals where human and livestock dung is easily available, it would come cheaper than using kerosene, firewood or charcoal, with their added labour and transportation costs. Although capital costs are relatively higher-about US 1,000 dollars for material, labour and accessories—biogas is cheaper in the long-run. Other technological innovations which could be used to reduce running costs in health care delivery include:

- use of solar energy for refrigeration, lighting and heating;
- water "harvesting" during the rainy season for hospitals and dispensaries in areas where water is scarce; underground storage of water has been found to be relatively cheap;
- use of Ventilated Improved Pit (VIP) latrines in areas where water supply is unreliable and where resources are inadequate for installing and maintaining flush water toilets; and
- avoiding recently introduced brand name drugs and relying instead on cheap generic products.

Dr. Nashara's five year experiences at the district hospital underline the importance of preventive rather than curative measures. He has seen a steady drain of the resources needed to treat patients suffering from preventable diseases.

"If the environment is kept clean, swamps are sprayed and water is treated, the incidence of diarrhoea can be kept low" he says confidently, since experience has shown him that diseases prevalent in the area have a devastating impact on the community and on available resources.

Health care is gaining acceptance as a strategy for bringing basic health services to all the people. Such programmes can have a significant impact on health by focussing on a carefully selected number of health problems that are preventable by means of simple, and relatively low cost, interventions.

Decisions concerning the health technology that is necessary and affordable should be made after evaluating the basic procedures to be carried out in the fields of medicine, surgery, paediatrics, obstetrics and so forth. There is no point in training "Cadillac mechanics" if they are to work on "motor scooters and bicycles." But man is not a machine and technology does not only mean "nuts and bolts." We need improved technologies and abilities to undertake health advocacy, to inform and communicate about health. We have to create social awareness about appropriate technologies, and to stimulate political will for appropriate decisions about the use of resources that will result in relevant technical solutions. But for all of this, we need to build a sound scientific and technological base in order to give credibility to our persuasion.

Eero Lehtinen and Daphne Fresle[3] in their article "Medical diagnostic ultrasound" rightly warn against the use of too much modern technology. To quote them:

> "New technologies in the field of radiology have sprung up like mushrooms after rain in the last decade."

Indeed, within the last ten to fifteen years medical technology has evolved with a sometimes bewildering rapidity, improving and creating new diagnostic tools which complement, or even compete with, each other. The difficult task for the doctor, health administrator and policy-maker is that of informed choice. Even the richest countries cannot possibly provide the total range of available technology, so high is the cost to patient and society. The key surely lies in the cost benefit risk equation in its broadest sense. And until we truly view health care and the medical technologies, not in isolation but as part of a total pattern of social and economic development, you shall be unable to use to real advantage the extraordinary advances in knowledge which make the present age so challenging and stimulating.

Professor H. Abrams, one of the most prominent radiologists in the United State, concluded his presentation at a symposium on the impact of the new imaging technologies on health care by stating:

> "In summary, we simply cannot afford the new technologies. They will cost a great deal and be overused. They will take resource from the poor and have little impact on the health of the sickest segment of the population. A paradox thus unfolds. On the one hand, a nation with high unemployment may well have better things to spend its resources on the computer topography scanning, nuclear magnetic resonance and digital radiography. On the other hand, the individuals who constitute the nation and are subject to illness want nothing less than the best and the newest, if there is the faintest possibility that it may affect their health."

Let us explain with an example. WHO has developed a kit for Dais for ensuring safe delivery. There is no more crucial passage in life than birth. Yet 60 per cent of the world's women do not have access to pregnancy care and safe delivery care, which would dramatically reduce the risk of maternal and newborn mortality. Making available this appropriate technology would be a decisive, step towards Health for All.

The basic kit is simple, inexpensive and can be made from locally available materials. It supports three essential factors that will dramatically reduce the risk of infection in mother and child; a clean delivery surface, clean hand (soap and a nail stick), clean cutting of the umbilical cord (a razor blade and cotton for tying-off the cord).

A tape measure enables the health worker to monitor the growth of the uterus regularly, in order to detect conditions that require special care. Newborn babies and infants can lose as much as 25 per cent of their body heat unless they are well wrapped up; a simple cap made from several layers of cloth can conserve a large part of their body heat and thus make them less vulnerable to diseases. This is another example of appropriate technology for birth.

There has been a great revolution in technology in medical sciences. Complicated machines to be handled by experts are available 21st century is going to be more explosive as far as the innovations in new technology are concerned. However, there is a need to simplify this highly complicated technology, which only a few can afford. We must develop simple technology, which people can afford and sustain, e.g. Oral Dehydration therapy.

Denise Ayres[4] rightly says, "Few health technologies have as great a potential as oral dehydration therapy (ORT) to make an impact on childhood mortality in developing countries. Simple, inexpensive and effective, ORT can be used not only throughout the health system but at home as well."

Robert J. Gerety[5] in his article, "A New Use for Yeast" said, Plasma-derived vaccines against hepatitis B cannot satisfy the needs of less affluent areas of the world where the disease is endemic. But vaccines produced in yeast by recombinant DNA technology seem likely to fulfil all the needs on a global scale.

Kirsten Staehr Johansen[6] in his article, "International Insulin Pump Study" rightly said, "One of the best examples of medical technology intended for home care of the patient is the miniature insulin pump. No larger than a pack of playing cards, it is usually secured by a belt to the chest or thigh of a diabetes sufferer. An imparted "shunt" (valve) releases insulin into the patient's vein in quantities that he or she can regulate according to need. Insulin is essential for diabetes victims to maintain their blood-sugar level, and without it they risk falling into a coma. The pump can be recharged manually from an external source, or by inserting a cartridge containing fresh insulin."

According to Jan Stjernsward and Peter Ozorio[7] there is the knowledge to prevent cancer pain, derived from several decades of clinical experience and research, and there are simple and inexpensive methods to ease pain. There are, as well, drugs to provide relief for patients, and to allow the incurably ill to die with dignity.

Yet despite the best intentions, what is known is not applied, and even though pain relief is the only human therapeutic alternative, it is not offered adequately to millions. There is a need of global commitment.[8]

Appropriate technology in health is going to be the greatest challenge of new millennium because of the following reasons:

1. Technology is becoming highly sophisticated with the passing of time.
2. It is highly costly to afford by developing countries on a large scale.
3. Manpower to make use of new technology is not available as it costs in their retention and training.
4. There are many inherent dangers in the new technology to have negative effects on health of the people.
5. Very less attention is being paid to develop appropriate technology to suit the needs of millions of people suffering from abject poverty and illness.
6. Complicated machines go out of order and we need highly trained specialists to maintain them.

Therefore, in the new millennium, we should focus attention on providing appropriate technology to suit majority of the population.

Health policy 1983 suggests that the frontiers of the medical sciences are expanding at a phenomenal pace. To maintain the country's lead in this field as well as to ensure self-sufficiency and generation of the requisite competence in the future, it is necessary to have an organised programme for the building up and extension of fundamental and basic research in the field of bio-medical and allied sciences. Priority attention would require to be devoted to the resolution of problems relating to the containment and eradication of the existing, widely prevalent diseases as well as to deal with emerging health problems. The basic objective of medical research and the ultimate test of its utility would involve the translation of available know-how into simple, low-cost, easily applicable appropriate technologies, devices and interventions suiting local conditions, thus placing the latest technological achievements, within the reach of health personnel, and to the front line health workers, in the remotest corners of the country. Therefore, besides devotion to basic, fundamental research, high priority should be accorded to applied, operational research including action research for continuously improving the cost effective delivery of health services. Priorities would require to be identified and laid down in collaboration with social scientists, planners and decision-makers and the public. Basic research efforts should devote high priority to the discovery and development of more effective treatment and preventive procedures in regard to communicable and tropical diseases—Blindness, Leprosy, TB, etc. Very high priority would also have to be devoted to contraception research to urgently improve the effectiveness and acceptability of existing methods as well as to discover more effective and acceptable devices. Equally high attention would require to be devoted to nutrition research, to improve the health status of the community. The overall effort should aim at the balanced development of basic, clinical and problem-oriented operational research.

Health Policy 2002 recommend that over the years, health research activity in the country has been very limited. In the Government sector, such research has been confined to the research institutions under the Indian Council of Medical Research, and other institutions funded by the States/ Central Government. Research in the private sector has assumed some significance only in the last decade. In our country, where the aggregate annual health expenditure is of the order of Rs. 80,000 crores, the expenditure in 1998-99 on research, both public and private sectors, was only of the order of Rs. 1150 crores. It would be reasonable to infer that with such low research expenditure, it is virtually impossible to make any dramatic break-through within the country, by way of new molecules and vaccines; also, without a minimal back-up of applied and operational research, it would be difficult to assess whether the health expenditure in the country is being incurred through optimal applications and appropriate public health strategies. Medical Research in the country needs to be focused on therapeutic drugs/vaccines for tropical diseases, which are normally neglected by international pharmaceutical companies on account of their limited profitability potential. The thrust will need to be in the newly-emerging frontier areas of research based on genetics, genome-based drug and vaccine development, molecular biology, etc. NHP-2002 will address these inadequacies and spell out a minimal quantum of expenditure for the coming decade, looking to the national needs and the capacity of the research institutions to absorb the funds.

B. APPROPRIATE RESEARCH FOR PRIMARY HEALTH CARE

W.A. Hassouna[9] in his article, "Solving People's Problems" has rightly said that, "Health services research is a relatively new field of scientific endeavour which achieved recognition in the 1960s. It seeks to identify ways and means of taking medical knowledge, expertise and technology out of laboratories, academic institutions and pilot projects, and applying it in order to solve the health problems of the people. It is an interdisciplinary approach which is mainly concerned with action involving all the factors that affect health status through the use of health resources. It assists decision-makers at various levels in making accurate assessments of the health services delivery system and in identifying and testing the changes that can be made so as to lead towards more effective and efficient methods of meeting people's real health needs."

George C. Salmond[10] discusses the need, meaning and scope of research for Primary Health Care. To many people the word "research" conjures up visions of laboratories, mathematical formulas and scientists in white coats. The work is thought to be complex, difficult to understand, and of little interest or concern to ordinary people. Health services research is not like this at all. It is best characterised by relatively simple studies of practical health problems, carried out in the community with the wide involvement, not only of those who organize and provide care, but also of those who use it.

Health services research can be defined as the systematic study of the means by which basic medical and other relevant health knowledge is brought to bear on the health of individuals and communities under a given set of conditions. Its aims is to provide new information and insights which will:

- permit a better understanding of health problems and the role and influence of health services;
- assist in more rational health planning;
- result in more effective and efficient health care, which at the same time is better attuned to the cultural and emotional needs of people; and
- by actively involving people in the study of their own problems, will encourage greater personal, family and community self-reliance in health matters.

Research has a particular contribution to make towards the development of strategies for primary health care. If systems are to be designed providing the essential care that people need, wide coverage and the people's full participation, all at a cost the community and country can afford, then research is needed to explore the possibilities, and to cost and test the various options. It is important for research efforts to focus on all points of the spectrum of services provided, and therefore, the effectiveness and efficiency of the whole referral system up to the big and specialised hospitals must also be considered.

The scope of the research is very wide, and may involve scientists and health workers from many disciplines. Research projects may range in size from major multinational collaborative studies to small studies involving one or to workers in a village or urban neighbourhood. But, regardless of the size and type of operation, the success of health services research must be measured not by the mere production of results but by whether those results are used to good effect to promote health and improve health services.

Incorporating community interests in health services research has brought benefits to both the researchers and the community. From the researchers' view-point, the priority health problems were identified and studied, and the results used to promote health and improve health services. Some compromises did have to be made. The research design was changed on a number of occasions to meet the requirements of the steering committee. The researchers' grew in their understanding of the ways of communities, and in their sensitivity to people's need for well definition. Without these insights such research must be limited in its success.

Huge sums of money are poured out annually on clinical hospital-based research in most States of India. One would not under-estimate the importance of this type of research because it adds to knowledge. However, one has to think in terms of defining the priorities of research. A State where the bulk of people are living in the rural areas, should normally involve the greater number of doctors doing researches in community health. India is one country which cannot boast of even a single good epidemiological study of such communicable diseases as tuberculosis, from which a sizable number of people suffer every year. In fact, the area of community health research does not encourage clinicians to work in the rural areas. The problems of community health, no doubt, are vast and intriguing. Yet, the state cannot afford to ignore them. India lives primarily in the villages and it is the villagers who are the recipients of probably the poorest quality of medical care. The future of the state also depends on the progress made in the villages, particularly in the area of health. One has to watch and see how different States plan and administer their health programmes so that their rural beneficiaries are not outnumbered by their urban beneficiaries. Thus, the present trend of our spending on curative medicine research has to change in favour of community health research particularly in the rural areas. This is a challenge which no State of India can afford to ignore.

B.O. Osuntokun[11] has rightly said, "We already know that health services research can produce impressive innovatory advances in health care services and a significant improvement in the health care of populations. The infectious disease yaws was eliminated from the forest belt of West African countries not by doctors but by "yaws scouts"—young illiterate men trained over periods of three to six weeks to recognize the early lesions, and armed and empowered to use the syringe, needle and penicillin-based drug. In Bangladesh, young women trained in a few weeks to carry out tubal ligation on women who chose this as a means of contraception achieved results as good or even better than those recorded by doctors. A glorious achievement of WHO's immunization programme is the worldwide eradication of smallpox, inspite of the various constraints including man-made ones such as wars."

Finally, epidemiological and health services research imply the establishment of a template of primary health care which is unchallengeably the ideal *modus operandi* by which WHO's goal of an acceptable level of health for all can be achieved. Developing countries must however bear in mind in supporting medical research that—as Daniel Coit Gilman, first President of the Johns Hopkins University, in Maryland, USA, expressed it, "Those ventures are not always most sagacious that expect a return on the morrow. It sometimes pays. ....to make investments with an eye to slow but sure returns."

Sir Gustav Nossal[12] in his article, "Global and regional strategy has rightly said, "The great strength of these expanding national efforts has been the fact that local experts, knowledgeable in the cultural traditions and practical constraints pertaining to particular regions, are addressing and solving local problems. This brings solutions adapted to the situation and applicable in the given socio-economic framework."

The weaknesses will differ from country to country, but four constraints are sufficiently widespread, and sufficiently soluble in principle, to warrant drawing to the attention of decision-makers.

Career structures for full-time medical research are non-existent or inadequate in many countries. In some countries where adequate number of posts do exist, the remuneration is so far below that available in private medical practice as to represent a serious disincentive.

- Specialized consumable supplies, such as enzymes, chemicals and biologicals, which require foreign currency and importation, are difficult to obtain on a regular basis, while maintenance of equipment represents a great problem.
- Training programmes available for younger scientists are poorly adapted to their needs, and to their future tasks. On many occasions, the researcher receives his training in a highly sophisticated overseas institution specializing in a complex line of fundamental experimentation. He soon becomes dependent on a vast infrastructure, and skilled in that ultra-specialized field. Returning home, he finds the simpler working conditions and the more applied nature of the problems frustrating.
- Communication links between scientists in developing countries and their counterparts in the developed nations are still far less evolved than they should be. Medical research is quite essentially international in character, depending on a network of communication and scholarship, each component part complementing every other one like the pieces of a huge and ever-growing jigsaw puzzle. Frequently the scientific literature cannot keep up with the pace of progress, and the chief operational tool guiding research consists of informal communication between members of a peer group (constituting an "invisible college"), or a small, specialized conference or symposium with participation by invitation only. It is vital that academics in the Third World be embraced in this network.

W.A. Hassouna,[13] has pointed out that, "It is my conviction that health services research should form the core of the WHO strategy to develop primary health care as a means of achieving Health for all by the year 2000, What will be essential will be to develop a clear understanding of the practical aspects of primary health care, and to support research activities that demonstrate the cost-effectiveness of this approach as an essential and integral part of a pyramidal health services system. It will be necessary to support the development of national capabilities in health services research, and to concentrate on small-scale activities at country level. An information education communications programme will have to be developed." Some areas for research are mentioned below:[14]

(a) Health manpower—their training, development, utilisation, availability, needs and demands, etc., including experimentation with the development of various categories of health manpower.
(b) Primary Health Care—their availability, utilisation, needs and demands.
(c) Organisational and management process in health and family welfare services, their linkages, etc., including referral systems.
(d) Perception, attitude, utilisation factors (promoters and barriers) effecting utilisation, etc. of population towards health and family welfare services.
(e) Problems and bottlenecks in the existing organisational systems and redesigning of existing systems to eliminate the same.
(f) Cost-benefit and cost-effectiveness analysis of health and family welfare services, programmes and projects.
(g) Development and testing of technology suited to the Indian health scene and needs.
(h) Studies focused on the interphase between community and health services organisations.
(i) Studies on health status and social and economic development.
(j) Enlisting of community participation.
(k) Identification of goals and priorities of the health services.

In the past, there has been little progress in the areas of research in vital areas affecting the health of the people. There has been research in high technology and sophisticated fields benefitting few people. In the new millennium, health research should become an indispensable part of other socio-economic research being carried out in universities and research institutes. In a WHO document, it has been realised that the universities can play a great role in conducting community researches.

Today, the universities must have a wider vision. Its three functions of teaching. research and service have to be reviewed in the light of a world blemished with gross inequalities and glamours with need. The winds of change must blow away the cobwebs of learning for its own sake (and of course Oxford itself is changing).

In the particular field of health; teaching is vital; but it must be directed towards all categories of health workers, including those in primary health care, not merely towards the medical specialist. And then research too is vital; but it should seek to resolve real problems, rather than being "pure research." And the service function of a university should surely rate top priority; in any country, whether developing or developed, there are serious gaps in the public health services which can only be filled through the efforts of well-motivated people who are keen to apply their talents and their hard-earned skills to serving the community.

Problem-based learning is seen as a powerful educational strategy to maximise students' achievement of relevant knowledge, skills and attitudes. Specific considerations include the following:

The systematic selection of problem and population-based concepts which represent health needs of the community. This will require a balanced understanding of:

- Scientific technological advances and social systems;
- The definition of relevant skills, including skills in problem-solving, independent learning, critical appraisal of evidence and teamwork;
- The strengthening of teaching staff capacities related to community-orientation and problem-based learning;
- The development of curriculum design methods and learning tools appropriate to a community-oriented and problem-based educational system;
- A system of selecting health professional students, if feasible;
- The design of procedures and tools for assessing student and graduate performance; and
- The evaluation of innovative programmes including their contribution to the development of effective, efficient and human health care, and the commitment to Health for All.

The Network attempts to establish health research programmes that include basic, applied and operational research that is relevant to health and health care problems of the community to be served. In the new millennium, we have to explore researches in health which can raise the quality of life of the people living in rural areas, urban slums and tribal areas.

CONCLUSION

Appropriate technology is one of the core components of primary health care. Appropriate technology includes practical, scientifically sound, health measures, for promotive, diagnostic, therapeutic or rehabilitative purposes, that are accessible and affordable to the community. Through this approach, technology is made to serve society's needs. Machinery or equipment, if involved, is simple to run and repair, and locally produced and maintained. It is used to develop self-reliance and self-determination. Examples of appropriate technology for health are:

(a) Home-based oral rehydration solutions (ORS) have proven efficacy to combat dehydration.
(b) Use of herbal and home remedies for treatment of minor ailments.
(c) Use of neem sticks for burshing teeth, massage of gums and gargling after every meal for promoting good oral health.
(d) Use of Jaipur foot as an aid for orthopaedically disabled persons.
(e) Intraocular lens at low cost and indigenously produced.
(f) Use of hay-boxes as incubators for newborns.
(g) Use of sputum microscopy for diagnosis of pulmonary tuberculosis, over chest X-ray, as was accepted by the National Tuberculosis Programme.
(h) Simple kits for Traditional Birth Attendants (dais) with a sterilized blade, clean tie, swab, soap and polythene sheet.
(i) 'Nutrition' bangles for detection of malnutrition in children.
(j) Dip sticks for urine testing of sugar and albumin in the field.
(k) Low cost, effective health education kits with messages painted on cloth and use of puppets.
(l) Bicycle driven ambulance.
(m) Low cost lightweight rehabilitation aids.[15]

Notes and References

1. Claudine Brelec, "Appropriate Technology for Health", in *World Health*, June 1985, p. 21.
2. Hakan Hellberg, "Technology for Health", in *World Health*, June 1985, p. 3.
3. Ero Lehtinen and Daphne Fresle, "Medical Diagnostic Ultrasound", in *World Health*, June 1985, p. 18.
4. Denise Ayres, "Oral Rehydration Therapy" in *World Health*, June 1985, p. 9.
5. Rober J. Gerety, "A New Use for Yeast", in *World Health*, June 1985, p. 12.
6. Kirsten Staehr Johansen. "International Insulin Pump Study", in *World Health*, June 1985, p. 15.
7. Jan Stjernsward and Peter Ozorio, "Why Not Freedom from Cancer Pain", in *World Health*, June 1985, p. 23.
8. Bui Duc Khanh, "Health Insurance in Vietnam", in *World Health*, Nov.-Dec., 1994, p. 21.
9. W.A. Hassouna, "Solving People's Problems", in *World Health*, April 1980, p. 27.
10. George C. Salmond, "New Problems New Strategies", in *World Health*, January 1980, p. 15.
11. B.O. Osuntokun, "Third World Needs", in *World Health*, April 1980, p. 9.
12. Sir Gustav Nossal, "Global and Regional Strategy" in *World Health*, April 1980, p. 20.
13. W.A. Hassouna, "Solving People's Problems", in *World Health*. April 1980, p. 27.
14. S.L. Goel, Public Health Administration, New Delhi, Sterling, 1984, p. 312.
15. Karnataka towards Equity, Quality and Integrity in Health, Final Report, Government of Karnataka, April 2001, pp. 19-20.

8
CHAPTER

Trained Birth Attendants (TBAs)

"Trained Birth Attendants promote safe reproductive and child health services and support MPW (F) and HS (F) in implementing National Health Programmes."

A. IMPORTANCE OF TBA IN REPRODUCTIVE AND CHILD HEALTH

Care of mothers and children—the most vulnerable sections of our society—occupies a paramount place in our health services delivery system. This is reflected from the fact that 9 out of the 17 goals listed in the National Health Policy (1983) related to Maternal and Child Health. Trained Birth Attendants can play a vital role in the promotion of health of mothers and children.

Prevailing ill-heath among women is a major concern. These are being addressed through several programmes, such as nutrition, RH, MCH and RCH. Accordingly, investment in women's health has been one of the actions identified in the Declaration for Health Development in the South-East Asia Region in the 21st Century. It has been recognized in the Declaration that since women's health is integral to development, a multi-sectoral approach would be needed through the development of partnerships with other relevant sectors.

Too many women still die needlessly due to complications during pregnancy and childbirth and too little attention is given to other aspects of women's health. Data clearly shows the link between low maternal mortality and a high proportion of deliveries by trained personnel, well established primary health care infrastructure and good referral system.

Findings from research in the early 1980s and the International Safe Motherhood Conference in 1987 drew the attention of the world community to maternal mortality. During this decade, countries adopted various tools for safe motherhood, including the district team problem-solving approach,

CHART 8.1

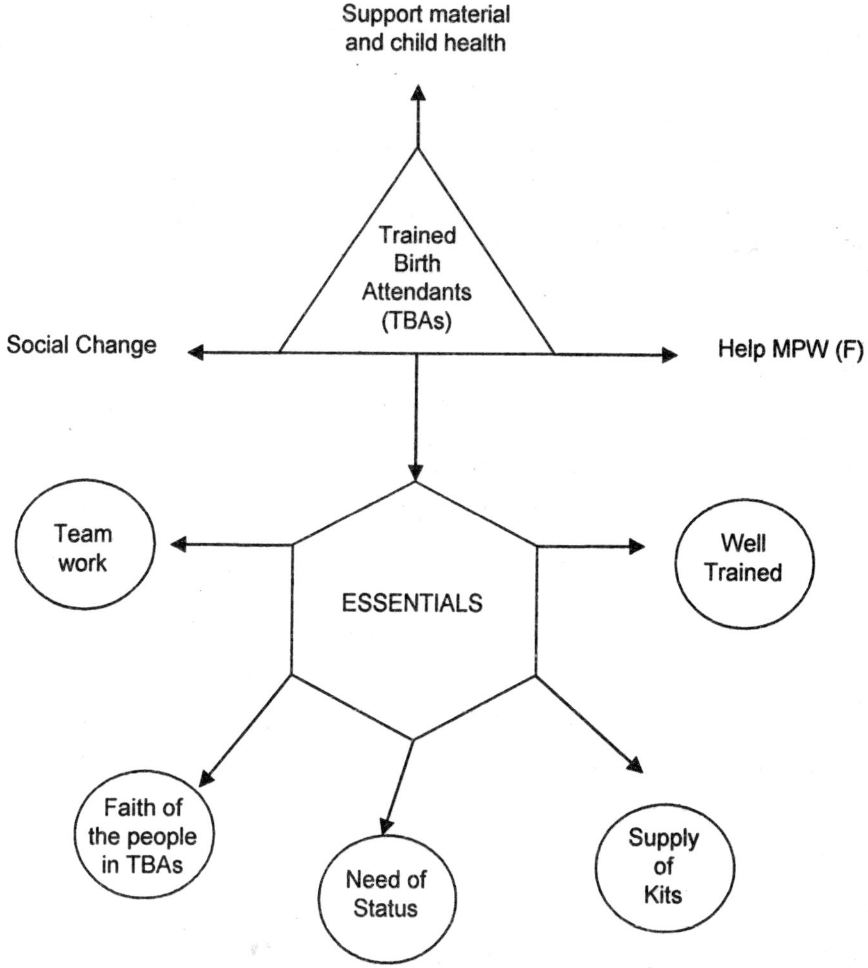

the partograph, safe delivery kits, and the Mother-baby Package—a strategic tool for planning safe motherhood programs.

Yet many problems remain. Most are due to socio-economic and cultural factors, and the failure of the health system to provide good quality services. The training and deployment of large number of auxiliary health workers and volunteers in the community contributed to significant reductions in infant mortality, but did not substantially reduce maternal deaths. During the past decade, midwives who were trained to provide care to pregnant women and to assist in deliveries were used as multipurpose health workers in some countries. The focus on their midwifery role was thus diluted, and maternity care was neglected. Efforts should be made to ensure that all deliveries are attended by Trained Birth Attendance, so that high rates of maternal mortality can be reduced.

Dai Training Programme

Maternal and Pre-natal mortality rates in the country are high due to lack of even the basic maternal and newborn care, to more than half the women at the time of labour. The SRS data for 1993 indicates that proportion of deliveries attended by untrained hands is still very high in the country. Currently, about one out of two women do not have access to trained personnel and deliver under conditions of high risk both for women and the newborn. Training of dais is a part of the overall effort to improve basic maternal and newborn care to ensure clean delivery practices, and to increase early referrals of high risk/complicated cases.

The National Health Policy (1983) envisaged that 100% deliveries will be conducted by trained personnel by the year 2000 A.D. This would mean training/retraining of at least one Dai for each of six lakh villages in the country.[1]

The need for bringing down maternal mortality rate significantly and improving maternal health in general has been strongly stressed in the National Population Policy, 2000. This policy recommends a holistic strategy for bringing about total intersectoral coordination at the grass root level and involving the NGOs, Civil Societies, Panchayati Raj Institutions and Women's Group in bringing down Maternal Mortality Ratio and Infant Mortality Rate.

In the last decades, the life expectancy of the population in India has shown remarkable improvement from 41 at birth in 1961 to 65 years at present. Yet, over a 100,000 women in India continue to die of pregnancy-related causes every year. The Maternal Mortality Ratio in India is 407 per 100,000 live births (SRS, RGI 1998). However, reliable estimates of maternal mortality are not available.

Maternal Mortality Ratio (MMR)

MMR is defined as the number of maternal deaths per 100,000 live births due to causes related to pregnancy or within 42 days of termination of pregnancy, regardless of the site or duration of pregnancy.

MMR India: The national average of MMR is 407 per 100,000 live births, which in itself is very high compared to the international scenario like Sweden (8), UK (10), Greece (2) and even in neighbouring countries like Sri Lanka (60), China (60) and Thailand (54). Within the country, the States above this average are:

- UP (707)
- Rajasthan (670)
- MP (498)
- Bihar (451)
- Assam (409)

Under the CSSM Programme, training of Dais is being undertaken in all the states. The training with emphasis on 'hands on' skill development for the Dais is imparted for 6 days in identified health facilities which have enough case loads.

During 1994-95 and 1995-96, and 1996-97 3,126,021,755 and 1,58,459 Dais have reportedly been trained. After completion of training each Dai is provided with a Dai kit (Centrally procured) to help her in conduct of safe and clean delivery.

Prevailing ill-health among women is a major concern. These are being addressed through several programmes, such as nutrition, RH, MCH and RCH. Accordingly, investment in women's health has been one of the actions identified in the Declaration for Health Development in the South-East Asia Region in the 21st Century. It has been recognized in the Declaration that since women's health is integral to development, a multi-sectoral approach would be needed through the development of partnerships with other relevant sectors.[2]

Too many women still die needlessly due to complications during pregnancy and child-birth and too little attention is given to other aspects of women's health. Data clearly shows the link between low maternal mortality and a high proportion of deliveries by trained personnel, well established primary health care infrastructure and good referral systems.

Findings from research in the early 1980s and the International Safe Motherhood Conference in 1987 drew the attention of the world community to maternal mortality. During this decade countries adopted various tools for safe motherhood, including the district team problem-solving approach, the partograph, safe delivery kits, and the Mother-Baby Package—a strategic tool for planning safe motherhood programmes.

Yet many problems remain. Most are due to socio-economic and cultural factors, and the failure of the health system to provide good quality services. The training and deployment of large numbers of auxiliary health workers and volunteers in the community contributed to significant reductions in infant mortality but did not substantially reduce maternal deaths. During the past decade, midwives who were trained to provide care to pregnant women and to assist in deliveries were used as multipurpose health workers in some countries. The focus on their mid-wifery role was thus diluted, and maternity care was neglected. Efforts should be made to ensure that all deliveries are attended by Trained Birth Attendants so that high rates of maternal mortality can be reduced.[3]

Besides social cost of maternal deaths is very high. The impact of maternal mortality on the individual, the family and society at large is like a pebble dropped into a pond, where the ripples of action and reaction reach out to all. Maternal mortality is therefore now recognized as a symptom of neglect and failure, the society's neglect of women's and girl's health, and failure of the health care system to meet their health needs. This situation has to change. A high level of political commitments, strengthening of the health infrastructure, and generation of societal, community and family support to pregnant women will improve the situation.[4]

A maternal death is defined as the death of a woman while pregnant or within 42 days of the termination of pregnancy, irrespective of the duration and site of the pregnancy, from any cause related to or aggravated by the pregnancy or its management but not from accidental or incidental causes.

Reducing maternal mortality is one of the most cost effective strategies in public health, bringing benefits to women, infants and communities as a whole. The goal of the WHO Safe Motherhood Initiative is to reduce maternal mortality to half of the 1990 levels by the year 2000.

When a mother dies, the effects on the family are often devastating. In Bangladesh, a study of children under 10 years of age has shown that over a period of two years following the death of a mother, mortality rates in her children were twice as high for boys and three times as high for girls, as compared to children with living mothers.[5]

The South-East Asia Region in fact accounts for about 40% of the world's maternal deaths. Maternal mortality ratios range from 40 to 539 per 1,00,000 live births, largely reflecting the varying social status of women and their access to essential obstetric care.

Where maternal mortality data are not segregated by socio-economic group and other relevant factors, national statistics can be misleading. For example, there are considerable variations between urban and rural areas. In India in 1995, an indirect estimate for the national maternal mortality ratio was 580, with 638 maternal deaths per 1,00,000 live births estimated for rural areas and 389 for urban areas. Different parts of the country also had different rates—the maternal mortality ratio was reported to be as low as 247 in the southern state of Kerala and as high as 1068 in the eastern state of Assam. In addition, maternal deaths are often under reported, especially those occurring outside of health facilities, in early gestation, in remote areas, and in those who die due to indirect obstetric causes.[6]

Most maternal deaths are preventable. The medical interventions necessary to prevent them are trained assistance at delivery, a well established primary health care infrastructure with a good referral system, and referral facilities (e.g. at district level) for managing complications. In most of the backward Districts of India with high maternal mortality, most women do not receive the services of a skilled attendant (mid-wife, nurse or doctor) at the time of delivery.

For example, the report of a three year study covering a population of 686,000 in a rural area of India showed that "delay in seeking care and too many and inappropriate referrals through lower levels of the health system not capable of dealing with the problem significantly increased the risk of dying. Similarly, residence in the village proper (which has better transport facilities) as compared to the hamlets had a protective effect. A trained attendant at delivery, presence of an ANM (Auxiliary Nurse Midwife) in the village, an educated husband (the usual decision-maker) and the social custom of migrating to the natal home for delivery, all had a protective effect. "

B. NEED AND ACTIVITIES OF TBA[7]

India can not afford highly sophisticated maternal and Child Health Services. The Birth Attendants, if adequately trained and supported can really help in mitigating high maternal and infant mortality rate.

The Dai is an important person in her village. She serves as a link between the families in her village and the ANM. These are some of the things she can do to improve maternal and child health in her village.

1. She should contact every pregnant woman in her area and see that she is registered at the sub-centre or primary health centre.
2. She should attend the weekly pre-natal clinic and assist ANM.
3. She should try to ensure that every pregnant woman in her area attends the pre-natal clinic at least three times, i.e., after the third month to confirm pregnancy, during the seventh month and during the ninth month.
4. She should try to ensure that every pregnant woman is immunized against tetanus (two doses—the last dose at least one month before the delivery and the first dose one month before the last).
5. She should try to ensure that every pregnant woman takes iron and folic acid tablets as prescribed.
6. If any abnormal pregnancy is detected she should show the case immediately to the ANM or LHV or refer the case to the PHC.
7. She should ensure that preparations for delivery are made either at home or at the PHC or hospital.
8. If she finds any abnormality during labour she must seek medical aid without delay.
9. When she receives a call for delivery:
   - She should take her kit with her.
   - She should watch the progress of labour carefully.
   - She should allow labour to progress normally without any unnecessary interference.
   - She should observe aseptic techniques while conducting the delivery.
10. She should see that her kit is always replenished, clean and ready for use during a delivery.
11. She should make the mother and baby comfortable and attend to the nutrition of both.
12. She should instruct the mother and the relatives as to when she should be called immediately, e.g., in case the mother has excessive bleeding or there is bleeding from the baby's cord.
13. In the post-natal period if she finds any complications in the mother, e.g., fever or foullochina, or in the baby, e.g., cord infection or jaundice, she should immediately inform the ANM or refer the mother or baby to the PHC.

14. She should try to ensure that all infants in her area are immunized with BCG, OPT and poliomyelitics vaccine.
15. She should motivate the eligible couples in her area to use a contraceptive method or to undergo sterilization.
16. She should distribute nirodh, foam tablets, and jelly to those couples who require these contraceptives.
17. She should report all births and deaths in her area to the health worker (male) or health worker (female)/ANM.

National Health Policy has also stressed the role of TBAs. A vicious relationship exists between high birth rates and high infant mortality, contributing to the desire for more children. The highest priority would, therefore, require to be devoted to efforts at launching special programmes for the improvement of maternal and child health, with a special focus on the less-privileged sections of society. Such programmes would require to be decentralised to the maximum possible extent, their delivery being at the primary level, nearest to the doorsteps of the beneficiaries. While efforts should continue at providing refresher training and orientation to the TBAs, schemes and programmes should be launched to ensure that progressively all deliveries are conducted by competently trained persons so that complicated cases receive timely and expert attention, within a comprehensive programme providing ante-natal, intra-natal and post-natal cares.[8] Care of mothers and children—the most vulnerable sections of our society—occupies a paramount place in our health services delivery system.[9]

C. FACTS AND SUGGESTIONS

1. Low Status of Trained Birth Attendants

Trained Birth Attendants are doing a good work but their status is very low. They are paid very less and treated like domestic servants. It is high time that the health department should treat them well and support them in their endeavour of safe delivery.

2. Illiterate and Poor Background

At present, most of the women engaged are both illiterate and belong to poor backgrounds. The health department should encourage young educated girls to take up this profession and fix good honorarium for them for delivery of safe babies as well as involve them in other national health programmes.

3. Inadequate Training

Training arrangements are not adequate. They are not trained properly. They attend the programme simply to get an honorarium. The training may be extended to at least 6 months.

4. Trainees lack Interest

Most of the trainees lack interest and thus do not take interest in training. It is a simple formality that the PHC staff want to complete.

5. No Support from Above

The health functionaries presently provide a casual supervision, support and guidance to the TTBAs. All levels of health system should ensure adequate supervision, support and guidance so that the TTBAs could help the Health Department in achieving the objectives of HFA by 2000 AD.

6. No Arrangements for Refresher Training

Keeping in view inadequate basic training, the importance of regular and repeated retraining cannot be overemphasized. A mechanism should be evolved, whereby, the TBAs receive at least one to two exposures per annum and the retraining should be arranged/organized as near to the residence of TBA as possible. During the retraining the TBA should be adequately compensated by way of per diem, etc.

7. No Interest shown by Voluntary Organisations

Voluntary organisations such as Mahila Mandals, Youth Clubs, FP Clubs, etc. should play enlarged role in propagating the importance of Dai training programme and utilization of the services of the TBAs. They should also cooperate in all the activities organized by the TTBAs.

8. Dai Kit not Replenished

Dai kit is not supplied in time and not replenished in time: Dai kit is very useful but this is not provided during the training causing difficulties in learning. It is not replenished in time. There is a need to develop a fool proof mechanism to ensure the availability of the kit with the Dai.

9. Old Manuals out of date

Manuals need updating: All Dais find the usefulness of the manual. However, all of them do not get it during the training period.

It must be made available to them before training so that it can serve as a reference material. The manual also needs thorough rewriting and revision to accommodate latest developments.[10]

D. CONCLUSION

Despite extensive development of health infrastructure in the rural areas, maternal health is still, by and large, being looked after by the TBAs (both trained and untrained).

We can increase their performance through a well designed training programme which can be a real weapon to improve the existing status of maternal and child health services.

Traditional mid-wives were once thought of as poor relatives in the family of health workers, but now, with training, they are slowly but surely winning favour with health administrations in developing countries, and WHO is advocating their use as one way of meeting basic health needs.

With good reason too, for traditional birth attendants—TBAs as they have come to be known—deliver from 60 to 80 per cent of all babies in the Third World. They also care for mothers before and after birth, and, if need be, help with household chores as well.

Not only are they being counted upon to perform traditional tasks, but also to take on new duties. In some countries they are charged with dispensing oral contraceptives, and with bringing mothers who wish to regulate births to clinics for counselling. In others, they promote breast-feeding.

Today TBAs are appreciated as never before, and people who formerly were sceptical of their worth now accept them as valued members of the health team, according to a report on ten-year trends carried in a recent issue of WHO's Chronicle.

The acceptance is reflected in the number of countries formally recognising the skills of traditional birth attendants through schemes of registration, certification, or licensure. It is also seen in the increase of training programmes run by health administrations for mid-wives.

To encourage training, many countries offer mid-wives incentives. Some pay stipends, and a few provide uniforms. UNICEF gives them a mid-wifery kit, which is prized most.

Above all, the most telling indication of the newly-won respect of TBAs is seen in the change of attitude towards them. In 1972, the majority of 37 administrations replying to a questionnaire thought of them as replaceable, and their services as an unavoidable interim measure.

Today that view is held by a minority, with 56 of 64 countries surveyed considering them as irreplaceable in the decades ahead. "While expanding professional training, countries are also expanding the training of traditional birth attendants," according to a report recently published that describes experiences in seven countries.

All of which makes good sense, for approximately half a million women dies every year, not of disease, but of the complications of child-bearing. And over 10 million children a year die before reaching their first birthday.

TBAs will continue to deliver most of the world's babies, whether they are trained or not. Training however is relatively inexpensive, costing, for instance, US $ 92 in Nicaragua, and $ 17 in Samoa, including the price of the mid-wifery kits.

It is thus a sound investment, for TBAs, by virtue of the service they render to communities, hold a high place in village societies, and thus can influence others. But even more important is their willingness to work with their people living in rural areas.

We can increase their performance through a well designed training programme which can be a real weapon to improve the existing status of maternal and child health services.[11]

Notes and References

1. GOI, Ministry of Health and Family Welfare, Annual Report, 1996-97, New Delhi, p. 25.
2. WHO: SEARO, Highlights of the works of WHO in the South-East Asia Region, New Delhi, 1998, p. 37.
3. WHO: SEARO, Regional Health Report, 1997, New Delhi, 1997, pp. 27-28.
4. *Ibid.*
5. WHO: SEARO, Regional Health Report, 1998, New Delhi, pp. 1-2.
6. *Ibid.*, p. 12.
7. National Institute of Health and Family Welfare, Management Training Modules for Dai (TBA), New Delhi, Year Not Mentioned.
8. Annual Report, 1996-97, Ministry of Health and Family Welfare, Government of India, New Delhi, 1997, pp. 29-30.
9. *Ibid.*, p. 30.
10. *Ibid.*, p. 8.
11. *World Health*, December, 1982, p. 30.

9

CHAPTER

Community Health Centres

Community Health Centre is the first referral institution to provide specialist services at a minimal cost near to their area of residence and relieve the urban hospitals of unnecessary rush.

INTRODUCTION

WHO defines Community Health Centre as Reference Health Centre. "The reference health centre differs from the generic health centre in that it is a functional concept that can be realized by strengthening one or more health centres to improve referral within the health system in rural areas. Thus, in addition to its generic health centre functions, it provides essential surgical, maternity and medical care, as well as carrying out preventive and promotive activities in the neighbourhood it serves. The reference health centre lightens the burden of the first referral hospital by taking over certain routine interventions, at the same time bringing appropriate care closer to the population at only a fraction of the cost of similar operations performed in local hospitals. Health centres, including reference health centres and hospitals, are components of a health care system, each playing a different but complementary role:" [1]

Dr. H. Mahler, former Director General of WHO said:[2] A health system based on primary health care cannot, and repeat, cannot be realized, cannot be developed, cannot function, and simply cannot exist without a network of hospitals functioning in a manner I have tried to describe. But hospitals have to change their ways so that they become one of the main flag-bearers of the most daring yet the most promising health movement in the history of humanity, the movement for health for all by the year 2000."

The concept of the "Community Health Centres" consists of interrelated components that contribute to health in homes, educational institutions, workplace, public places, and communities as well as in the

CHART 9.1

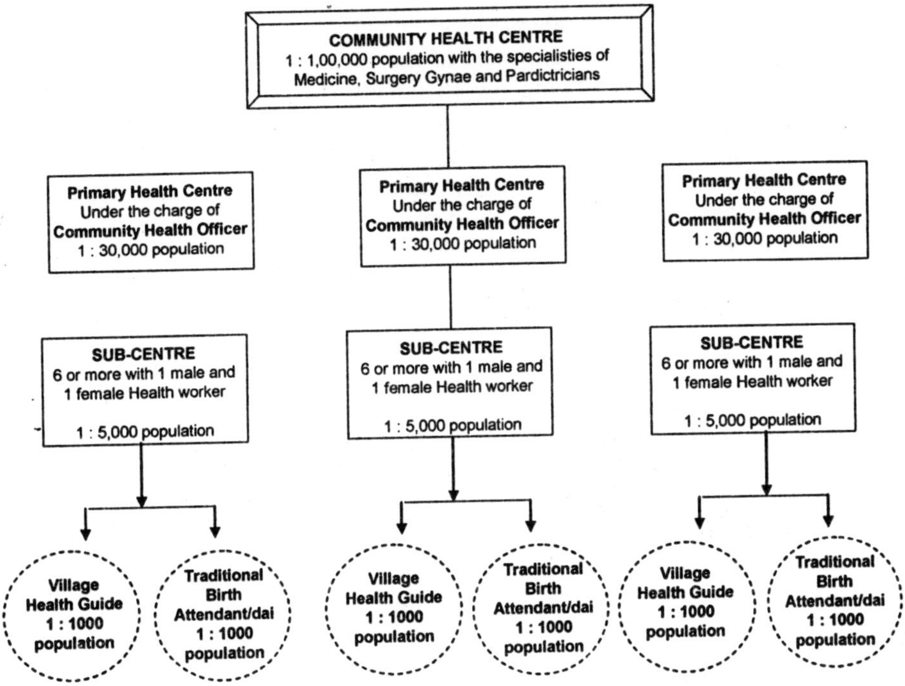

physical and psychological environment in the health and related sectors, like agriculture, education, environment, continuity of care, etc. A health system is usually organized at various levels, starting at the most peripheral level, also known as the community level or the primary level of health care, and proceeding through the intermediate (district, regional or provincial) level to the central level. At the same time it includes individuals and families participating in taking an active interest in solving their own health problems, thus becoming full members of the health care team. The intermediate and central levels deals with those elements of the health system for which they are given responsibility by the country's administrative organisation, and they also provide progressively more complex and more specialized care and support.

A community health centre is the main institution linking the health services with the people; has the responsibilities, and unique potential for providing people with the ability and confidence to solve their own problems; it provides a full range of health promotion and preventive services including mother and child care; it provides curative care primarily to ambulatory patients and those with selected conditions. It has a multidisciplinary team providing a range of services and with doctors, specialists, Nurses, Pharmacists and Technicians.[3]

A WHO document also mentions the role of first referral hospital as:[4]

> The hospital at first referral level, whether serving an urban or a rural population, is an integral part of the district health system with a key role to play in achieving health for all. It can function not only as a place to which patients with complex medical conditions are referred for diagnosis, treatment, and care, but also as a resource centre for health promotion in the district and for the planning and delivery of primary health care. This report of a WHO Study Group considers the responsibilities of the first referral hospital in its district setting, identifying its specific tasks in the provision of health care, training, and hospital support services, and defining its relationship both with the community and with health centres and other components of the district health system. Management principles for the first referral hospital are also discussed, in the context of the national health programme, with emphasis on decentralization, planning, and the efficient use of human and financial resources. The report concludes with recommendations for action by WHO, governments, and hospitals themselves, stressing the need for a change in approach if the first referral hospital is to fulfil its functions within a district health system based on primary health care.

The same document indicates the importance of first referral hospital in a district health set-up. To quote:[5]

> Half of the world's people live in villages, where the organisation of health services may be hampered by remoteness, adverse climate conditions, poor communications, and poverty, and perhaps by illiteracy and superstition. The first referral hospital may be very small, with a tiny staff that is limited in experience and expertise. The other half of the world's people live in cities, some of enormous size, where poverty is again a factor and where overcrowding, pollution, and stress may be overwhelming.

The problems that city hospitals must face are different from those of village hospitals, yet both types of hospitals provide essential services and it is important to see how they can be incorporated into the district health system.

In the past century medicine has grown increasingly scientific and hospitals have tended to become technological workshops for the diagnosis and treatment of disease. The trend will undoubtedly continue, but at the same time, the functional integration of hospitals into district health services is of vital importance, if they are to provide efficient, effective, affordable, and equitable services to their communities. This is not to underrate good clinical care and diagnosis, which are still the bedrock of hospital practice at the first referral level, but rather to emphasize the importance of making such care available to those most in need of it.

Within a district health system, there has to be a place to which patients with complex medical conditions can be referred for diagnosis, treatment, and care, and which can act as a resource centre for the health work of the district. This place is the first referral hospital.[6]

Out of four Primary Health Centres, one community health centre has been created with 30 beds in rural areas and 50 beds at taluk level to serve as referral hospital for the rural population. The purpose is to provide second tier referral services near their place and with better facilities so that their unnecessary approaching district hospitals may be avoided to save cost and provide better services to the rural population. Facilities required for 30 bedded/50 bedded hospitals have been provided in the Primary Health Centres upgraded in terms of infrastructure, personnel, equipment, etc. so that these institutions can handle cases coming to them directly or referred from Primary Health Centres.

These centres offer considerable advantages to both patients and Society, from the point of view of society, hospitalization both protects the family from many of the disruptive effects of caring for the ill in the home and operates as a means of guiding the sick and injured in medically supervised institutions where their problems are less disruptive for society as a whole. To quote Perry, "the success with which, a hospital contributes towards meeting the patients needs can be measured by the fullness of the life he is able to lead on leaving it."[7]

Community Health Centre provide good life to the people and social services to develop modern society. It has also included some important activities like:

(a) Community services including community planning;

(b) The organisation of local voluntary services and village or area councils of social services;

(c) The extension of organized social and community health services to rural areas;

(d) The organisation of citizens committees for community health care and social action.

(e) For adequacy and well-being of the community, there is community coordination, social security and family centres are needed.

Comprehensive definition of Hospital has been given by WHO which needs to be adopted by the CHCs. Hospital is an integral part of a social and medical organisation, the functions of which are to provide for the complete health care of the population—both curative and preventive and whose out-patients services reach out to the family and its home environment; the hospital is also a centre for training of health workers and for bio-social research.[8]

ORGANISATIONAL STRUCTURE

Personnel

The CHC is headed by Senior Medical Officer (SMO) who is generally a medical officer with 20-25 years of experience. He is the chief executive and has to ensure the smooth functioning of CHC. The other staff in CHC is as given below:

Staff for Community Health Centres

1.	Medical Officer	4
2.	Nurse Mid-Wives	7
3.	Dresser	1
4.	Pharmacist/Compounder	1
5.	Laboratory Technician	1
6.	Radiographer	2
7.	Ward Boys	1
8.	Dhobi	2
9.	Sweepers	1
10.	Mali	2
11.	Chowkidar	1
12.	Aya	1
13.	Peon	1
	Total	25

CHCs are being established and maintained by the State Government under MNP/BMS programme. It is manned by four medical specialists, i.e. Surgeon, Physician, Gynecologist and Pediatrician supported by 21 paramedical and other staff. It has 30 in-door beds with one OT, X-ray, Labour Room and Laboratory facilities. It serves as a referral centre for 4 PHCs and also provides facilities for obstetric care and specialist consultations. As on September, 2005, there are 3346 CHCs functioning in the country. This increased as to 3910 as on March 2006. It increased to 22669 as on March 2006.

As on March 2006 there are 3910 Community Health Centres. These have increased from 761 in Sixth Plan to 3910 as on March 2006 giving a rise of more than five times. Maharashtra with a strength of 407 is number one while there is none in Delhi (Refer Table 9.1)

Out of 3910 Community Health Centres, information about buildings is available only for 3753. Out of 3753, 3467 were functioning in Government buildings, 75 in rented buildings, 260 were in rent free buildings while 416 buildings were under constructions (Refer Table 9.2)

As on March 2006, 15640 specialists were required while 9071 were sanctioned. Even out of these, 3979 specialists were in position while 4681 posts were lying vacant giving a short fall of 9413 (Refer Table 9.3)

The population covered by a community health centre was less than 1 lakh in 11 states/UTs, the population varied between 7 lakh and 3 lakh in 20 states/UTs, 3-5 lakhs in 2 states/UTs and in one state 5-7 lakhs. The all India average was 189895 (Refer Table 9.4) p. 61 report

Table 9.5 reveals the following: Average coverage for one CHC is 163 villages, 20, 6 PHC ; Each PHC has 6 sub-centres, Each CHC has 6 PHC.

Building Environment comprises of the following:

Components for good health facilities for health staff and patients:

1. Adequate lighting;
2. Cleanliness;
3. Good Equipment;
4. Congenial Atmosphere and temperature;
5. Optimum utilization of space;
6. Noise control;
7. Proper Ventilation;
8. Safety Requirement;
9. Security and secrecy
10. Interior Decoration.

TABLE 9.1

Establishment of Community Health Centres during Five Year Plans

S. No.	State/UT	Community Health Centres functioning at the end of				Tenth Plan Target	Community Health Centres Functioning[1] as on Sept. 2005
		Sixth Plan [1981-85]	Seventh Plan [1985-90]	Eigth Plan [1992-97]	Ninth Plan [1997-2002]		
1	2	3	4	5	6	7	8
1.	Andhra Pradesh	27	46	207	219	208	167
2.	Arunachal Pradesh	0	6	9	20	0	31
3.	Assam	12	60	100	100	81	100
4.	Bihar	52	147	148	148	403	70
5.	Chhattisgarh					26	118
6.	Goa	3	5	5	5	1	5
7.	Gujarat	22	143	185	252	4	273
8.	Haryana	2	41	63	65	39	82
9.	Himachal Pradesh	28	35	42	65	0	66
10.	Jammu and Kashmir	19	33	45	53	0	80
11.	Jharkhand					122	197
12.	Karnataka	98	156	242	249	19	254

(Contd.)

1	2	3	4	5	6	7	8
13.	Kerala	4	54	80	105	75	107
14.	Madhya Pradesh[2]	58	172	198	342	100	229
15.	Maharashtra	147	290	300	351	88	407
16.	Manipur	6	10	16	16	0	16
17.	Meghalaya	3	3	10	13	6	24
18.	Mizoram	1	4	6	9	0	9
19.	Nagaland	1	4	5	9	5	21
20.	Orissa	59	92	157	157	108	231
21.	Punjab	10	70	105	105	14	126
22.	Rajasthan	76	185	261	263	49	325
23.	Sikkim	0	2	2	2	2	4
24.	Tamil Nadu	30	72	72	72	237	165
25.	Tripura	3	8	11	11	13	10
26.	Uttaranchal					36	49
27.	Uttar Pradesh[2]	74	177	262	310	588	386
28.	West Bengal	23	87	89	99	332	346
29.	A & N Islands	0	3	4	4	0	4
30.	Chandigarh	1	1	1	1	0	1
31.	D & N Haveli	0	0	0	1	1	1
32.	Daman and Diu	0	0	1	1	0	1
33.	Delhi	0	0	0	0	8	0
34.	Lakshadweep	1	1	3	3	0	3
35.	Pondicherry	1	3	4	4	0	4
All India		**761**	**1910**	**2633**	**3054**	**2565**	**3910**

Notes: 1. There is a reduction in the number of Centres functioning as on March 2006.
2. As compared to those functioning at the end of Ninth Plan due to the division of State.

Source: Bulletin on Rural Health Statistic in India, Ministry of Health and Family Welfare, 2006, p. 26.

TABLE 9.2

Building Position for Community Health Centres (As on March 2006)

Sl. No.	*State/UT*	*Total Number of CHCs functioning*	*Number of CHCs for which information on building is available*	*Sub-Centres functioning in Government Buildings*	*Rented Buildings*	*Rent Free Panchayat/ Vol. Society Buildings*	*Buildings under construction*	*Buildings requried[1] to be constructed*
1.	Andhra Pradesh	167	167	167	0	0	0	0
2.	Arunachal Pradesh	31	-	NA	NA	NA	NA	NA

3. Assam	100	100	100	0	0	0	0
4. Bihar	70	70	70	0	0	0	0
5. Chhattisgarh	118	118	116	0	2	23	0
6. Goa	5	5	5	0	0	0	0
7. Gujarat	273	273	226	0	47	44	3
8. Haryana	82	82	82	0	0	8	*
9. Himachal Pradesh	66	66	65	0	1	0	1
10. Jammu and Kashmir	80	80	79	1	0	22	*
11. Jharkhand	194	194	170	21	3	0	24
12. Karnataka	254	254	207	0	47	0	47
13. Kerala	107	107	107	0	0	0	0
14. Madhya Pradesh	229	229	229	0	0	83	*
15. Maharashtra	407	407	297	4	106	38	72
16. Manipur	16	16	8	0	8	5	3
17. Meghalaya	25	25	25	0	0	7	*
18. Mizoram	9	9	9	0	0	0	0
19. Nagaland	21	21	21	0	0	0	0
20. Orissa	231	231	231	0	0	0	0
21. Punjab	126	-	NA	NA	NA	NA	NA
22. Rajasthan	325	325	279	0	46	8	38
23. Sikkim	4	4	4	0	0	1	*
24. Tamil Nadu	165	165	165	0	0	0	0
25. Tripura	10	10	10	0	0	1	*
26. Uttaranchal	49	49	49	49	0	0	0
27. Uttar Pradesh	386	386	386	0	0	176	*
28. West Bengal	346	346	346	0	0	0	0
29. A & N Islands	4	4	4	0	0	0	0
30. Chandigarh	1	1	1	0	0	0	0
31. D & N Haveli	1	1	1	0	0	0	0
32. Daman and Diu	1	1	1	0	0	0	0
33. Delhi	0	0	0	0	0	0	0
34. Lakshadweep	3	3	3	0	0	0	0
35. Pondicherry	4	4	4	0	0	0	0
All India[2]	**3910**	**3753**	**3467**	**75**	**260**	**416**	**188**

Notes: NA: Not available

1. Required number = Total functioning – (Government Buildings + Under Construction) (ignoring excess).

* States having construction in excess of the number required to be constructed.

TABLE 9.3

Total Specialists at CHCs (as on March 2006)

S. No.	State/UTs	Required[1] [R]	Sanctioned [S]	In Position [P]	Vacant [S—P]	Shortfall [R—P]
1.	Andhra Pradesh	668	406	224	182	444
2.	Arunachal Pradesh	124	4	0	4	124
3.	Assam	400	NA	NA	NA	NA
4.	Bihar	280	280	88	192	192
5.	Chhattisgarh	472	700	49	651	423
6.	Goa	20	14	7	7	13
7.	Gujarat	1092	322	84	238	1008
8.	Haryana	328	112	37	75	291
9.	Himachal Pradesh	264	NA	NA	NA	NA
10.	Jammu and Kashmir	320	276	142	134	178
11.	Jharkhand	776	63	146	*	630
12.	Karnataka	1016	843	691	152	325
13.	Kerala	428	424	115	309	313
14.	Madhya Pradesh	916	253	49	204	867
15.	Maharashtra	1628	1628	448	1180	1180
16.	Manipur	64	30	3	27	61
17.	Meghalaya	100	2	1	1	99
18.	Mizoram	36	0	0	0	36
19.	Nagaland	84	0	0	0	84
20.	Orissa	924	496	NA	NA	NA
21.	Punjab	504	343	177	166	327
22.	Rajasthan	1300	870	592	278	708
23.	Sikkim	16	16	4	12	12
24.	Tamil Nadu	660	NA	NA	NA	NA
25.	Tripura	40	2	2	0	38
26.	Uttaranchal	196	163	71	92	125
27.	Uttar Pradesh	1544	1110	413	697	1131
28.	West Bengal	1384	692	624	68	760
29.	A & N Islands	16	12	0	12	16
30.	Chandigarh	4	4	4	0	0
31.	D & N Haveli	4	2	2	0	2
32.	Daman & Diu	4	0	0	0	4
33.	Delhi	0	0	0	0	0
34.	Lakshadweep	12	0	0	0	12
35.	Pondicherry	16	4	6	*	10
	All India[2]	**15640**	**9071**	**3979**	**4681**	**9413**

Notes: NA: Not Available.

*: Surplus.

1 One per each Primary Health Centre.

2 For calculating the overall percentages, the States/UTs for which manpower position is not available, should be excluded.

TABLE 9.4

Classification of States/UTs According to Average Population covered by a Community Health Centre (As on March 2006)

Sl. No.	Population Covered (Range)	Number of States/ UTs	Name of States/UTs	Average population (2001) covered
1.	Less than 1 lakh	11	Lakshadweep	11228
			Arunachal Pradesh	28067
			Mizoram	49730
			A & N Islands	59989
			Meghalaya	74588
			Nagaland	78440
			Pondicherry	81432
			Himachal Pradesh	83065
			Chandigarh	92120
			Jammu and Kashmir	95338
			Manipur	99426
2.	More than 1 lakh and less than 3 lakhs	20	Daman and Diu	100856
			Jharkhand	108000
			Gujarat	116267
			Sikkim	120245
			Punjab	127750
			Uttaranchal	128781
			Rajasthan	133209
			Goa	135418
			Orissa	135443
			Maharashtra	137046
			Karnataka	137358
			Chattisgarh	141085
			West Bengal	166904
			D & N Haveli	170027
			Haryana	183284
			Madhya Pradesh	193803
			Tamil Nadu	211647
			Kerala	220322
			Assam	232163
			Tripura	265345
3.	3-5 Lakhs	2	Andhra Pradesh	331743
			Uttar Pradesh	341084
4.	5-7 lakhs	1	Bihar	1061667
	All India	**34**	**All India**	**189895**

TABLE 9.5

Average Number of Villages covered by a Sub-centre/PHC/CHC and Number of Sub-centres per PHC and Number of PHCs per CHC (As on March 2006)

Sl. No.	State/UTs	Average Number of villages covered by a			Number of Sub-Centres per PHC	Number of PHCs per CHC
		Sub-Centre	PHC	CHC		
1.	Andhra Pradesh	2	18	168	8	9
2.	Arunachal Pradesh	11	48	131	4	3
3.	Assam	5	43	263	8	6
4.	Bihar	5	27	644	5	23
5.	Chhattisgarh	4	39	172	9	4
6.	Goa	2	19	72	9	4
7.	Gujarat	3	17	68	7	4
8.	Haryana	3	17	85	6	5
9.	Himachal Pradesh	10	46	305	5	7
10.	Jammu and Kashmir	4	18	83	5	5
11.	Jharkhand	8	99	168	12	2
12.	Karnataka	4	18	116	5	7
13.	Kerala	0	2	13	6	8
14.	Madhya Pradesh	6	46	242	7	5
15.	Maharashtra	4	24	107	6	4
16.	Manipur	6	33	149	6	5
17.	Meghalaya	15	60	241	4	4
18.	Mizoram	2	14	91	6	6
19.	Nagaland	3	16	63	5	4
20.	Orissa	9	40	222	5	6
21.	Punjab	4	26	101	6	4
22.	Rajasthan	4	24	127	6	5
23.	Sikkim	3	19	113	6	6
24.	Tamil Nadu	2	12	87	7	7
25.	Tripura	2	12	87	7	7
26.	Uttaranchal	10	76	343	7	5
27.	Uttar Pradesh	5	29	278	6	9
28.	West Bengal	4	44	118	11	3
29.	A & N Islands	5	29	278	6	9
30.	Chandigarh	2	0	24	0	0
31.	D & N Haveli	2	12	70	6	6
32.	Daman and Diu	1	8	23	7	3
33.	Delhi	4	21	0	5	0
34.	Lakshadweep	2	6	8	4	1
35.	Pondicherry	1	2	23	2	10
	All India	**4**	**28**	**163**	**6**	**6**

Note: NA: Not Available.

EQUIPMENT

Specialists have identified the minimum essential requirements of Equipment for Community Health Centres to provide 2nd tier of health services. We may mention here the list of important categories as these would help us in assessing their availability and utilisation. The equipment has been broadly classified under the following heads:

1. Imaging
2. Electro-medical
3. Pneumatic-hydraulic and sterilization
4. Laboratory
5. Air conditioning and refrigeration
6. Hospital utility support systems
7. Administration
8. Minor equipment and furnishings
9. Surgical instruments and packs

The equipment mentioned here is not supplied to CHC resulting in unsatisfactory services. The state health department must ensure the availability of all equipment in functional condition to ensure the benefits of referral system.

FACILITIES

Following facilities should be provided in a CHC:

1. Radiological investigations
2. Laboratory Investigations
3. Surgery
4. Trauma and Life Support
5. Chest
6. Surgery
7. Urogenital
8. Surgical Conditions Abscess
9. Ophthalmology
10. Gastro Enterology
11. Thoracic
12. ENT
13. Obs. and Gynaec
14. Use of drugs causing Analgesis
15. Regional Anesthesia.

NORMS OF SERVICES

If we want to run CHCs successfully then we must imbibe ethical values among doctors. Smith also observes "..... I felt that if you are really going to run an ethical institution, set high standards, you have to set them from top."[9]

Being Government run institutions, the staff has to follow the civil service rules and also to honour the norms, values and ethics of the profession, which are helpful in policy making and planning for setting up the new CHCs. Some steps in this direction are given below:

1. Create an environment for progress;
2. Build effective processes for work;
3. Help in education and training;
4. Help in policy planning;
5. Prepare guidelines for decision-making and conflict resolution;
6. Accept its own accountability and responsibility;
7. Duties towards patients;
8. Duties towards profession; and
9. Doctor to doctor relationship.

Government has developed Norms of Services for CHC to avoid confusion. These norms help the health department and CHC staff to maintain standards and ensure quality health care. These norms also help in policy-making and planning for the new CHCs to be established.

The CHC staff should not restrict themselves only to the technical aspects of effectiveness but to such other aspects as well, like comparability of services and work environment, communication with patients and their relations and promotion of collective responsibility for medicare and health of the community. The success of these norms depends upon the availability of facilities in good condition.

FUNCTIONS

1. It acts as a referral centre. All those who are referred from PHC or sub-centre are attended here with more facilities and by qualified personnel. It provides good examination facilities or gets it done from district hospital at higher level.
2. It serves as a part of district health system, thereby getting the benefits of exchange of services.
3. It should be an integral part of the primary health care and should support all activities of primary health centres and sub-centres.
4. It should provide training to its staff to make them more and more professional and dynamic.
5. It should have intimate contact with the people. The communities and involve them in their own health promotion.

Thus, community health centre should be looked at from a wider angle and not merely from curative aspect of a higher degree. It should encompass all aspect of health care and should promote and coordinate all health activities as a part of district health system to provide better health care to the people. However, when first referral, level is not competent. the case be referred to district hospital.

ASPECT OF CHC SERVICES

(i) OPD Functions

The patient either referred from below or approached directly by CHC should be received well. However, preference may be given to referred patients coming from a long distance. The patient needs the following services:

(a) Diagnosis by the specialists with the help of laboratory tests and electronic equipment supplemented by clinical sense of the doctor. This should be done thoroughly. Well begun is half done.

(b) Treatment—Diagnosis is followed by treatment which can take any of the following form:

  (i) Sending the patient back home after prescribing treatment. This can be followed at later dates convenient to doctor and patient.
  (ii) Treatment in the OPD.
  (iii) Admission and treatment in a CHC ward.
  (iv) Refer to District/Specialist hospital.
  (v) Refer to PHC back to be followed by PHC Doctor.

The patient needs good care, courteous behaviour, prompt services and clear communication. He would judge the CHC from the care given to him and not by the technical details. However, in practice, we find that the patients feel lot of discomforts and complain of apathy of CHC staff. Let us mention some of the common problems.

Problems of OPD

(a) Lack of proper seating arrangements.

(b) Delays resulting into time wastage, it takes 2-3 hours for a patient to get his/her turn.

(c) Lack of punctuality—Doctors on duty are not in time resulting into rush and impatience among patients.

(d) Lack of proper examination—Patients feel that they are not properly examined and that is why they prefer private doctors resulting in the mushroom growth of Nursing homes and private practitioners.

(e) Doctors lack social conscience—Doctors do not havé concern for social justice, compassion for underprivileged.

There is lack of strong commitment and spirit of service, vital for the success of medical profession—

(a) Discourteous behaviour.
(b) Non-availability of medicine.
(c) Fear of hospital infection because of poor cleanliness.

Thus, there is a need of far reaching improvements in the management of OPD services to ensure optimisation of resources and satisfaction of patients. Author has rightly said that "We should not be contended merely with the availability and accessibility of health services in OPDs but rather in their acceptability and acceptance."[10]

A special out-patient clinic that sees only referred cases can be a great help to both hospital and health centre as well as achieve the objective of management by exception. Many patients can be diagnosed and treated without the need for admission when the absence of overcrowding allows the doctor to give enough time to each of them, since these patients have already been examined and their detailed history is with them. Wherever possible, medical and surgical patients should be separated. The referred note, including relevant comments and advice, should always receive a proper reply, and the patient should be referred back as soon as possible for continued treatment either at the health centre or at home to avoid confusion.

(ii) Ward

Ward is the heart of CHC where patient comes in direct and intimate contact with the staff and services of CHC. After the patient has been examined in the OPD or the emergency area, he may be advised admission in the ward. Ward management is the undivided responsibility of the ward sister concerned. Specialists visit the ward as and when necessary. A ward is that area of the hospital where all the amenities—physical, social and especially medical care—are made available to make the patients feel at home till they are discharged. In other words, a ward is a temporary home for the patients admitted there. Evidently, there is a need to ensure a healthy environment to help early recovery of the patients and to win their confidence. In each ward, there is a nursing unit to take care of the patients for all the 24 hours. The efficient planning of this unit would ensure maximum care of the patient. The broad categories of functions that should be discharged by the nursing units are:

(a) Meeting personal needs of the patients.
(b) Efficient ward management.
(c) Proper maintenance of records of the patients.

(d) Provision of basic institutional services.
(e) Availability of diagnostic and treatment equipment,
(f) Arranging formal and informal health education of the patients and their relatives.

(iii) Specialities

CHC is provided to take care of the following specialities:

(a) Medical Core

Medical and nursing staff should make themselves available to provide services for chronic illness like asthma, diabetes, hypertension, chronic obstructive pulmonary disease, tuberculosis, heart ailment. The patient should be monitored frequently to arrive at conclusions. If controlled, patient can be referred back to primary health centres. If serious, they may be referred to specialists at higher levels.

(b) Obstetric Care

CHC must have arrangements for complicated delivery cases. CHC should provide quality maternity and child health services.

(c) Pediatric Care

There should be good arrangements for the care of children to reduce infant mortality rate. There should also be arrangement for the education of mothers who accompany the child.

(d) Surgery

Since at primary health centre, there is no arrangement for surgery, CHC must take care of minor operations. The performance of surgery requires a medical doctor with surgical background who should either be familiar with local anaesthesis techniques or work with a competent anaesthetist and trained nursing staff. It requires a suitable minor operating theatre and sterile instruments and supplies. An additional room for post-operative recovery is essential. Surgery should not be performed unless there are suitable arrangements. Minor surgery may be performed at CHC, if the responsible surgeon considers that the person performing it has had a firm grounding in the basics of surgery and in the appropriate diagnostic and surgical techniques. All such minor surgery must be carefully monitored by the senior surgeon. There must be strict rules concerning permitted procedures and a regular and rigorous review of faults and failures. CHC should ensure good arrangements for surgical cases.

(iii) Emergency Services

The image of the CHC depends upon the type, quality and speed with which emergencies are attended to. S.K. Garg has nicely explained the need and requirements of emergency services. To quote him:[11]

"Causality, means—a patient who comes to the hospital unannounced with accidental injury and is seen and treated otherwise than at a consultative session."

Every hospital, big or small, therefore, requires to set-up a well organised emergency unit, because the image of hospital mainly depends upon the quality and type of treatment a hospital can provide to a patient suffering from any medical or surgical complications, requiring immediate care. Emergency Department of a hospital, therefore, means a section or a part of hospital to which persons injured in road accidents or those suffering from serious complications are taken for urgent treatment. The Emergency Department provides round the clock, immediate diagnosis and urgent treatment for illness of emergent nature and injuries from accidents. It is in this context that the Emergency Department of the hospital is often the point of major public impact, even more than the out-patient department, providing every important service and at the same time being the most vulnerable to criticism and censure. The department is meant to provide round the clock immediate diagnosis and best possible treatment for illness of emergency nature and injuries from accidents.[12]

To ensure that the emergencies are attended to quickly and effectively, it is necessary to have an efficient set-up well knit with other departments of the CHC with well laid out procedures and work distribution. It is to act as information centre, i.e. to reply to public queries on telephone or otherwise about first-aid, treatment of accident cases, antidotes of various poisons, etc.

- To handle medico-legal cases.
- To manage ambulance services.
- To manage a disaster.
- To carry out Research, i.e. Pathogenesis of accidents.
- To achieve all this, there is a need of competent staff to manage the emergency department.

To quote C.S. Balaraman:

"The patient and his relatives accompanying are considerably excited and tense and land at the casualty office under the premise of being attended right away and given relief and solace as soon as possible. The demands on the working staff are very exacting and need to be managed in a very critical manner envisaging a competent staff pattern in the doctor, nurse and attendant to manage these problems."[13]

(iv) Laboratory and X-ray Facilities

For proper diagnosis of ailments of patients it is necessary to have diagnostic laboratory facility properly manned. It is important that all laboratory investigations be adequately controlled, and useful records kept of results which should be reported without delay. The data collected should be standardized and presented in reports that can be used by health authorities and epidemiologists in health planning. Equipment should be adequately maintained. There must be an effective system for the decontamination of infected material' and the safe disposal of laboratory waste. The success of medical prescription would depend upon proper laboratory diagnosis. Laboratories for routine blood, urine, microbiology, X-ray, etc., should provide round the clock service. It is desirable to locate the laboratory block and X-ray block in between the OPD and indoor area to be able to serve both the areas.

We must ensure that the technicians are really doing the job because a minor mistake on their part may ruin the life of the patients. There is a need for constant supervision over the functioning of these laboratory services.[14]

Besides, in CHC, there is reception counter, small operation theater, injection room, dental clinic, dispensary, lounge for OPD patients and office records room.

CRITICAL APPRAISAL

We present here various facts which if taken care of, can make CHCs efficient and effective.

I. Poor Quality of Service

Quality of care is very important for patient's health. Quality assurance means making sure that the services provided by the hospital are the best possible. Quality assurance is vital for the hospitals' clinical support services (X-ray, laboratory, pharmacy, central sterile supplies) which have an obligation to maintain high standards. However, there is no quality care in CHC. This indicates the carelessness of the CHC staff. The DHO must exercise his authority to ensure good quality of services if not excellent. K.G. Aggarwal has rightly said that, "Hospital effectiveness which can be measured in terms of patient's satisfaction does not depend on the improvement of hospital services aspect alone but on the medical care aspect."[15]

Goel suggests, "Effective coordination should be established between the medical services and the supportive services to ensure promptness and clarity."[16]

Kulwinder Sanga in his article relating to an excellent hospital (CHC) newly built in Punjab, "Hospital Services Poor" has found highly unsatisfactory services based on actual facts. To quote him, attendants of patients are forced to convert ordinary school exercise books purchased from the canteen from the premises into indoor patient files. . . . Most of the beds are empty. Patients complain that although antenatal check up is done, aid at delivery time is uncertain. They say doctors in the department are not available at night. Patients also complain that when an operation has to be performed doctors give a list of items, including cotton gloves, to be purchased The area around the hospital building is full of congress grass and other wild growth."[17]

2. Quality of Behaviour

It is generally believed that many patients can be cured simply by courteous, soft and healing tongue of the CHC staff. Behaviour is an important variable though intangible in the treatment of patients. CHC staff especially the Class IV staff behaves rudely with patients as they want to extract money from patients. They forget that the patients are already in trouble. They lack the art of communication.

There is a need to inculcate among the CHC Staff the techniques of interacting with the patients who are already agitated with their sufferings. C.N. Ray in his Article, "Citizen's Charter in India: An Overview" rightly suggests the need of framing citizens' charter by CHC to maintain their dignity and honour. To quote him, "If the spirit of a charter is to prevail, the lower level officers need to be exposed and convinced of its benefits through training and orientation programmes. . .[18] We must ensure and encourage courteous behaviour by the medical team to patients to create good relationship.

Mary D. Shanks and D.A. Kennedy have rightly emphasized the need of human approach. To quote: "The hospital today is more than the combination of medical and therapeutic treatments by specialists, greater and refined medical and surgical knowledge and ever better and more effective facilities and equipment. It includes these factors as the care of its efficient operation but an additional dimension—one which is too often ignored or at least minimized—is the human and social element in the structure of the organisation."[19]

3. Quality and Availability of Medical Facilities

Quality of medical facilities is extremely poor or rather hopeless. Most of the facilities are non-functional. Medicines are not available. Infections are very high. We must be clear that the efficiency of CHC depends not only on the competence of medical personnel but also on the availability of drugs in right quantity and quality.

4. Infrastructural Facilities Inadequate

Linen, urinals, latrines, bathrooms were extremely hopeless which is a very sad reflection on the functioning of CHCs. Cleanliness is the first and most important aspect of a CHC as it affects the organisational climate. This is more a question of attitude and not much of resources. Patients and relatives feel suffocated with stinking smell all around. CHCs must give top priority to keep the premises clean to promote both preventive and curative health care. People are the true measure of success of policies and programmes. At the same time, people are the determinants of success. In brief, we can say that in the past, beneficiaries of CHCs were passively receiving CHC Services, A trend has emerged where in the beneficiaries and the community at large wish to participate in the programme of delivery of health services which must be kept in mind by CHCs and other staff members. All the functionaries of the CHCs must keep the importance of the patient in mind.[20]

We may also suggest that the Government must prepare a patient's charter wherein provisions should be made to compensate patients for the wrongs done by Medical Staff.

5. Referral Services not Functioning

The real purpose of creating CHCs was to provide efficient referral services within rural areas at a lower cost and with the best treatment, CHCs have failed to serve as a referral centre both up and down and thus defeating the purpose for which these were created.

The state health department should review this and find out the reasons for such lapses. However, there are very few referred patients who come to CHCs because:

(a) Referral services are not known to people.
(b) There is no well defined procedure for reference.
(c) Those who come go dissatisfied.
(d) Beds remain vacant.
(e) No feed back of the referred patients.
(f) Lack of adequate facilities as per norms mentioned earlier.

On the basis of our discussion, observation, and analysis, we suggest the following to make referral system from PHC and CHC a real success:

1. Norms of services at each level to be clearly defined, i.e. primary, secondary and tertiary. The community and the providers should know about this.
2. Quality of services at each level is to be maintained in order to build and promote confidence among patients and the community. There is need to develop confidence. that the patient shall be referred and promptly transferred to higher level of health care, as required.
3. Some procedures need to be designed, so that patients do not by-pass lower level of facilities
4. Renovating and upgrading hospital buildings to provide appropriate space for services.
5. Upgrading and updating clinical skills of medical officers and staff nurses through an effective training programme.
6. Providing ambulance for transporting critical patients.
7. Installing phone, fax and paging systems in hospitals.

8. Financial powers to Senior Medical Officers incharge of the hospitals to purchase individual items upto Rs. 5,000.
9. The user charges should be retained at the site of collection. These should be used by the Senior Medical Officer in-charge of the hospital for patient's benefit.
10. Referral and feed back cards need to be introduced.
11. Referral guidelines that specify the 'what' and 'how' of implementing the referral system need to be provided.
12. An incentive system for patients who follow referral procedures should be envisaged.
13. Linkages and communications between the first referral hospitals and primary health care facilities through regular training and out reach visits should be established.
14. Intensive information, education and communication (I.E.C.) targeted at providers and the community should be initiated.
15. District Health Committees should monitor the implementation of the referral system at district level.
16. It must be ensured that all the vacant posts are filled and mismatching is reduced to nil. All equipment should be available and be kept in working order 24 hours a day and 365 days a year.

It is expected that with these measures, there will be better functioning of the CHCs. The patients and the community will gain confidence. These CHCs will become referral points for the PHC level patients.

6. Poor Quality of Medical Record Keeping

Medical record is a scientific, clinical, administrative and legal document relating to patient's care in which is recorded sufficient data to justify diagnosis, treatment and results. Good record-keeping is essential. If medical records are illegible, incomplete, ambiguous, and incorrectly filled, they affect medical care. The quality of medical records is an important managerial and medical consideration. When a patient gets discharged from hospital, an accurate summary of his or her record should be made and retained and a copy sent to the source of referral for future reference.

A unit system of record keeping should be practiced. Each patient should have a permanent number and is assigned a folder containing all relevant records, past and present, medical or surgical inpatient or outpatient indexed by a summary sheet.

- The responsibility of completing the medical records accurately and adequately should lie with the treating physician.
- Diseases should be classified (coded) according to international classification of diseases.

- Medical Record should be easily accessible and retrievable. The efficiency and working of a hospital can be judged from its record maintenance quality.

Analysis of records by the author revealed the following:

(a) Medical Record keeping is not taken seriously resulting in poor quality of health services.

(b) Decision-making by a Doctor who has not examined him in first instance becomes difficult and irrational.

(c) It causes complications in Medico-legal cases.

(d) It avoids the evaluation of medical competence of the MO/SMO concerned.

(e) It is a major hurdle in making referral system a success for which these CHCs have been created.

Rajneesh Goel in his study of 50 sheets of patients in 10 CHC found: In 85.4 percent cases, the patients name was not available, 87 percent had no C.R. number and 56.6 percent cases did not have name of attending medical officer. In 84 percent cases, there was no diagnosis, in 84.2 percent cases, no medication was mentioned, while in 86.7 percent cases, no follow-up details were given. Further, in 89.4 cases, entries were legible and 65.8 percent cases were complete. In 82.7 percent cases, physical examination and history was complete on admission. However, discharge summary was absent in as many as 84.9 percent. Even the front sheet has been signed by MO/SMO is only in 31.7 percent cases. It was very disheartening to find that there was no certification of time and date of death in 92.5 percent cases and cause of deaths in 92.9 percent cases. However, the operation sheet was complete in 69.5 percent cases. (See graphic representation Appendix 9.3 and Table 9.1)

We, therefore, suggest that MO/SMO/CMO should be made legally and morally responsible to ensure completion of medical record sheets. They may be provided training and instructions to ensure its compliance. A column in ACR may also be made for quality of records maintained to make them realise its importance.

Storage of Medical records should be done at a place where proper conditions of temperature and a circulation of air and humidity are provided. After storing the records, indexing is necessary to locate the record for retrieval.

Unfortunately this vital area has not received adequate attention. But for few exceptions, the system of medical records is very rudimentary in most of the CHCs. Trained medical record personnel are not posted in our hospitals, and it will be unrealistic to expect hospitals to make progress in this field without them in near future.

TABLE 9.6

Analysis of "Medical Record Evaluation" in CHC Karnataka—Total Records Analyse: 50

	% Yes	% No	% NA/ DNR
1. Are all pages of the cases notes correctly identified with:			
(a) Patient's Name	13.2	85.6	1.4
(b) C.R. Number	11.6	67.0	1.4
(c) Attending medical Officer	41.6	56.6	1.6
2. Is there an entry on discharging containing:			
(a) Diagnosis	11.1	84.0	4.9
(b) Medication	10.8	84.2	5.0
(c) Follow-up (by whom and when)	8.7	86.7	5.5
3. Are entries:			
(a) Legible	89.4	7.8	2.8
(b) Complete	65.8	29.0	5.2
4. Was a physical examination and history completed on admission	82.7	16.2	1.1
5. Is the Discharge summary present?	13.8	84.7	1.3
6. Has the front sheet been correctly completed with?	31.7	68.0	0.3
7. Was death certified in the medical record including:			
(a) Time and date	7.5	92.5	—
(b) Cause of death	7.1	92.9	—
8. Has the operation sheet been correctly complete?	69.5	30.5	—

7. Nurses Involved only in Clinical Activity

The real foundation of health can be laid if nursing is properly developed for Primary Health Care. This is meant to provide preventive and promotive health education. The objective of nursing in PHC may include:

(1) health counselling to individuals, families and community groups in promoting health;
(2) provision of nursing care when necessary, and teaching and supervision of others providing nursing care;
(3) active involvement in the National Health Programmes;
(4) promotion of environmental sanitation in homes, schools, industry;
(5) case-finding related to the agency's programmes, and participation in epidemiological investigation;
(6) cooperation in community studies and other special research of the agency;
(7) participation in educational programmes for nurses, other professionals and members of the community; and
(8) educating patients in preventive health care.

CHART 9.2

Medical Record Evaluation

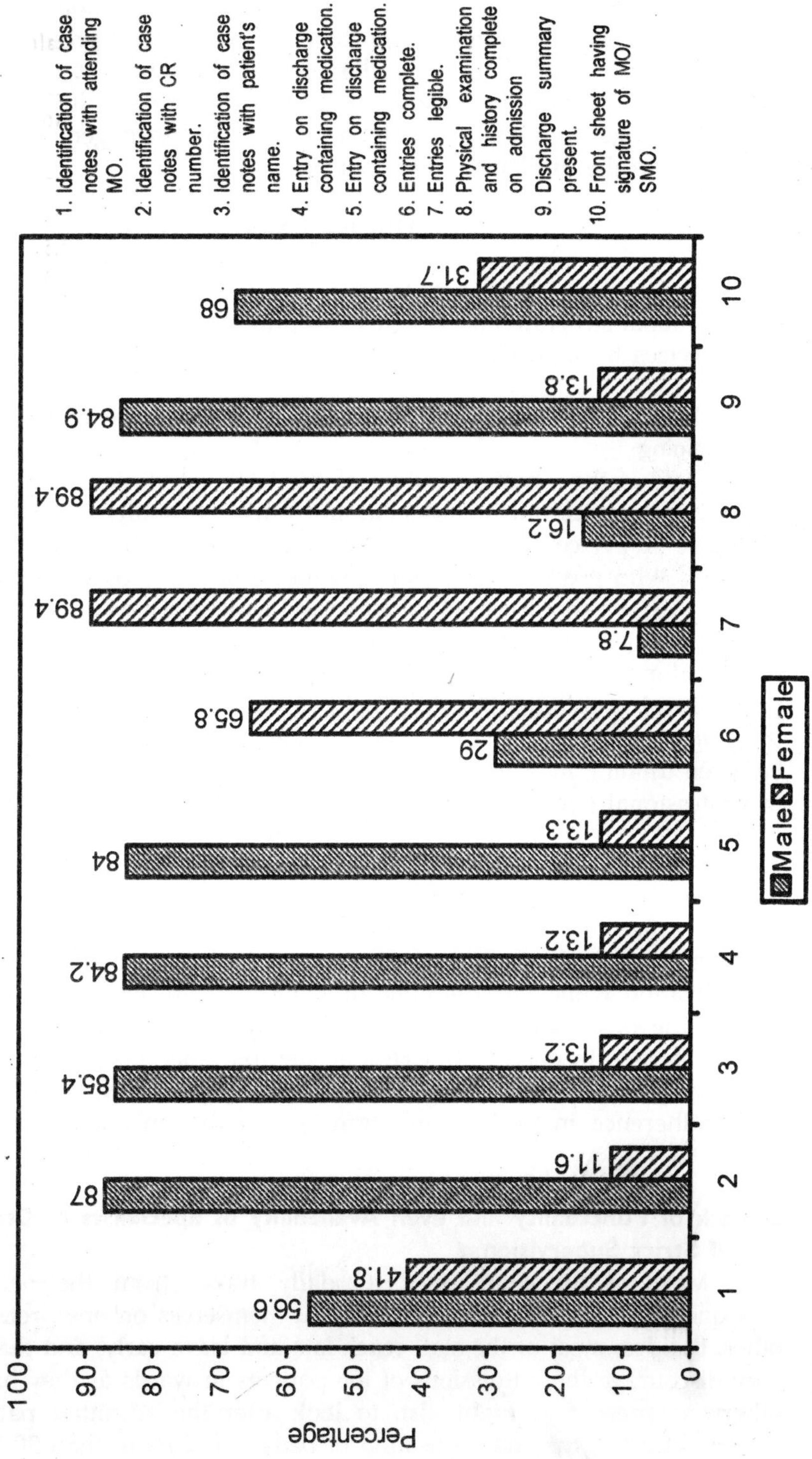

Besides, we must plan the use of nurses in the promotion of primary health care. The International Council of Nurses (ICN) representing nurses throughout the world, supports the present (WHO/UNICEF concept of Primary Health Care). In so doing, ICN affirms the commitment of nurses to effect changes in nursing education, practice and management, which are conducive to the implementation of PHC.

SUGGESTIONS

We present here the facts and suggestions to improve upon organisational structure and resources to provide decent second level health care services through CHCs.

1. SMO Lacks Administrative Skill and Competence: Need for Imparting Training

SMO is the Chief Executive of the CHC appointed on the basis of seniority in service but he lacks administrative capability for which he has to devote 50 per cent of his time. We should appoint those doctors to head the CHC who possess leadership qualities and are good at working with a team. A CHC should select dynamic and adequately qualified person and then offer them opportunities though training and work experience and self-development as professional leader who have competence in both professional and administrative field as well as high motivation. It is, therefore essential that medical personnel engaged in administration should be given training in administration so that they can become competent both in professional knowledge as well as in administrative competence.

2. Mismatching of Resources: Need for Strict Policy of Posting and Transfer

We have mentioned the need of four specialities in a CHC but in practice, we find that there is more than one consultant in one specialization while there is none in some of them. Besides about 40 per cent of the posts sanctioned are lying vacant. Even sanctioned posts fall short of target. In one of the CHCs all the four specialists were from skin. It is a very sad reflection on the State Health Department. We must ensure strict adherence in posting and transfers so that mismatching does not occur.

3. Lack of Punctuality and even Availability of Specialists in CHC: Need of Strict Supervision

Most of the Staff in CHC daily travel from the nearby city headquarters. Most of them try to absent themselves on one pretext or the other. Besides, most of the staff reach late and leave early, and that is why, they discourage the admissions of the patients in wards as they have to be otherwise present at night also to look after the admitted patients. Its indirect effect is that the utilisation of beds is not more than 30 to 40 per cent, thus incurring heavy cost and defeating the purpose for which CHCs were created. The health department must ensure the compulsory stay of the SMa and other consultants either by constructing good accommodation or by hiring good houses for them.

4. Vacant Posts: Need for Timely Appointments

Many posts of Staff Nurses, Technicians and others remain vacant affecting the services of CHC. Hospital services can't be run without the required staff. The state health department must ensure the availability of the staff to ensure optimum utilisation of CHC.

5. Equipment is Either not Available or Non-functional

A physical verification of the equipment revealed that 50 per cent of the essential equipment listed earlier has not been provided to these CHCs while a lot of equipment is out of order needing repair and maintenance. One of the SMOs told that the Staff using these instruments do not handle and maintain them properly. There is a need to inject proper culture to keep their instruments clean and in working order. The health department must also be quick in replacing them with new ones.

6. All the Services Entrusted to CHC not Available

We have listed the services which need to be provided by CHC but in practice, they are not able to meet even 50 per cent of these because of physical and financial constraints. There is a need to ensure availability of all equipment in functional form and availability of personnel through strict supervision and control. In one of the CHCs, there was a Dental Chair and other equipments but no dental surgeon but in another CHC, there was no Dental Chair but the Dental Surgeon was in position. Such glaring wastages should be curbed and supervisory personnel should be held responsible for such lapses.

We may also mention here the problems mentioned by CHC staff which need consideration and analysis:

(i) DHO and district staff do not take keen interest in removing the problems of CHC promptly.

(ii) There is always a financial constraint which affects the functioning of CHC.

(iii) Shortage of medicine continues even after reminders.

(iv) No formal linkages between PHC/CHC/Civil Hospital. District Hospital except through DHO/District Surgeon.

(v) Lack of adequate planning and monitoring by District staff and State Health Departments.

In brief, the following actions should certainly see the system functioning more efficiently:

1. The staff members of CHC must be made aware of their responsibilities to make the Primary Health Care and district health system a success.
2. The CHC should constantly engage itself in staff development through motivation and training.
3. The CHC should ensure that its staff members should provide integrated health care and not simply remedy for diseases.
4. The CHC should continuously appraise performance particularly its quality of care in terms of humanity, effectiveness and efficiency.
5. The CHC should continuously monitor its infrastructure and health facilities to ensure that these are properly maintained.
6. The CHC should devote time and resources to action-oriented health services research.
7. The CHC should look for additional sources of funds which should be spent equitably and efficiently.
8. The CHC must design its referral system clearly.
9. CHC must engage itself constantly in improving its services and performance. Simple commitment by CHC staff is not enough. The improvement process must become basic and continuous. If we want to safeguard the future, it is high time that all those who are serving CHC should get concerned with creativity and change—take a second look at their work system and style and evolve an appropriate work method, upholding the new criteria of promoting creativity and total change—if not a total revolution. Tarun Bahl in his article: "Truthful Living" in *The Tribune,* dated January 16, 2000, rightly says about basic values which must be cherished by CHC staff. "Truthful living is nothing out living by convictions, standing up for "that one believes to be correct, taking up the cause of the downtrodden, continuing to do the right things even when one is not being watched."
10. The CHC should ensure excellent internal working environment wherein the staff feel happy in providing services.

CONCLUSION

We can conclude by saying that CHCs are not serving the purpose for which these were created to provide referral services to PHCs. CHCs have also failed to provide even basic preventive, curative and promotive health care. It is high time for the State Health Department of Government to evaluate the functioning of CHCs and revamp them to make them fit for the delivery of health care services, otherwise, the resources invested in them would go waste as is happening at present. There is a need to provide quality health care at CHC level, which means to deliver and maintain a safe, sure and effective health care to patients.

In the new millennium, we must equip these first referral level institutions within rural set-up and ensure availability of all the specialists so that they can meet the needs of the rural people in their vicinity and at an affordable cost. In this way, we are sure to make primary health care a great success.

NOTES AND REFERENCES

1. WHO, District Health Systems: Global and Regional Review Based on Experience in Various Countries, Geneva, 1995, p. 18.
2. H. Mahler, The Role of Hospitals in Primary Health Care, Report of a conference sponsored by the Aga Khan foundation and the World Health Organisation, 22-26 Nov. 1981, Karachi, Pakistan, Geneva, Aga Khan Foundation. 1981, Pan II, p. 5.
3. WHO: The Health Centres in District Health System; Geneva, 1994, p. 6.
4. WHO, Technical Report Services 819, Geneva. 1992 (back cover).
5. *Ibid.*, p. 11.
6. WHOs Technical Report Series. 395, 1968, p. 6.
7. Elen B. Perry. Ward Management, Balliere, London, 1978, p. 2.
8. WHO, Technical Report Series, 395, 1968, p. 1.
9. S.K. Bhatia, Business Ethics and Managerial Values, New Delhi, Year 2002, p. 72.
10. S.L. Goel and R. Kumar (Ed.), Hospital Administration and Management, New Delhi, Deep &. Deep, year not mentioned, Vol. 2, p. 13.
11. S.K. Garg, Emergency Services in General Hospital in Hospital Administration and. Management, S.L. Gael and. R. Kumar (Ed.), New Delhi, Deep &. Deep, Vol. 2, pp. 28-29.
12. S.K. Garg, *Ibid.*, pp. 28-29.
13. C.S. Balaraman. "Emergency Services in Hospitals" quoted in S.L. Goel and R. Kumar, *op. cit.*, p. 21.
14. S.L. Goel, Public Health Administration, New Delhi, Sterling, 1984, pp. 388-89.
15. K.G. Aggarwal. "Managing Patient Satisfaction in Hospitals", in *Indian Journal of Public Administration*, Vol. XXII, No. 2, April-June 1976, p. 154.
16. S.L. Goel, Public Health Administration, New Delhi, Sterling, 1984, p. 401.
17. *The Daily Tribune*, Chandigarh, Aug. 13, 1999. p. 3.
18. C.N. Roy, "Citizens Charters in India: An Overview" in *IJPA*, Vol. XLIV, October-December 1998, p. 814.
19. Mary D. Shanks and Dorothy A. Kemedy, The Theory and Practice of Nursing Service Administration, McGraw Hill, London, 1965, p. 95.
20. Edy the Alexander, *et al.*, Nursing Service Administration, (ed.) New York, Mosby, 1962, p. 63.

APPENDIX 9.1

STAFFING PATTERNS

A	STAFF FOR SUB-CENTRE	1
1.	Health Worker (Female)/ANM	1
2.	Health Workers (Male)	1
3.	Voluntary worker (Paid @ Rs. 100 p.m. as honorarium)	1
	TOTAL	3
B.	STAFF FOR NEW PRIMARY HEALTH CENTRE	
1.	Medical Officer	1
2.	Pharmacist	1
3.	Nurse Mid-wife (Staff Nurse)	1
4.	Health Workers (Female)/ANM	1
5.	Health Educator	1
6.	Health Assistant (Male)/LHV	1
7.	Health Assistant (Female)/LHV	1
8.	Upper Division Clerk	1
9.	Lower Divison Clerk	1
10.	Laboratory Technician	1
11.	Driver (Subject to Availability of Vehicle)	4
12.	Class IV	15
C.	STAFF FOR COMMUNITY HEALTH CENTRE	
1.	Medical Officer #	4
2.	Nurse Mid-Wife (Staff Nurse)	7
3.	Dresser	1
4.	Pharmacist/Compounder	1
5.	Laboratory Technician	1
6.	Radiographer	2
7.	Ward Boys	1
8.	Dhobi	3
9.	Sweepers	1
10.	Mali	1
11.	Chowkidars	1
12.	Aya	1
13.	Peon	25

APPENDIX 9.2

RURAL HEALTH INFRASTRUCTURE—NORMS AND LEVEL OF ACHIEVEMENTS (ALL INDIA)

Sl. No.	*Indicator*	*National Norms*		*Achievements*
1.	**Rural Population (2001) covered by a:**	**General**	**Tribal/ Hilly/ Desert**	
	Sub-Centre	5000	3000	5085
	Primary Health Centre (PHC)	30000	20000	31954
	Community Health Centre (CHC)	120000	80000	2.21 lakhs
2.	Number of Sub-Centres per PHC	6		6
3.	Number of PHCs per CHC	4		7
4.	**Rural Population (2001) covered by a:**			
	MPW (F)	5000	3000	5574
	MPW (M)	5000	3000	11994
5.	Ratio of HA (M) to MPW (M)	1:6.0		1:3\
6.	Ratio of HA (F) to MPW (F)	1:6.0		1:8
7.	**Average Rural Area (Sq. Km) covered by a:**			
	Sub-Centre	—		21.35
	PHC	—		134.20
	CHC	—		931.95
8.	**Average Radial Distance (Kms) covered by a:**			
	Sub-Centre	—		2.61
	PHC	—		6.53
	CHC	—		17.22
9.	**Average Number of Villages covered by a:**			
	Sub-Centre	—		4
	PHC	—		27
	CHC	—		19

APPENDIX 9.3

The Community Health Centres provide specialized medical care in the form of facilities of Surgeons, Obstetricians and Gynaecologists, Physicians and Paediatricians.

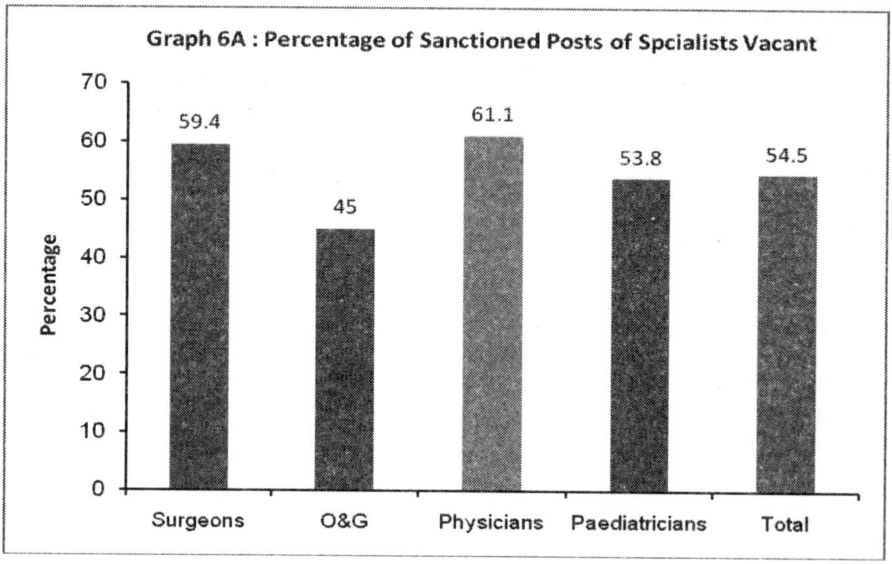

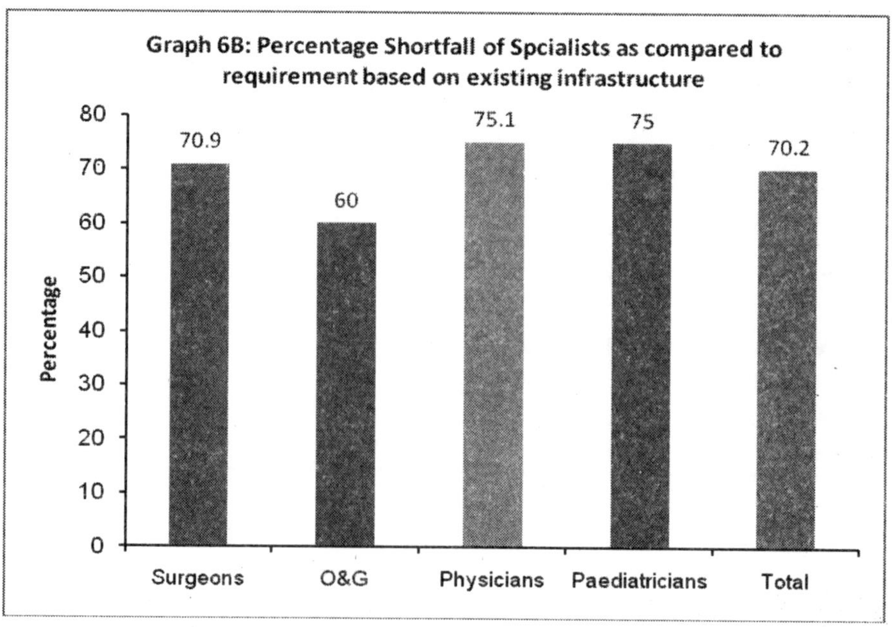

The current position of specialists manpower at CHCs reveal that out of the sanctioned posts, about 51.8% of Surgeons, 43.6% of Obstetricians and Gynaecologists, 56.5% of Physicians and about 56% of Paediatricians were vacant. Overall about 49.9% of the sanctioned posts of specialists at CHCs were vacant. Moreover, there was a shortfall of 6110 specialists at the CHCs as compared to the requirement for existing infrastructure on the basis of existing norms.

10

CHAPTER

Organisation and Working of Primary Health Centres

(A) RATIONALE AND PHILOSOPHY

Primary Health Centre is the pivot around which the success of Primary Health Care system revolves as it is first level of Primary Health Care

WHO has defined the health centre as that which covers all health facilities other than hospitals. It is usually the facility at the first contact level and has a unique potential, as well as responsibility, for increasing people's ability to solve their own problems with confidence. It provides a full range of health promotion and preventive services, as well as curative care limited mainly to ambulatory patients. It has multi-disciplinary team capable of providing the range of services mentioned above.[1]

The term health centre signifies the essential facilities for the promotion and protection of the health of the people. Primary health centres are to provide health education or preventive health services to rural people who suffer because of their old beliefs and superstitious.

In the district health system, each health centre should be responsible for a defined population so that no groups or families are left without a health team to provide care. The care should include accountability for outreach for essential public health and clinical services. In most countries this population will reside in a geographically defined area. If the boundaries relate to other functions of government, it is likely that the total population will be included in planning and implementation and this increases the potential for intersectoral collaboration. A major advantage is the much greater potential for sustainability and equity.[2]

A health centre is the main institution linking the health services with the people, it has the responsibility and unique potential for providing people with the ability and confidence to solve their own problems; it provides a full range of health promotion and preventive services including mother and child care; it provides curative care primarily to ambulatory patients and those with selected conditions. It has a multi-disciplinary team providing a range of services and may or may not have a doctor.[3]

The concept of the PHC as an institution to provide both curative and preventive services can be traced to the report of the consultative council on Medical and Allied Services, held in 1920, in England, under the Chairmanship of Lord Dawson of Penn.[4] In this region, the PHC was established at Kalutura, Ceylon, in 1926 with the assistance of Rockefeller Foundations.[5] The services offered at the centre were mainly preventive: health examinations of mothers and babies, imnunizations, environmental sanitation, health education, and mid-wifery. Little attention was paid to curative medical care, on the ground that such care was the function of outpatient departments at hospitals. In addition, it was felt that the provision of curative services would so overwhelm the staff that preventive care would be neglected.

One of the fathers of the health centre movement during this period was John Grant of the Rockefeller foundation who was Professor of Public Health at the Peking Union Medical School in 1920s where he based much of the teaching and research on an Eastern Health District Centre patterned on the one in Baltimore.

Another expert of primary health care was Andrija Stampar of Yugoslavia. He was a contemporary of Grant and they worked closely together over many years. He developed a nation-wide system of health centres.

Many developing countries especially in Asia, have felt the need to provide a model for their own planning of integrated health centres. Much of the thinking current during the 1940s and 1950s can be found in a report of the WHO Expert Committee on Public Health Administration, which mentions the basic services that should be offered by rural health units, the personnel needed for local health work, the cost and financing of local health programmes, and the planning of integrated health services.

Provision of Rural Health

Services through Rural Health Centres was recommended by the European Conference on Rural Hygiene of Geneva, in 1931 under the Health Organisation of League of Nations. It defined the "Rural Health Centres" as:

> "An institution for the promotion of the health and welfare of the people in a given (rural) area, which seeks to achieve its purpose by grouping under one roof or coordinating in some other manner, under the direction of a health officer, all the health work of that area, together with such welfare and relief organisations as may be related to the general public health work."[6]

A working group on the role and functions of Health Centres in District Health System met in Geneva from 12 to 16 July 1993 with participants from Dominica, Indonesia, Nigeria, Philippines and Senegal, who defined the concept as "The Generic Health Centre is a self-contained segment of the national health system guided by the district health service, of which it is a part. It comprises a variety of interrelated components that contribute to health in homes, schools, workplaces and the community, including support for self-care administered at home. These components are supported by a professional staff, together with appropriate diagnostic, laboratory and logistical services and coordinate in a dedicated management structure.[7]

The concept gathered momentum in socialist countries. The Inter-governmental Conference for Eastern countries, convened at Bandung under the auspices of League of Nations recommended the integration of preventive and curative services in preference to curative services. Similar developments took place in Eastern European countries that have come under the influence of socialism.[8] This concept spread to other countries after World War II.

The underlying idea of such thinking was to give priority to preventive health care as 75 per cent of diseases are preventable and the cost of prevention is much less than the cost for curative care.

(B) GENESIS AND GROWTH

Let us discuss in detail about the development of this concept in India. The Bhore Committee (1946) recommended that a Primary Health Centre should be set-up to serve as the focal point for providing comprehensive, curative and preventive health services in the rural areas. The report, in its long-term programme, recommended a primary health unit for a population of 20,000, a secondary unit for a population of 6,00,000 and a district headquarter's organisation for a population of three million. The committee in its short-term programme recommended a primary unit for a population of 40,000, a secondary unit for a population of one and a half million, and a district headquarter's organisation for a population of three million. To improve the operation of primary health centres, this committee recommended a reduction in the population covered by them, expansion and strengthening of district hospitals, and introduction of mobile teams of specialists to provide necessary supervisory and consultancy services to the periphery.

To cope with the family planning services required to control the rising population trend, the Government of India planned an expansion of facilities at Primary Health Centres and an increase in the number of sub-centres under each Primary Health Centre. Similarly, many health workers were provided to help in control of other endemic diseases. In this way, there was a great deal of proliferation of facilities and services. All these programmes were being run independent of each other by staff recruited under each programme. There was practically no co-ordination either at the field level or supervisory level. Such an isolated approach led to duplication, wastage of resources and poor impact on beneficiaries. This prompted the need for effective integration of services. To quote the first meeting of the executive committee of the Central Family Planning Council held on 20 September 1972: "Steps should be taken for the integration of medical, public health and family planning services at the peripheral level."[9]

The Planning Commission was also seized of the problem and in the report of the steering group on health, family planning and nutrition for the Fifth Five Year Plan, the following observations were made: "Family planning and nutrition have been in operation for a long time. These programmes are mostly vertically conceived and are being implemented at the field level by the staff deployed to implement these programmes individually, with little co-ordination or integration of the services. The steering group felt that the proper integration of health, family planning and nutrition programmes is highly desirable as it would be more economical and effective. This could be possible only by converting unipurpose workers into multipurpose workers. It may be appreciated that the multipurpose health worker (who may be designated as health auxiliary for convenience of reference) would be entrusted with carrying out integrated functions and would have greater rapport with the people in rural areas who would naturally look to him for all their needs in the field of naturally reinforcing components of health, family planning and nutrition."

In pursuance of these recommendations, the Government of India appointed a committee on multipurpose workers under the health and family planning programmes in October, 1972. The committee submitted its report in September, 1973 recommending: (i) Multipurpose workers for the delivery of health, family planning and nutrition services to the rural community, (ii) one PHC for every 50,000 population, (ii) each PHC to be divided into 16 sub-centres each having a population of 3,000-3,500 depending on topography and means of communication; (iv) each sub-centre to have a team of one male and one female worker; (v) one male and one female supervisor to supervise the work of four sub-centres; (vi) the doctors at PHC to divide the population on a geographical basis for their field visits; (vii) for effective integration of workers engaged in vertical programmes of health and family planning, the concept of integration to be extended to the district and state levels. The committee also suggested the job responsibilities and training progamme for various categories of health workers.

The Government of India accepted the recommendations of the committee except the ones in respect of one PHC for every 50,000 population and one sub-centre for 3,000 to 3,500 population; instead it was agreed to have a sub-centre for 5,000 population.

(C) STRENGTHENING OF INFRASTRUCTURE

The rural health infrastructure was to be further strengthened in the Sixth Plan to achieve the objective of Health for All by 2000 A.D. The norms elivisaged were: (i) one community health volunteer for every village for a population of 1,000 chosen by the community to form the base unit; (ii) one sub-centre for a population of 5,000 in the plains and 3,000 in the hilly and tribal areas; (iii) one PHC for 30,000 population in the plains and 20,000 in the hilly and tribal areas; (iv) one community health centre (CHC) for a population of one lakh or one community development block.

Health infrastructure in rural areas is of prime importance for realisation of the objectives set forth in the National Health Policy and for attaining the goal of 'Health for All' by the Year 2000 A.D. Co-ordinated efforts under various Rural Health Programmes are essential to provide effective and efficient services to the people in the rural areas.

Numerous programmes and schemes are being implemented under the Minimum Needs Programme to provide Primary Health Care relevant to the actual needs of the community in the rural areas. The status of establishment of the Sub-Centres, PHCs and Community Health Centres under the Minimum Needs Programme, has been of great significance. This development is in consonance with the thrust of all plans for Rural Development.

(D) EXTENT AND FUNCTIONS

Primary Health Centres

As on March 2006, 22669 Primary Health Centres were functioning. These increased from 9115 in Sixth Plan (1981-85) (Refer Table 10.1) to 22669 as on March 2006. Out of 22669 PHCs information about building position was available for 22584. Out of these, 17002 were functioning in the Government buildings, 3437 in rented buildings, 2145 rent free, 1838 buildings under constructing (See Table 10.2)

Out of 22669 doctors required for PHCs, 27927 post of Doctors have been sanctioned. There were 22273 doctors in position while 5801 were vacant giving a short fall of 1793 (Refer Table 10.3) . Out of 22669 Health Assistant, male required 24207 posts of Health Assistant, male were sanctioned, 18228 were in position, 5984 vacant posts giving a short fall of 7169 posts (refer table 10.4). Out of 22669 required Health Assistant (Female)/LHV, 19487 were sanctioned, 17107 were in position, 2871 vacant posts, giving a shortage of 5941 (Refer Table 10.5).

Table 10.6 depicts number of PHC with Doctors, Technicians and Pharacist. Out of 22669 PHCs, 419 have 4 doctor, 8483 doctors, 4702 have only 2 doctors, 10586 with one doctor, 1213 without doctor and 7284 with one lab technician and 3200 without pharmacist, 3019 with only one lady doctor. Table 10.7 examines block extension educator. Out of Sanctioned posts 5609 posts, 3165 were in position while 2447 were vacant.

CHART 10.1

Organsiational Structure of Primary Health Centre

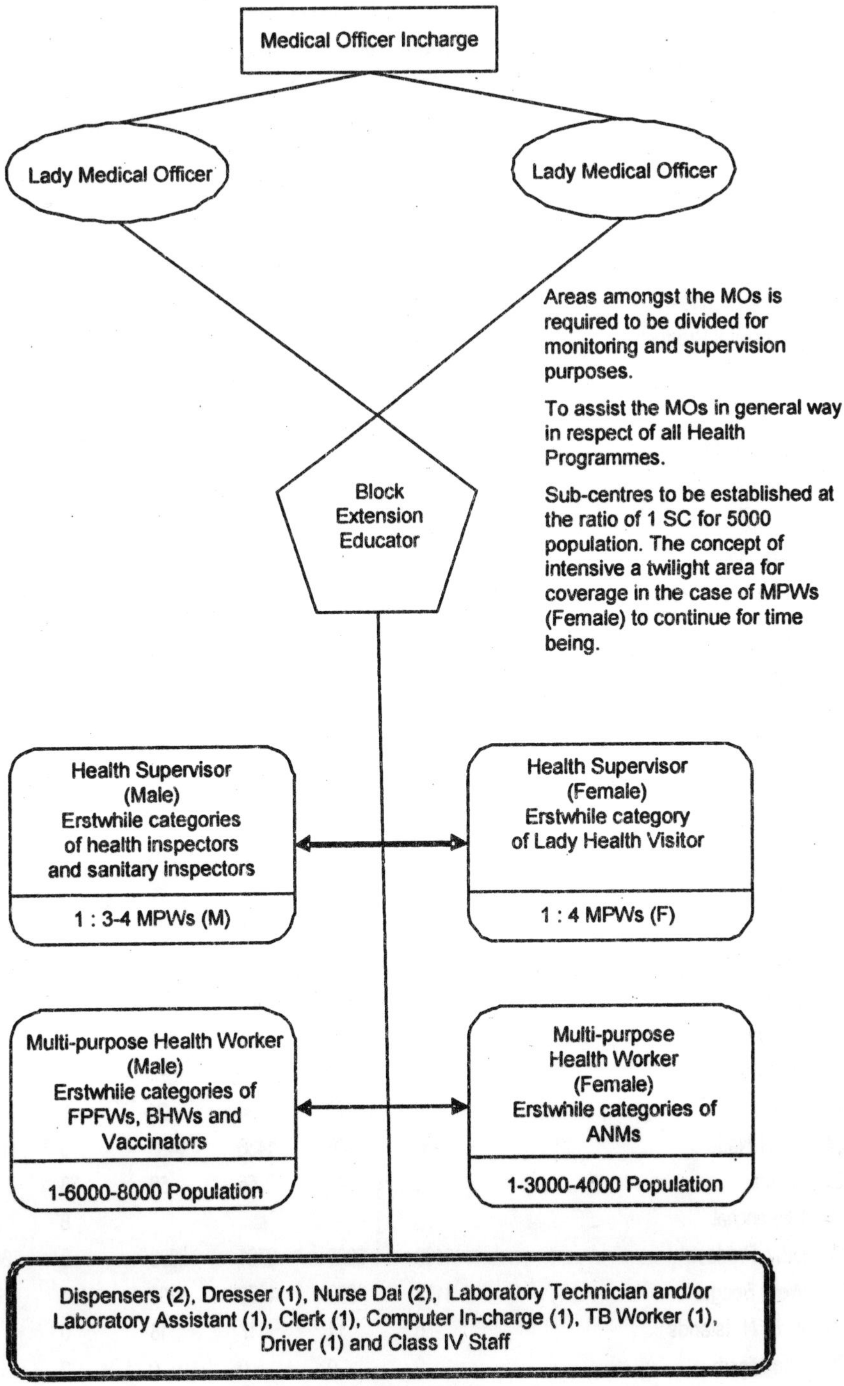

TABLE 10.1

Establishment of Sub-centres during Five Year Plans

Sl. No.	State/UT	Sub-Centres functioning at the end of					
		Sixth Plan [1981-85]	Seventh Plan [1985-90]	Eight Plan [1992-97]	Ninth Plan [1997-2002]	Tenth Plan Target	Sub-Centres Functioning[1] as on Sept. 2006
1.	Andhra Pradesh	555	—	1335	1386	321	1570
2.	Arunachal Pradesh	0	24	45	65	0	85
3.	Assam	237	449	610	610	116	610
4.	Bihar[1]	796	2001	2209	2209	319	1641
5.	Chhattisgarh					159	518
6.	Goa	13	17	17	19	4	19
7.	Gujarat	310	842	960	1032	0	1072
8.	Haryana	163	366	399	403	12	408
9.	Himachal Pradesh	106	190	260	302	0	439
10.	Jammu and Kashmir	123	266	335	337	0	374
11.	Jharkhand					115	330
12.	Karnataka	365	1142	1601	1676	0	1679
13.	Kerala[2]	199	908	938	944	0	909
14.	Madhya Pradesh[1]	680	1181	1690	1690	123	1192
15.	Maharashtra	1539	1671	1695	1768	0	1800
16.	Manipur	31	64	69	69	0	72
17.	Meghalaya	32	56	81	85	0	101
18.	Mizoram	19	35	55	58	0	57
19.	Nagaland	21	33	33	46	8	84
20.	Orissa	484	875	1102	1352	0	1279
21.	Punjab	130	460	484	484	0	484
22.	Rajasthan	448	1048	1616	1674	0	1713
23.	Sikkim	18	20	24	24	0	24
24.	Tamil Nadu	436	1386	1436	1436	0	1252
25.	Tripura	32	49	55	58	38	71
26.	Uttaranchal					8	222
27.	Uttar Pradesh[1]	1169	3000	3761	3808	0	3600
28.	West Bengal	1172	1250	1262	1262	464	922
29.	A & N Islands	6	14	17	18	0	20
30.	Chandigarh	0	0	0	0	2	0

31. D & N Haveli	3	5	6	6	1	6
32. Daman and Diu	2	2	3	3	0	3
33. Delhi	8	8	8	8	24	8
34. Lakshadweep	4	4	4	4	0	4
35. Pondicherry	14	22	39	39	0	39
All India	**9115**	**17388**	**22149**	**22875**	**1714**	**22669**

Notes: 1. There is a reduction in the number of centres functioning as on March 2006 as compared to those functioning at the end of Ninth Plan due to the divisionof state.

2. The number of Primary Health Centres reported functioning in Kerala has reduced as compared to that in 2002 because some PHCs are now falling in the urban area.

The number of Primary Health Centres reported functioning in some States has reduced as compared to that in 2002 due to upgradation of centres to CHCs.

Table 10.8 examines Pharmacist at PHC and CHC. Requirement in 26579 posts sanctioned in 22816, 18419 in position, 4445 vacant and short falls are 4389.

TABLE 10.2

Building Position for Primary Health Centres (As on March, 2006)

Sl. No. State/UT	Total Number of PHCs functioning	Number of PHCs for which information on building is available	Sub-Centres functioning in: Govt. Buildings	Rented Buildings	Rent Free Panchayat/ Vol. Society Buildings	under construction Buildings	Buildings requried[1] to be constructed
1. Andhra Pradesh	1570	1570	1281	289	0	194	95
2. Arunachal Pradesh	85	NA	NA	NA	NA	NA	NA
3. Assam	610	610	610	0	0	0	0
4. Bihar	1641	1641	842	286	513	23	776
5. Chhattisgarh	518	518	326	0	192	96	96
6. Goa	19	19	18	1	0	0	1
7. Gujarat	1072	1072	721	0	351	50	301
8. Haryana	408	408	290	0	118	41	77
9. Himachal Pradesh	439	439	312	46	81	40	87
10. Jammu and Kashmir	374	374	219	155	0	83	72
11. Jharkhand	330	330	117	185	28	0	213
12. Karnataka	1679	179	1439	90	150	92	148
13. Kerala	909	909	831	31	47	4	74
14. Madhya Pradesh	1192	1192	746	446	0	270	176
15. Maharashtra	1800	1800	1493	37	270	133	174
16. Manipur	72	72	39	0	333	8	25

(Contd.)

Sl. No.	State/UT	Total Number of PHCs functioning	Number of PHCs for which information on building is available	Sub-Centres functioning in Govt. Buildings	Rented Buildings	Rent Free Panchayat/ Vol. Society Buildings	under construction Buildings	Buildings requried[1] to be constructed
17.	Meghalaya	101	101	101	0	0	7	*
18.	Mizoram	57	57	57	0	0	0	0
19.	Nagaland	84	84	84	0	0	0	0
20.	Orissa	1279	1279	1279	0	0	0	0
21.	Punjab	484	484	409	0	75	1	74
22.	Rajasthan	1713	1713	1468	0	245	63	182
23.	Sikkim	24	24	24	0	0	0	6
24.	Tamil Nadu	1252	1252	1206	4	42	9	37
25.	Tripura	73	73	73	0	0	2	*
26.	Uttaranchal	222	222	182	40	0	14	26
27.	Uttar Pradesh	3660	3660	1835	1825	0	584	1241
28.	West Bengal	922	922	922	0	0	122	*
29.	A & N Islands	20	20	20	0	0	122	*
30.	Chandigarh	0	0	0	0	0	0	0
31.	D & N Haveli	6	6	6	0	0	0	0
32.	Daman and Diu	3	3	3	0	0	0	0
33.	Delhi	8	8	8	0	0	0	0
34.	Lakshadweep	4	4	4	0	0	0	0
35.	Pondicherry	39	39	37	2	0	2	0
	All India	**22669**	**22584**	**17002**	**3437**	**2145**	**1838**	**3875**

Notes: NA:Not available

1. Required number = Total functioning—(Government Buildings + Under Construction) (ignoring excess)

* States having construction in excess of the number required to be constructed.

TABLE 10.3

Doctors at PHCs (as on March 2006)

S. No.	State/UT	Required[1] [R]	Sanctioned [S]	In Position [P]	Vacant [S-P]	Shortfall [R-P]
1.	Andhra Pradesh	1570	2497	2202	295	*
2.	Arunachal Pradesh	85	78	78	0	7
3.	Assam	610	NA	NA	NA	NA
4.	Bihar	1641	2078	1606	472	35
5.	Chhattisgarh	518	1542	1154	388	*
6.	Goa	19	56	53	3	*
7.	Gujarat	1072	1070	907	163	165
8.	Haryana	408	570	433	137	*
9.	Himachal Pradesh	439	354	467	*	*

10. Jammu and Kashmir	374	668	643	25	*
11. Jharkhand	330	3906	2332	1574	*
12. Karnataka	1679	2237	2041	196	*
13. Kerala	909	1345	1151	194	*
14. Madhya Pradesh	1192	1278	839	439	353
15. Maharashtra	1800	1800	1191	609	609
16. Manipur	72	62	96	*	*
17. Meghalaya	101	127	106	21	*
18. Mizoram	57	57	35	22	22
19. Nagaland	84	53	53	0	31
20. Orissa	1279	1353	1353	0	*
21. Punjab	484	634	350	284	134
22. Rajasthan	1713	1525	1316	209	397
23. Sikkim	24	48	48	0	*
24. Tamil Nadu	1252	3089	2537	552	*
25. Tripura	73	161	152	9	*
26. Uttaranchal	222	272	182	90	40
27. Uttar Pradesh	3660	NA	NA	NA	NA
28. West Bengal	922	922	811	811	*
29. A & N Islands	20	36	36	0	*
30. Chandigarh	0	0	0	0	0
31. D & N Haveli	6	6	6	0	0
32. Daman and Diu	3	5	5	0	*
33. Delhi	8	31	23	8	*
34. Lakshadweep	4	4	4	0	0
35. Pondicherry	39	63	63	0	*
All India[2]	**22669**	**27927**	**22273**	**5801**	**1793**

Notes: NA: Not Available.

*: Surplus.

1 One per each Primary Health Centre.

2 For calculating the overall percentages, the States/UTs for which manpower position is not available, should be excluded

The broad functions of a PHC are: (1) Medical Care, (2) Maternal and Child Health Services, (3) School Health Services, (4) Family Planning, (5) Control of Communicable Diseases, (6) Environmental Sanitation, (7) Health Education, and (8) Vital Statistics. The staff to provide these services would comprise a medical officer, a woman physician, a public health nurse, a health educator, a statistical clerk, a clerk-stenographer, a mid-wife, a health inspector (Sanitarian), a laboratory technician, and several family planning field workers, with health assistant to assist the staff members. Similar range of health services has been mentioned in a "Guide to rural health centre work" issued by the Government of Burma.[10]

CHART 10.1

Buiding Position for PHC on March 2006

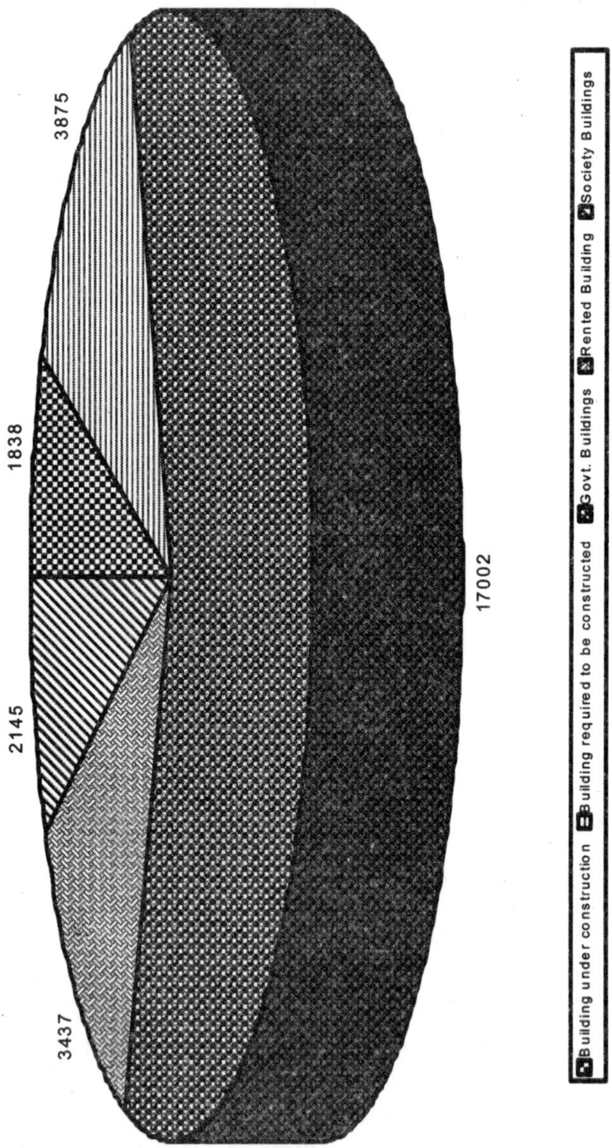

TABLE 10.4

Health Assistants (Male) at PHCs (as on March 2006)

S. No.	State/UT	Required[1] [R]	Sanctioned [S]	In Position [P]	Vacant [S-P]	Shortfall [R-P]
1.	Andhra Pradesh	1570	2162	1814	348	*
2.	Arunachal Pradesh	85	26	26	0	59
3.	Assam	610	NA	NA	NA	NA
4.	Bihar	1641	649	323	326	1318
5.	Chhattisgarh	518	3551	2940	611	*
6.	Goa	19	22	15	7	4
7.	Gujarat	1072	1265	616	649	456
8.	Haryana	408	416	256	160	152
9.	Himachal Pradesh	439	413	361	52	78
10.	Jammu and Kashmir	374	334	334	0	40
11.	Jharkhand	330	272	118	154	212
12.	Karnataka	1679	1302	837	465	842
13.	Kerala	909	802	796	6	113
14.	Madhya Pradesh	1192	1192	1168	24	24
15.	Maharashtra	1800	1800	1800	0	0
16.	Manipur	72	62	52	10	20
17.	Meghalaya	101	102	87	15	14
18.	Mizoram	57	57	57	0	0
19.	Nagaland	84	15	15	0	69
20.	Orissa	1279	176	168	8	1111
21.	Punjab	484	289	208	81	276
22.	Rajasthan	1713	938	714	224	999
23.	Sikkim	24	30	8	22	16
24.	Tamil Nadu	1252	384	303	81	949
25.	Tripura	73	153	152	1	*
26.	Uttaranchal	222	552	417	135	*
27.	Uttar Pradesh	3660	5712	4061	1651	*
28.	West Bengal	922	1496	550	946	372
29.	A & N Islands	20	0	0	0	20
30.	Chandigarh	0	0	0	0	0
31.	D & N Haveli	6	6	3	3	3
32.	Daman and Diu	3	3	3	0	0
33.	Delhi	8	NA	NA	NA	NA
34.	Lakshadweep	4	4	4	0	0
35.	Pondicherry	39	22	17	5	22
	All India[2]	**22669**	**24207**	**18223**	**5984**	**7169**

Notes: NA: Not Available.
*: Surplus
1. One per each Primary Health Centre
2. For calculating the overall percentages, the States/UTs for which manpower position is not available, should be excluded.

TABLE 10.5

Health Assistants (Female)/LHV at PHCs (as on March 2006)

Sl. No.	State/UT	Required[1] [R]	Sanctioned [S]	In Position [P]	Vacant [S-P]	Shortfall [R-P]
1.	Andhra Pradesh	1570	1614	1564	50	6
2.	Arunachal Pradesh	85	16	16	0	69
3.	Assam	610	NA	NA	NA	NA
4.	Bihar	1641	850	491	359	1150
5.	Chhattisgarh	518	779	709	70	*
6.	Goa	19	18	11	7	8
7.	Gujarat	1072	1227	862	365	210
8.	Haryana	408	231	101	130	307
9.	Himachal Pradesh	439	350	348	2	91
10.	Jammu and Kashmir	374	120	62	58	312
11.	Jharkhand	330	461	278	183	52
12.	Karnataka	1679	1209	1170	39	509
13.	Kerala	909	830	740	90	169
14.	Madhya Pradesh	1192	1192	1074	118	118
15.	Maharashtra	1800	1800	1718	82	82
16.	Manipur	72	41	55	*	17
17.	Meghalaya	101	85	75	10	26
18.	Mizoram	57	57	57	0	0
19.	Nagaland	84	15	15	0	69
20.	Orissa	1279	726	726	0	553
21.	Punjab	484	291	264	27	220
22.	Rajasthan	1713	1358	1358	0	355
23.	Sikkim	24	25	23	2	1
24.	Tamil Nadu	1252	1994	1734	260	*
25.	Tripura	73	69	62	7	11
26.	Uttaranchal	222	185	181	4	41
27.	Uttar Pradesh	3660	2535	2128	407	1532
28.	West Bengal	922	1726	1227	499	*
29.	A & N Islands	20	20	20	0	0
30.	Chandigarh	0	0	0	0	0
31.	D & N Haveli	6	7	5	2	1
32.	Daman and Diu	3	3	3	0	0
33.	Delhi	8	26	19	7	*
34.	Lakshadweep	4	0	0	0	4
35.	Pondicherry	39	14	11	3	28
	All India[2]	**22669**	**19874**	**17107**	**2781**	**5941**

Notes: NA: Not Available.

*: Surplus

1. One per each Primary Health Centre.
2. For calculating the overall percentages, the States/UTs for which manpower position is not available, should be excluded.

TABLE 10.6

Number of PHCs with Doctors and without Doctors/Lab Technician/Pharmacist

Sl. No.	State/UT	Total PHCs functioning	With 4 + Doctors	With 3 doctors	With 2 doctors	With 1 doctor	Without doctor	Without lab tech.	Without pharma.	With lady doctor
1	2	3	4	5	6	7	8	9	10	11
1.	Andhra Pradesh	1570	0	71	221	983	295	161	67	644
2.	Arunachal Pradesh	85	0	0	0	78	0	78	78	0
3.	Assam	610	26	80	314	190	0	185	0	NA
4.	Bihar	1641	141	137	317	925	121	810	686	74
5.	Chhattisgarh	518	0	0	518	0	0	249	157	80
6.	Goa	19	13	0	0	6	0	1	0	12
7.	Gujarat	1072	0	0	0	907	165	330	427	0
8.	Haryana	408	0	100	254	54	0	130	49	112
9.	Himachal Pradesh	439	0	4	51	373	11	35	125	67
10.	Jammu and Kashmir	374	0	26	308	0	0	0	NA	308
11.	Jharkhand	330	NA	NA	NA	NA	NA	NA	NA	NA
12.	Karnataka	1679	0	34	197	1448	0	452	375	360
13.	Kerala	909	28	201	70	591	19	633	24	392
14.	Madhya Pradesh[2]	1192	0	0	86	839	253	1106	412	22
15.	Maharashtra	1800	0	0	1366	392	42	886	210	503
16.	Manipur	72	3	7	19	33	10	39	32	22
17.	Meghalaya	101	2	2	15	82	0	1	11	48
18.	Mizoram	57	0	0	0	37	20	36	22	48

(Contd.)

TABLE 10.6 (Contd.)

1 2	3	4	5	6	7	8	9	10	11
19. Nagaland	84	0	0	0	60	27	83	23	0
20. Orissa	1279	0	0	120	1113	46	1162	48	62
21. Punjab	484	0	117	14	293	60	62	23	81
22. Rajasthan	1713	193	4	148	1238	130	113	245	68
23. Sikkim	24	0	0	24	0	0	0	24	23
24. Tamil Nadu	1252	NA	NA	NA	NA	NA	374	62	72
25. Tripura	73	10	11	25	25	2	40	25	7
26. Uttaranchal	222	0	42	45	135	0	35	9	11
27. Uttar Pradesh[1]	20	0	0	16	4	0	0	0	16
28. West Bengal	0	0	0	0	0	0	0	0	0
29. A& N Islands	6	0	0	2	41	0	0	0	0
30. Chandigarh	3	0	0	2	1	0	0	0	2
31. D & N Haveli	8	1	2	4	1	0	2	0	6
32. Daman and Diu	3	0	0	2	1	0	0	0	2
33. Delhi	8	1	2	4	1	0	2	0	6
34. Lakshadweep	4	0	0	2	0	2	0	0	0
35. Pondicherry	39	2	4	17	16	0	24	0	16
All India	**22669**	**419**	**848**	**4202**	**10586**	**1314**	**7284**	**3200**	**3019**

Notes: Figures are provisional.

In many states the total of the break of PHCs with 4+, 3, 2, 1 or no doctor do not tally with the total number of PHCs in the State.

NA: Not applicable.

For calculating the overall percentage, the States/UTs for which manpower position is not available, should be excluded.

1. One per each Primary Health Centre.
2. For calculating the overall percentages, the States/UTs for which manpower position is not available, should be excluded.

TABLE 10.7

Block Extension Educator (as on March 2006)

Sl. No.	State/UT	Sanctioned [S]	In Position [P]	Vacant [S-P]
1.	Andhra Pradesh	NA	NA	NA
2.	Arunachal Pradesh	2	0	2
3.	Assam	NA	NA	NA
4.	Bihar	394	80	314
5.	Chhattisgarh	210	183	27
6.	Goa	17	0	17
7.	Gujarat	251	251	0
8.	Haryana	90	62	28
9.	Himachal Pradesh	NA	NA	NA
10.	Jammu and Kashmir	123	67	56
11.	Jharkhand	NA	NA	NA
12.	Karnataka	531	428	103
13.	Kerala	161	256	16
14.	Madhya Pradesh	313	239	74
15.	Maharashtra	339	286	53
16.	Manipur	8	11	*
17.	Meghalaya	23	23	0
18.	Mizoram	20	12	8
19.	Nagaland	15	14	1
20.	Orissa	320	284	36
21.	Punjab	142	39	103
22.	Rajasthan	232	15	217
23.	Sikkim	9	3	6
24.	Tamil Nadu	383	273	110
25.	Tripura	18	14	4
26.	Uttaranchal	84	13	71
27.	Uttar Pradesh	1008	110	898
28.	West Bengal	900	600	300
29.	A & N Islands	0	0	0
30.	Chandigarh	1	1	0
31.	D & N Haveli	4	4	0
32.	Daman and Diu	2	2	0
33.	Delhi	9	6	3
34.	Lakshadweep	0	0	0
35.	Pondicherry	0	0	0
	All India[2]	**5609**	**3165**	**2447**

Notes: NA: Not Available.

*: Surplus.

1 One per each Primary Health Centre.

2 For calculating the overall percentages, the States/UTs for which manpower position is not available, should be excluded.

TABLE 10.8

Pharmacists at PHCs and CHCs (as on March 2006)

Sl. No.	State/UT	Required[1] [R]	Sanctioned [S]	In Position [P]	Vacant [S-P]	Shortfall [R-P]
1.	Andhra Pradesh	1737	1704	1637	67	100
2.	Arunachal Pradesh	116	31	31	0	85
3.	Assam	710	NA	NA	NA	NA
4.	Bihar	1711	989	291	698	1420
5.	Chhattisgarh	636	749	467	282	169
6.	Goa	24	28	27	1	*
7.	Gujarat	1345	1363	7987	566	548
8.	Haryana	490	517	439	78	51
9.	Himachal Pradesh	505	505	375	130	130
10.	Jammu and Kashmir	454	456	456	0	*
11.	Jharkhand	524	689	310	379	214
12.	Karnataka	1933	1935	1880	55	53
13.	Kerala	1016	1038	1012	26	4
14.	Madhya Pradesh	1421	1419	216	1203	1205
15.	Maharashtra	2207	2367	1976	391	231
16.	Manipur	88	26	65	*	23
17.	Meghalaya	126	145	113	32	13
18.	Mizoram	66	69	35	34	31
19.	Nagaland	105	85	85	0	20
20.	Orissa	1510	2040	1984	56	*
21.	Punjab	610	736	680	56	*
22.	Rajasthan	2038	2375	2355	20	*
23.	Sikkim	28	28	0	28	28
24.	Tamil Nadu	1417	1442	1380	62	37
25.	Tripura	83	47	56	*	27
26.	Uttaranchal	271	290	287	3	*
27.	Uttar Pradesh	4046	NA	NA	NA	NA
28.	West Bengal	1268	1614	1341	273	*
29.	A & N Islands	24	28	28	0	*
30.	Chandigarh	1	2	2	0	*
31.	D & N Haveli	7	8	8	0	*
32.	Daman and Diu	4	4	4	0	0
33.	Delhi	8	13	11	2	*
34.	Lakshadweep	7	11	11	0	*
35.	Pondicherry	43	63	60	3	*
	All India[2]	**26579**	**22816**	**18419**	**4445**	**4389**

Notes: NA: Not Available.

*: Surplus

1 One per each Primary Health Centre.

2 For calculating the overall percentages, the States/UTs for which manpower position is not available, should be excluded.

PHC is supposed to provide the following functions:

1. to provide preventive, promotive, curative and rehabilitative services with emphasis on preventive health care,
2. to meet local needs based on largely local resources,
3. to function as a unit for the promotion of positive health and not merely serve as a dispensary,
4. to ensure equitable and qualitative services and not merely rudimentary and traditional services,
5. to join with other sectors of socio-economic development to optimise benefit for the promotion of health services,
6. to make frequent visits to the community in order to develop sound relationships,
7. to make community surveys to locate critical areas and people needing their help,
8. to arrange exhibitions to make people aware of health developments and educate them in health education measures.
9. to provide training to workers in the centre,
10. to keep in constant touch with district, state and central health authorities, health research institutions to get advice and guidance,
11. to develop team work,
12. to encourage community leaders to support health development activities of health centres, and
13. health centres should empower community to take decisions with the support of PHC.

After all, moving towards greater equity is the first key principle in the PHC strategy. "PHC needs to redress the imbalance created by inbuilt biases in favour of high technology medicines and affluent urban dwellers, and against the poor anywhere. Reorientation towards PHC, therefore, involves centering attention on resource allocation among different types of activity, levels of care and geographical areas."[11] Let us understand the role of Primary Health Centre *vis-a-vis* secondary and tertiary hospitals.

Primary Health Care is the first level of contact between the individual and the health system where essential health care (primary health care) is provided. A majority of prevailing health complaints and problems can be satisfactorily dealt with at this level. This level of care is closest to the people. In the Indian context, this care is provided by the primary health centres, with community participation.

Secondary Health Care deals with more complex problems. This care comprises essentially curative services and is provided by the district hospitals, sub-divisional hospitals, area hospitals, and community health centres. This level serves as the first referral level in the health system as the patients are referred to such medical institutes from the Primary Health Centre.

Tertiary Health Care offers superspecialist care. This care is provided by the regional/central hospitals, teaching hospitals and superspeciality hospitals. These institutions provide not only highly specialized care, but also planning and managerial skills and teaching for specialized staff.

There is a Need of Making Primary Health Centres functional to inject economy and efficiency in health system. Hospitals provide a wide variety of services, from basic care to highly specialized diagnosis and treatment, depending on the technological capacity of a specific hospital. There is considerable duplication of services provided at different levels. Tertiary hospitals though equipped with highly sophisticated equipment with advanced technical capacity have to devote considerable time and resources to deliver basic secondary and even primary health care as there is lack of confidence in the system for secondary and primary health care or the people don't feel satisfied with them. Tertiary hospitals, however, are designed to treat only complicated cases, and because of their composition of skilled staff and medical equipment, the cost of treating a patient is much higher than the cost would be for the same type of patient in lower level or specialized alternative facilities. This undesirable use of the capacity of tertiary hospitals affects our patient and inpatient services. The outpatient departments of large tertiary care hospitals often suffer from overcrowding; this situation is exacerbated by the presence of a large number of patients who require only basic curative care that could be provided in a lower cost setting such as a district hospital or health centre like sub-divisional hospitals, CHCs or other lower run medical centres. If patients requiring basic care could be shifted to medically appropriate lower level or alternative treatment facilities, health system costs would be reduced and economic efficiency improved as the per capita cost of both outdoor and indoor patients is too high in these hospitals.

Analysis of discharge information by cause and severity of the illness or condition is needed to assess the potential for reallocation of the case load within different hospital systems. In large tertiary facilities, perhaps 75% of outpatient care and 30% to 50% of inpatient care could be easily and effectively delivered in district hospitals or at lower levels, i.e. PHCs. A comparison of the cost per outpatient visit or inpatient day between varying levels of hospital suggests that the savings could be of the order of 50% of current costs per patient. PHCs can take care of 75 per cent of diseases at their levels. Therefore, there is a need of assessment of working of Primary Health Centres to make them effective and efficient.

ORGANISATIONAL STRUCTURE OF PHC

(a) Organisation

The PHC functions with a Medical Officer of Health or Administrative Medical Officer as the chief of the PHC, and a Lady Medical Officer (LMO) as the second medical officer. One Block Extension Educator, one Pharmacist, a Para-Medical Worker and two Senior Health Assistants (a male and a female) function under the Medical Officer's supervision. Seven Male Multipurpose workers are under the supervision of the Senior Health Assistant (Male) and seven Female Multipurpose workers work under the supervision of the Senior Health Assistant (Female). Three staff members in the category of Group D (Class IV) form the lowest staff category of PHC. In the sub-centre, trained dais (TBAs), who are not government employees, help multipurpose worker (Female) when required.

The buildings of PHC are not adequate to meet the needs. The infrastructure generally includes a hall, 5 rooms and two inpatient wards. The hall serves as the outpatient ward, where the Administrative Medical Officer (AMO) examines the patients. The room adjacent to the right side of the hall is being used as Injection room. The room to the left of the hall is supposed to be 'Dispensary' where the pharmacist is expected to dispense medicines/drugs as per doctor's prescriptions.

In the other wing are two rooms and an inpatient ward. The first room is occupied by the Lady Medical Officer (LMO) who examines the patients there. The room adjacent to this room is the rest room as well as the staff room. Another inpatient ward is built opposite the room of the Lady Medical Officer.

Though two rooms with six beds each are provided for inpatients, due to lack of residential quarters and basic facilities, admission of inpatients is a rare phenomenon. Only emergency delivery cases and asthma cases are admitted for 2-3 days. Patients with severe weakness are admitted just for the day (working hours) to administer glucose drips and later discharged the same evening.

Let us now analyse the duties and responsibilities of important functionaries of PHC.

(b) Role of the Doctor (Administrative)

The PHC team is led by a Medical Officer (Administrative) of Health. Generally a lady medical officer acts as the second medical officer. While the role of the Medical Officer of Health (also called Administrative Medical Officer, AMO) includes the management of the PHC (all administrative aspects) besides attending to patients, the function of a Lady Medical Officer (LMO) is basically attending to patients alone. Only when the AMO is on leave, or is away on official work, the LMO acts as the Officer Incharge of the PHC. We now discuss the responsibilities of medical officer in-charge of the PHC.

The Medical Officer of primary health centre is responsible for providing direction and guidance in all the health activities radiating from the health centre. He keeps himself fully conversant with the area, topography, demography, community health needs and public health problems. Being the chief-executive of health of the area, he undertakes promotive, preventive and curative work in an integrated manner. For this purpose, the medical officers in the primary health centre divide the area amongst themselves on a geographical basis and are responsible for all the health programmes in their respective areas.

One of the very important tasks of the medical officer is to supervise, direct and control the performance of the sub-centres organisation within the scope of law, policy and regulations already established. He can achieve effective supervision through a number of methods, viz. setting of service standards, budgetary control; reporting system, inspections, etc. In order to be effective as a supervisor, he must possess three qualities, job competence, the ability to guide the subordinates and the personal traits like ability to cooperate and motivate others.

The Chief Executive is to ensure participation of people in the formulation and implementation of plans and programmes. Imaginative measures are needed on the part of the medical officer to promote and sustain the interests of the citizens in the administration to give them a sense of participation in the decisions that immediately affect them and to enable them to contribute to better administration.

Implementation of Programmes

Words, written or spoken, are of no use unless they are put into action. The emphasis should be more on performance rather that paper planning. Khalid Gibran has rightly said, that "believing is a fine thing, but placing those beliefs into execution is a test of strength. Many are those who talk like the roar of the sea, but their lives are shallow and stagnant, like the rotting marshes. Many are those who lift their heads above the mountain tops, but their spirit remains dormant in the obscurity of the caverns."

Walter R. Sharp has also mentioned the importance of the personnel in the organisation. He says: "Even poorly devised machinery may be made to work if it is manned with well-trained, intelligent, imaginative and devoted staff. On the other hand, the best planned organisation may produce unsatisfactory results if it is operated by mediocre or disgruntled people."[12]

Besides, the doctors must have faith in the ideals of the PHC programmes, be willing to accept hardships and be prepared to work in the spirit of service. Their ambition and enthusiasm should not be dampened by local conditions which may not provide them with the necessary facilities.

Unfortunately, the sense of dedication has been the crassest casualty of the prevailing atmosphere of cynism bred by increasing propensity towards expediency.[13]

(c) Role of Block Extension Educator[14]

The Block Extension Educator functions under the technical supervision and guidance of District Extension and Media Officer. However, he is under the immediate administrative control of the Medical Officer in-charge of PHC. One of his primary responsibilities is to promote community participation for ensuring self-reliance in the community. He is responsible for providing support to and National Health and Family

Welfare Programmes in the PHC but the main function relates to the promotion of FW and MCH programmes.

Role of Senior Health Assistants

Health Assistants (Male and Female) have separate headquarters and work separately. They are not supposed to issue any instructions to the multipurpose health workers who report weekly to the BHO/MO who in turn, issue necessary instructions to the multipurpose health workers. In MCH clinic, ante-natal and post-natal clinics are attended by the health assistant (female) and concerned multipurpose health worker (female). The number of such clinics under the supervision of health assistants (female) has been increased to 20 clinics in a month instead of 4 earlier. The worker (female) attends to the clinic and the pregnant and other female patients and children in the village. In the clinic, all the women in the area are to be given TT irrespective of the fact whether they are pregnant or not. The children are given immunisation against six deadly diseases, namely, diphtheria, pertussis, tatanus, tuberculosis and polo myelitis. The health assistant (f) are to supervisor the Anganwadis and ensure that children are being given protected water and clean food supplements.

An analysis of work of senior health assistants male and female revealed the following:

(a) Their supervision of sub-centres is not adequate. No report of visits was available resulting in inaction.
(b) Multipurpose workers have poor perception of their professional skills. They need to be given refresher courses.
(c) They lack in communication skills vital for such programmes. They may be trained in the art and science of communication.
(d) They lack the art of health education, vital for the success of all programmes.

The senior health assistants, alongwith multipurpose workers, should devote personal attention to health education and not leave it to media alone.

Sociologists have categorised diffusion process, which leads to a widespread acceptance of the programmes, into five critical stages; awareness (the individuals first introduction to a new idea or practice), interest (the stage at which he actively seeks further information and background data), evaluation (the stage of assessment on critical grounds), trial (a limited phase of experiment), and finally, acceptance or adoption. These processes have been occurring for centuries. The need of the present day health administration is to accelerate adoption of the health programmes and to control diffusion process in a short span of time to achieve effective implementation of health programme"[15]

Alastair Metheson, Deputy Director of UNICEF's division remarks on the basis of his research that, "To get people to act in ways that conform to new values almost always requires that mass communications be reinforced by personal influence."[16]

Role of Pharmacist

A pharmacist in PHC is normally appointed to: (i) dispense medicines/drugs as per the prescriptions given by the medical officers, and (ii) maintain a record of No. of outpatients treated (as also the no. of inpatients, where beds are provided and inpatients treatment is given).

It was observed that the pharmacist spent very little time on dispensing drugs. He was generally found to be busy with office correspondence or certificate work. He was sent to the treasury to submit the pay bill of the PHC staff and later to collect the salary cheques. This could be attributed to the fact that PHCs have no clerical staff to perform these functions.

CRITICAL APPRAISAL

Creation of Primary Health Centres has not served its real purpose as health care activities are not being provided properly at this level, resulting in great rush at secondary and tertiary level. Besides, it is causing great hardships to rural population and urban slums as well as wastage of colossal amounts aimed at providing adequate and efficient health care. Since the success of secondary and tertiary care depends upon the soundness of Primary Health Care, therefore, it is essential to ensure its fruitful functioning.

Neither the infrastructure nor the personnel working here are satisfactory resulting in unsatisfactory functioning at this level. In most of the states, there were bitter complaints about Government run PHCs. It was mentioned in the consolidated reports from various states that PHCs are disgustingly dirty, patients are lying on the floors, there is even lack of elementary articles like spirit and cotton sheets are drenched in blood. There were complaints about the corruption and indifference of doctors and Class IV employees. Medicines meant for free distribution are reported to be illegally sold.

Dr. M.D. Saigal, Deputy Director General of Health Services also mentioned that out of the 4,500 PHCs, 700 are without any buildings while 2,620 have no staff quarters; out of the 39,000 sub-centres functioning today, 15,000 have no buildings.[17] We give some of the facts and suggestions which can help in improving the performance of the Primary Health Centres.

1. Lack of Coordination among the Developmental Agencies

There are a large number of developmental agencies working at block level and villages under its jurisdiction. We have already discussed that health affects and is affected by all other sectors of development. We find no coordination among these agencies. It is suggested that all the developmental agencies in a particular area must promote the process of development simultaneously to produce sustained impact on the population inhabiting these areas.

2. Absence of Organised Structure for People's Participation

We do not find any organised structure in a block at any level to involve the beneficiaries and utilise their potential energy profitably. It is very difficult for the government to contact all the individuals/families through their paid employees. There is a need for some structure or groups of people to help themselves under the guidance of the expert advice offered by the government. We have already witnessed the failure of the Community Development Programmes as we could not associate the people with our programmes. It is suggested that the Health Department may try to set-up voluntary organisations of the people in collaboration with other developmental agencies to ensure effective communication and understanding.

3. Poor Quality of Service

Most of the people complain of very poor quality of services at PHC. A frequent question in many countries in relation to health centres is: why are people bypassing them? The answer is usually to be found in the poor quality of care. Quality is a complex notion not connected merely with technical procedures, expensive drugs, and sophisticated apparatus. It has perhaps more to do with the reliability of services and with the provision of those services in a way that ensures an equitable approach, accessibility, accountability, and continuity. Understanding any concern on the part of health personnel would add sufficiently to confidence in health centres services to make people feel secure and satisfied. Frequent staff changes, an excessive burden of tasks, and poor motivation worsen the perceived quality of services. However, the main problem more often lies in inappropriate technologies, inadequacy and unreliability of supplies, poorly trained health workers, deficient referral systems and poor organisation of work.

4. Absence of Linkages with Cultural, Social and Religious Institutions

We know that the success of health programmes depends upon their acceptance by the people. It was found that the health personnel do not try to go into the cultural, religious and social factors affecting the health of the people. These are very subtle factors which need our attention and care. The health personnel must try to enlist the cooperation of informal leaders who can help in accelerating the acceptance of these programmes. Customs and conventions of the area must be studied which can throw light on the behaviour of the people. It would be very easy to help the people provided we understand their attitude and preferences.

5. Absence of Political Will and Direction

We already know of the political crisis in the country and absence of rationality among the political leaders at the block and the lower levels. There is a need to create political will and sensitivity towards development. The Department of Health should motivate the local political leaders to associate them in the developmental tasks.

6. Absence of Missionary Spirit among the Health Personnel

The problems of public health are challenging as can be gauged from the statistics already enumerated. It is very difficult to solve these problems with bureaucratic and inhuman attitudes. It requires hard work, sympathy, and tolerance on the part of the health, personnel engaged in this arduous and challenging task. Most of the people felt that the personnel working are fulfiling only their legal duties that too reluctantly. We do not need highly specialized people in these areas. We, however, require dedicated people with missionary zeal to serve the people suffering from abject poverty. We must ensure the people of their full involvement in their own welfare.

7. Non-Involvement of the Universities in the Planning and Implementation of the Programme

It is a matter of great regret that no attempt is being made to associate the faculty members of the universities and colleges to involve them with these programmes. The teachers through their knowledge and influence can help a lot in this direction if they are given due status. Some of them can take up such studies as research projects or encourage their research students to undertake such problems. Such studies can be of great use in improving the implementation and the future planning.

8. Absence of Informal Supervision through Medical Colleges/Institutes

There is no involvement of the medical colleges/institutes in the area. There must be a regular dialogue between these institutions and the persons responsible for the planning and implementation of the programme of Primary Health Care. Student doctors may be encouraged to take interest in such projects. This would ensure the quick success and the future benefits in other areas.

9. Absence of Research in the Flora and Fauna of the Area

The health department is providing allopathic medicines to the people. These medicines have side effects and are costly. No attempt is being made to encourage research in the flora and fauna of the area which can provide cheap and effective medicine without side effects. The flora and fauna of the area is full of promise. This would encourage the development of the area also indirectly. We may extract medicines from plants and animals available in the area. This would be possible only if our research in the medical colleges/institutes is relevant to the area rather than only of theoretical significance and utility.

The need for research to improve health centre function is especially acute at present because for at least two decades the role and function of health centres has been largely ignored. From the past 50 years of experience worldwide have come strong but often invalid assumptions about the functions and approaches to be used in health centres. Traditional work patterns have been solidly bureaucratized in many health systems so that one of the first issues to be confronted is the explicit need to create an intellectual climate to encourage change and improvement. The concept of primary health care, the types of interventions now available, the interactions with the rest of the health systems, and the potential for communicating with and mobilizing the community are, so different from what they were when the health centres were originally set-up in developing countries that it is time for a major process of reappraisal.

The fundamental need is to encourage a spirit of problem -solving among both the health centre staff and the community. Systematic problem-solving can be organised best through applied field research. Health systems research, to systematize problem solving, is becoming more important as health centres search for ways to improve access, utilisation, and quality of care. If health centres make community diagnoses, then the most elementary research is already a component of existing activities. Likewise, if health centres can develop adequate information systems, then simple applied research will follow naturally. Health centres should ensure that problem-solving is a routine daily activity.

Author conducted a research study in Haryana on 20 PHC and 100 respondents (5 from each PHC).

They were asked about their awareness of PHC, 95 percent of them were aware of these facilities. When they were asked about their functioning, they came out with the following facts:

TABLE 10.9

Reactions of the villagers about the working of the Primary Health Centres (Percentage)

S. No.	Activities	Yes	No
1.	Punctuality of the PHC staff	X	100
2.	Equipment in Working Order	40	60
3.	Proper examination of Patients and Delays	60	40
4.	Prompt and Courteous Behaviours	50	50
5.	Availability of Medicine	30	70
6.	Arrangement for Indigenous system of medicine	X	100
7.	Health Education Services	70	30
8.	Involvement of the people	50	50
9.	Well designed referral systems	X	100

FINDINGS OF THE STUDY[18]

The author conducted the research study of Primary Health Centres in Punjab. The results are as follows:

1. Inadequate PHC Buildings

All the Primary Health Centers were functioning in buildings whether Government or rented which have limited available space. Besides there is not sufficient availability of residential accommodation in remote rural areas, which is acting as a great deterrent in motivating medical officers to work in such areas.

There is an urgent need of providing adequate building accommodation in each centre to provide good environment for service. Besides, the construction of houses for the staff should be taken up as it will increase the morale and efficiency of the personnel working there.

2. Public Health Facilities

The PHCs are supposed to provide health education to the people. This would be possible only if the premises of the PHCs are clean and well equipped. It was found that most of the centres had no public health facilities, like flush latrines, piped water supply and electricity.

3. Medicines and Equipment

The supply of medicines and equipment was inadequate in most of the health centres due to the paucity of resources. Besides, there was no regular supply. The stock of medicines was inadequate in all the centres.

Steps may be taken to ensure adequate and timely supply of medicines and equipment to health centres. They should maintain adequate stock of at least life saving drugs. This will raise the confidence of the people in PHCs and the people would not rush, unnecessarily to city hospitals. Medicine may not be provided according to quota system but should be given according to the needs of the people.

For efficient discharge of curative functions, the Primary Health Centres should be provided sufficient equipment like refrigerators, X-ray and laboratory facilities, oxygen cylinders, operation tables and surgical instruments. It may also be ensured that X-ray plants and laboratories remain in working condition. The existing laboratories should be suitably strengthened with equipment.

Each Primary Health Centre in the State had been provided laboratory under National Malaria Eradication Programme for the examination of malaria cases. But many of these laboratories were not equipped to handle cases for investigation of general diseases.

4. Health Education

Dissemination of health education among the masses is an important function of the health workers. It was found that health education of the people was not being done scientifically since the villagers were found ignorant about the basic health and hygienic practices.

5. Indoor Beds

Indoor beds in PHCs generally remain unutilized. It would be worthwhile if some of these beds were transferred to the nearest referral hospitals and reserved for patients referred to it by the Primary Health Centres. These beds may be utilised for other patients in case these remain unutilised. This arrangement would serve a dual purpose of reserving beds for the PHCs and also increasing the bed strength in referral hospitals.

6. Location not Ideal

While opening a new Primary Health Center care may be taken in selecting such a site which should be easily accessible to the largest number of villages in the block as it was revealed that only those people who are within 2-3 Kms. of the PHCs, are the frequent visitors to the PHC.

7. Administrative Powers of Medical Officers not Sufficient

For efficient functioning of the centres, the administrative powers should be decentralised. The Medical Officer of the PHC is supposed to be the planner, the manager, the supervisor, the coordinator as well as the Public Relation Officer, besides being a technical expert. Is he well equipped to discharge all these functions entrusted to his care? At present, all the incumbents possess no administrative competence which is essential to administer the PHC complex. It is suggested that the officers of the PHCs may be got trained in health administration either at NIHFW or some special course may be arranged for them at the State headquarters. In order to supervise and inspect sub-centres, transport facilities should be provided.

8. Linkage between Community and PHC

There are very poor linkages between the PHC staff and the community. The staff rarely find time to visit the community and diagnose its problems to ascertain its needs. The Medical Education Committee appointed by the Government of India observed that medical education should produce a basic doctor. The Committee defined: "A basic doctor is one who is well conversant with the day-to-day health problems of the rural and urban communities and who is able to play an effective role in the curative and preventive aspects of the regional and the national health problems." It is suggested that the PHC staff must visit once a week to provide health education through well arranged lectures in school building/panchayat ghars or arrange exhibitions. This would lay the foundation of health care administration.

There is a need of courteous behaviour with the patients who are already troubled with their sufferings. They can be made at ease through courteous behaviour. Tarun Bahl in his article, "Courtesy as a habit" in the *Daily Tribune*, Oct. 10, 1999 rightly stresses the value of courtesy. To quote him, "The good thing about practising courtesy is that while it costs nothing, it can bring rich dividends. No one is too big or too busy to be courteous. It enhances others self-worth and prods them to be good in return. Many brilliant and talented people were obnoxhus, pig-headed, insolent, ungrateful and ill-mannered. Their prosperity clouded their judgement and they forgot that they had to treat others with respect, dignity and humility before they can be accorded the same regard."

9. Vacant Posts Need to be Filled

Immediate steps may be taken to fill up the vacant posts of doctors and other para-medical staff to provide health care to the people. One lady doctor may be posted in each Primary Health Center, since rural women generally prefer to be examined by a lady doctor. Besides, the PHC may be put under the control of medical colleges to make the services more effective. This would also provide opportunity to undergraduate medical students to ascertain the health needs of the population.

The Fifth Plan (Approach Papers) also emphasised that the main thrust may be directed at making up the deficiencies in building staff, equipment and drugs and medicines in a coordinated way. Such studies and evaluation may be encouraged by the Health Department on institutional basis to provide clues for the effective functioning of PHCs. There is a need to invest funds to evaluate the functioning of these centres. If inadequate funds are invested, the entire effort may well be wasted whereas properly designed and supported research may yield the answer to this important question. The purpose of the study should be to ensure that PHCs and sub-centres are giving the best possible coverage in preventive and curative services within the resources available.

In the new millennium, we have to strengthen the local health system. Dr. Hiroshi Nakajima, Director-General of World Health Organisation in his Editorial "50 years of making people healthier" rightly stresses that: "Building up integrated health services at local level continues to be a major strategy, and has been the key to success in many areas. It has played a leading role in improving health status and increasing the life expectancy. In recent years, the Organisation has moved to broader family health approaches to provide people with a continuum of essential care at all stages of their lives and in their communities. These approaches can be traced back to the inclusive definition of health adopted in our Constitution, as well as to the primary health care strategy. But our new policy reflects a change in focus: attention now centres not so much on structures as on the people they exist to serve. In the future an even greater effort will be needed to understand users' needs, expectations and potential to contribute to the definition and implementation of health priorities and interventions.

This change in perspective reflects a growing awareness of the importance of developing an open and mutually respectful dialogue between health professionals and the public. Empowering people, especially women, in all cultures and segments of society with the necessary information and opportunities for health development is both an ethical and a technical imperative.

CONCLUSION

The success of the Primary Health Centre depends, to a great extent, upon the harmonious relationships between the citizens and health administration. Health administration should not function as a machinery but in a humane and purposeful way. The people in health administration should have a sense of dedication, responsibility, and be responsive and alert to the aspirations of the citizens. Citizens, on the other hand, should also provide meaningful cooperation to health administration. Under such an atmosphere, it would be very easy to provide health care to meet the needs of the people. The strengthening of primary health care system has to be attained through the participation of the people.

Good citizens and the health system relationship would:

(a) Encourage people's participation—a *sine quo non* for development and modernization of health system.
(b) Kindle the potential energy of the citizens into kinetic energy to accelerate health development;
(c) Supplement the efforts of the health system in the conduct of its affairs.
(d) Strengthen the values of democracy in the minds and spirit of the people;
(e) Enlist respect in the health system which is vital for the success of health system.
(f) Develop bonds of friendship and goodwill between citizen and health care system and *vice versa*.

Health system is never something apart from people and their needs, rather it is the means by which these needs are met and the health administrator who thinks of his organisation as something apart from the community will fail to recognize significant problems of the citizens and the health administration will not be in a position to deliver the goods.

Besides, the Government through its health department must be serious in overseeing the implementation of health policy at Primary Health Centres earnestly, otherwise every good intention for the promotion of health care would remain on the paper only. In the Third Five Year Plan, it has been rightly commented that "Nevertheless, without a concerted attempt to make the administration much more action-oriented than at present, these may not yield enough results."

The widespread visibility and feeling of inefficiency of Health Administration machinery of PHC has caused great damage to the delivery of good health care to the people. That is why, there is a disconcerting gap between intention and action of health services. To bridge this gap, we should boldly adopt whatever far reaching change in administration may be found necessary. We must introduce new organisational patterns and modern tools and techniques of management and administration. We should instill into the health system greater efficiency and a sense of urgency and make it more responsive to the need of the people.[19]

We can say that the success of health care system depends on impartial honest, efficient, dedicated, and action-oriented health administration. Words written or spoken are of no use unless put to action.

We may sum up in the words of A.P. Barnabas: For democracy to be successful at the national level, the grassroots organisations have to be strong. The local authorities have to respond to the felt needs of the people. The citizens have to have faith in the efficacy of the administrative system so that the distance between people and the government is reduced. The administration, for good governance, has to be accessible. In developing countries, it is the government, which initiates and implements development programmes. It must gain support of the people in the discharge of these programmes, particularly at the cutting edge. Such support would strengthen democracy as well as a positive response of the community to development programme, which should be the ultimate goal of good governance."[20]

Notes and References

1. WHO, District Health Systems: Global and Regional Review Based on Experience in Various Countries, Geneva, 1995, p. 18.
2. WHO: The Health Centre in District Health System, Geneva, 1994, p. 5.
3. *Ibid.*
4. League of Nations Health Organisation, European Conference on Rural Hygiene (1931), Recommendations on the Principles Governing the Organisation of Medical Assistance, The Public Health Services and Sanitation in Rural Districts of Geneva
5. W.G. Wickremesingh, The Premier Health Unit in Ceylon, Colombo, 1951.
6. League of Nations Health Organisation, European Conference on Rural Hygiene (1931), Recommendations on the Principles Governing the Organisation of Medical Assistance, The Public Health Services and Sanitation in Rural Districts of Geneva.
7. WHO: District Health System: Global and Regional Review, Based on Experience in Various Countries, Geneva, 1995, p. 18 (WHO/SHS/DHSI 95.1).
8. R.R. Veinerman, Social Medicine in Eastern Europe, Cambridge, Mass, Harvard University Press, 1935, p. 5, quoted in S.L. Goel, Public Health Administration, New Delhi, Sterling, 1984, p. 418.
9. Annual Report, Ministry of Health and Family Welfare, GOI, New Delhi, 1971-72, p. 35.
10. Government of Burma, A Guide to Rural Health Centre Work in Burma, Rangoon, Printing and Stationery.
11. WHO, Strengthening Ministries of Health for Primary Health Care, Geneva, 1984, p. 9.
12. Walter R. Sharp, Field Administrative in the UN System, London, 1961, p. 119.
13. Speech delivered by Chief Minister of J & K, at the joint meeting of the Central

Council of Health and Family Planning Council on 1974-75, held at Vigyan Bhavan, New Delhi.

14. Based on the document, prepared by NIHFW, Training Management Modules for Medical Officers.
15. S.L. Goel, Health Care Administration, Vol. III, New Delhi, Sterling, 1984, p. 127.
16. UNICEF, UNICEF News, "Communication: A tool for Development", Issue 84/1975/2, p. 18.
17. *Indian Express,* Chandigarh, 28 August, 1978.
18. S.L. Goel, Health Care Administration, Levels and Aspects, Sterling, 1981.
19. Government of India, Publication Division, All India Radio Broadcast, June 26, 1966, Selected Speeches of Mrs. Indira Gandhi, New Delhi, March 1971.
20. A.P. Barnasbas, Good Governance at Local Level, in *IJPA,* July-Sept. 1997, p. 453.

Appendix 10.1

Duties and Responsibilities of Medical Officer (Administrative)

Administrative

1. Supervise the work of staff working under him.
2. Scrutinize the programmes of his staff and suggest changes, if necessary, to suit the priority of work.
3. Prepare and display charts in his office to explain clearly the geographical area, location of peripheral health units, morbidity and mortality, health statistics and other important information about this area.
4. Hold monthly staff meetings with his staff for evaluating the progress of work and suggesting steps to be taken for further improvements.
5. Receive reports from the periphery, get them compiled and submit the returns regularly to the district health authorities.
6. Keep notes of the field visits he makes in his area and submit every month his tour reports to the CMO.
7. Ensure general clines inside and outside the primary health centre and also proper maintenance of all the equipment under his charge.
8. Keep the inventory and stock register of all the stores and equipments supplied to him up-to-date and will be responsible for its correct accounting.
9. Prepare indents for drugs, instruments, linen, etc. sufficiently in advance and will submit them to the appropriate health authorities.
10. Ensure the regular supply of medicines to health guides and disbursement of honorarium to health guides.
11. Maintain the prescribed records at the PHC level.
12. Discharge the financial duties entrusted to him.
13. Discharge the day-to-day administrative functions pertaining to the primary health centre.

Preventive Work

1. As an expert in health he is to ensure that health assistants, health workers, health guides and trained dais are fully conversant with the health programmes to be implemented in the villages where they work.
2. Supervise their work regularly, both in the clinics and in the community setting, and give them necessary guidance and direction.

3. Visit each sub-centre in his area at least once in a week on a fixed day not only to check the work of the staff but also to provide services on the spot guidance to health assistants, health workers, health guides and trained dais.
4. Provide technical guidance to health guides and encourage them to participate in promotive and preventive health activities.
5. Visit schools in his area at least once in a year for medical check-up, immunization, and health education. He also makes arrangements for the treatment of those students found with defects.
6. Carry out MCH services and actively involve health assistants, health workers, health guides and trained dais in the effective implementation of MCH, family planning and nutrition programmes.
7. Ensure that all steps are being taken for the control of communicable diseases and proper improvement of sanitation in the villages.
8. Take necessary action in case of any outbreak of epidemic in his area.

Curative Work

1. As an expert in health he is to organize the dispensary, out-patient department and in-patient wards and will allot duties to ensure smooth running of the same.
2. Make arrangement for distribution of work in the treatment of emergency cases which come outside the normal OPD hours.
3. Organize laboratory services for proper diagnosis of doubtful cases.
4. Make arrangements for rendering services for the treatment of minor ailments at community level and at the PHC through the agency of health assistants, health workers and health guides, and trained dais.
5. Attend to cases referred to him by health assistants, health workers, health guides and trained dais.
6. Screen case needing specialized medical attention and nursing care and refer them to referral institutions.
7. Provide guidance to the health assistants, health workers, and health guides in the treatment of minor ailments.
8. Cooperative and/or coordinate with other institutions providing health services in the Block.

Promotive Work

1. He has to organize/participate in village health committee/ village panchayat meetings to discuss health programmes with the public and enlist their cooperation.

2. Keep close liaison with the block development officer and his staff, community leaders and various social welfare agencies in his area and involve them to the best advantage in the promotion of health programmes.
3. Organize camps, meetings, health education talks and demonstrations, display of posters, exhibitions and films with the assistance of the block extension educator, health assistants and health workers.
4. Conduct field surveys to identity local health problems, and then, based on these health problems to devise a strategy for effective delivery of health services in his area.

Training

1. He is also to organize training programmes, including continuing education, with the assistance of the block extension educator and under the guidance of the district health authorities and Health and Family Welfare Training Centres (HFWTCs) under the multipurpose worker scheme.
2. Educate the community as to the selection of health guides and take necessary steps to train health guides from his area.
3. Provide assistance to the health assistants (F); and health workers (F) in organising training programmes for indigenous dais practicing in the area.

Source: NIHFW—Management Training Modules for Medical Officer.

APPENDIX 10.2

Duties and Responsibilities of Block Extension Educator.

Duties and Function: Maintenance of Data

To have with him all information on women and child development, Rural development, education and non-conventional energy programmes and activities in the block and utilize the same for programme planning.

He will collect and utilize data about the infant and maternal mortality, crude death and birth, literacy, couple protection and immunization rates and age at marriage at the block level.

To be responsible for regular maintenance of records of educational programmes daily dairies and other registers and ensure preparation and display of relevant maps and charts in the PHC.

Training

To organize in cooperation with local voluntary agencies, orientation training for Health and Family Welfare workers, opinion leaders, anganwadi workers, members of women groups, local medical practitioners, school teachers, dais and others involved in Health and Family Welfare work.

To maintain a complete set of educational aids for his own use and for training purposes.

Inter-sectoral Coordination

To be a member of the local Block level Family Welfare Committee and act as a resource person.

To ensure proper functioning of all Family Welfare Committees in the catachment area of PHC.

To maintain liaison with media units of other departments, including those of voluntary organisations and organize mass communication programmes like, Film shows, exhibitions, lectures and dramas with the help of District, Extension and media officer.

IEC Work

To be responsible for all educational, motivational and communication programmes in PHC area.

Assist the M.O. PHC in staff development programmes for the Health Assistants and Health Workers, at the PHC as well as in the field.

Be actively involved in the training of Health Assistants, Health Workers, and other health personnel at the Community Health Centre level.

Assist the M.O. PHC in monthly group activities at the PHC, sub-centre and community levels.

Be actively involved in the field training components of basic and refresher training programmes conducted by the institutes for basic training of various categories of health personnel.

Be actively involved in the field training components of training programs conducted by the Health and Family, Welfare Training Centres of various categories of health personnel.

Management and Supervision

Assist the M.O. PHC in conducting field investigations to delineate local health problems for planning changes in the strategy for effective delivery of health services.

Ensure that the sub-centres are properly maintained and managed by the Health Workers and Health Assistants.

Ensure that the supplies and equipment such as drugs, contraceptives, vaccines, nutritional supplements, bleaching powder, health educational materials, etc. are supplied in time to the sub-centres to enable the Health Assistants and Health Workers to carry out their functions effectively.

Ensure the regular replenishment of kits and the supply of drugs and dressings for the Health Guides, primary School Teachers and trained Dais and ensure regular disbursement of stipends/honorarium to the health Guides, Primary School Teachers and Dais.

Scrutinise the work plans of the health Assistants and Health Workers.

Supervise the maintenance of the prescribed records at sub-centre level.

Obtain the reports from the periphery, analyse and interpret the data available, and utilize the finding for improving the implementation of the health programmes in the PHC area.

Organise monthly staff meetings, not only for evaluating the progress of work and suggesting steps to be taken for further improvement, but also as a means of staff development and continuing education.

Organise meeting at regular intervals with the community level workers for discussing their activities and for providing continuing education.

Keep notes of his activities in the PHC area and to submit his tour report at regular intervals to the M.O. PHC.

Carry out any other duty assigned by the Medical Officer.

Source: NIHFW—Management Training Modules for Medical Officer.

Appendix 10.3

Detailed duties of Senior Health Assistants

3(a) Health Assistant (Male)

The health assistant (Male) will carry out the following functions:

1. Supervision and Guidance

1.1 Supervise and guide the health worker (male) in the delivery of health care services to the community.
1.2 Strengthen the knowledge and skills of the health worker (male).
1.3 Help the health worker (male) in improving his skills in working in the community.
1.4 Help and guide the health worker (male) in planning and organising his programme of activities.
1.5 Visit each health worker (male) at least once a week on a fixed day to observe and guide him in his day-to-day activities.
1.6 Assess periodically the progress of work of the health worker (male) and submit an assessment report to the medical officer of the primary health centre.
1.7 Carry out supervisory home visits in the area of the health worker (male).

2. Team Work

2.1 Help the health workers to work as part of the health team.
2.2 Coordinate his activities with those of the health assistant (female) and other health personnel.
2.3 Coordinate the health activities in his area with the activities of workers of other departments and agencies; and attend meetings at block level.
2.4 Conduct regular staff meetings with the health workers in coordination with the health assistant (female).
2.5 Attend staff meetings at the primary health centre.
2.6 Assist the medical officers of the primary health centre in the organisation of the different health services in the area.
2.7 Participate as a member of the health team in camps and campaigns in health programmes.

3. Supplies and Equipment

3.1 In collaboration with the health assistant (female) check at regular intervals the stores available at the sub-centre and indent to procure the supplies and equipment in good time.
3.2 Check that the drugs at the sub-centre are properly stored and that the equipment is well maintained.

3.3 Ensure that the health worker (male) maintains his kit in the proper way.

4. Records and Reports

4.1 Scrutinise the maintenance of records by the health worker (male) and guide him in their proper maintenance.
4.2 Maintain the prescribed records and prepare the necessary reports.
4.3 Review reports received from the health worker (male), consolidate them, and submit periodical reports to the medical officer of the primary health centre.

5. Malaria

5.1 Give radical treatment to all cases when blood smears are positive for malaria.
5.2 Supervise the spraying of insecticides during local spraying.

6. Communicable Diseases

6.1 Be alert to the sudden outbreak of epidemics of diseases such as diarrhoeal diseases, polio myelitis, ineffective hepatitis, encephalitis, plague and take all necessary remedial measures.
6.2 Take necessary control measures when any notifiable disease is reported to him.
6.3 In cases with continued fever, or prolonged cough, or spitting of blood, take sputum smears and send them for examination.
6.4 In cases suspected of having leprosy, take skin smears and send them for examination.
6.5 Carry out the destruction of stray dogs.

7. Environmental Sanitation

7.1 Help the community in the construction of: (a) soakage pits; (b) kitchen gardens; (c) manure pits; (d) compost pits; (e) sanitary latrines; (f) smokeless chulas; and supervise their construction.
7.2 Supervise the chlorination of water sources including wells.

8. Immunization

8.1 Conduct immunization of all school going children with the help of health worker (male).
8.2 Supervise the immunization of all children from one to five years.

9. Family Welfare

9.1 Personally motivate resistant cases for family planning.

9.2 Guide the health worker (male) in establishing make depot-holders for the distribution of conventional contraceptives and train the depot-holders with the assistance of the health worker (male).

10. Nutrition

10.1 Identity cases of malnutrition among infants and young children (zero to five years), give the necessary treatment and advice and refer various cases to the primary health centre.

11. Vital Events

11.1 Report births and deaths occurring in his area to the medical officer of the primary health centre.

12. Primary Medical Care

12.1 Provide treatment for minor ailments, provide first-aid for accidents and emergencies, and refer cases beyond his competence to the primary centre or nearest hospital.

12.2 Attend to cases referred by the health workers and refer cases beyond his competence to the primary health centre or nearest hospital.

13. Health Education

13.1 Carry out educational activities for control of communicable diseases, environmental sanitation, MCH, family planning, nutrition, immunization, and the need for registration of vital events.

13.2 Arrange group meeting with leaders and involve them in spreading the message for various health programmes.

13.3 Organize and conduct training of community leaders with the assistance of health worker (male).

Source: NIHFW—Management Training Modules for Medical Officer.

APPENDIX 10.4

Health Assistant (Female)

The health assistant (Female) will carry out the following functions:

1. Supervision and Guidance

1.1 Supervise and guide the health worker (male) in the delivery of health care services to the community.
1.2 Strengthen the knowledge and skills of the health worker (female).
1.3 Help the health worker (female) in improving her skills in working in the community.
1.4 Help and guide the health worker (male) in planning and organising his programme of activities.
1.5 Visit each health worker (male) at least once a week on a fixed day to observe and guide him in his day-to-day activities.
1.6 Assess periodically the progress of work of the health worker (female) and submit an assessment report to the medical officer of the primary health centre.
1.7 Carry out supervisory home visits in the area of the health worker (female).

2. Team Work

2.1 Help the health worker to work as part of the health team.
2.2 Coordinate her activities with those of the health assistant (male) and other health personnel including the dais.
2.3 Coordinate the health activities in her area with the activities of workers of other departments and agencies, and attend meetings at block level.
2.4 Conduct regular staff meetings with the health workers in coordination with the health assistant (male).
2.5 Attend staff meetings at the primary health centre.
2.6 Assist the medical officers of the primary health centre in the organisation of the different health services in the area.
2.7 Participate as a member of the health team in mass camps and campaigns in health programmes.

3. Supplies, Equipment and Maintenance of Sub-centre

3.1 In collaboration with the health assistant (male), check at regular intervals the stores available at the sub-centre and help in the procurement of supplies and equipment.
3.2 Check that the drugs at the sub-centre are properly stored and that the equipment is well maintained.

3.3 Ensure that the health worker (female) maintains her general kit and mid-wifery kit in the proper way.
3.4 Ensure that the sub-centre is kept clean and is properly maintained.

4. Records and Reports

4.1 Scrutinize the maintenance of records by the health worker (female) and guide her in their proper maintenance.
4.2 Maintain the prescribed records and prepare the necessary reports.
4.3 Review reports received from the health workers (female), consolidate them, and submit periodical reports to the medical officer of the primary health centre.

5. Training

5.1 Organise and conduct training for dais with the assistance of the health worker (female).

6. Maternal and Child Health

6.1 Conduct weekly MCH clinics at each sub-centre with the assistance of the health worker (female).
6.2 Respond to calls from the health worker (female) and trained dais, and from the health worker (male) in the twilight area and render necessary help.

7. Family Welfare and Medical Termination of Pregnancy

7.1 Conduct weekly family welfare clinics (along with the MCH clinics) at each sub-centre with the assistance of the health worker (female).
7.2 Personally motivate resistant cases for family planning.
7.3 Provide information on the availability of services for medical termination of pregnancy and refer suitable cases to the approved institutions.
7.4 Guide the health worker (female) in establishing female depot-holders for the distribution of conventional contraceptives and train the depot-holders with the assistance of the health worker (female).

8. Nutrition

8.1 Identify cases of malnutrition among infants and young children (zero to five years), give the necessary treatment and advice and refer serious cases to the primary health centre.

9. Immunization

9.1 Supervise the immunization of all pregnant women and infants (zero to one year).

10. Primary Medical Care

10.1 Provide treatment for minor ailments, provide first-aid for accidents and emergencies, and refer cases beyond her competence to the primary health centre or nearest hospital.

10.2 Attend to cases referred to by the health workers and refer cases beyond her competence to the primary health centre or nearest hospital.

11. Health Education

11.1 Carry out educational activities for MCH, family planning, nutrition and immunization with the assistance of the health worker (female).

11.2 Arrange group meetings with leaders and involve them in spreading the message for various health programmes.

11.3 Organize and conduct training of women leaders with the assistance of health worker (female).

11.4 Organize and utilize mahila mandals, teachers and other women in the community in the family welfare programmes.

Source: Ibid.

11

CHAPTER

Organisation and Working of Sub-Centres

Multipurpose worker should be equal in excellence to a five star hotel, but should be accessible to everyone from the richest to the poorest

Sub-centre is the most important institution in providing health care. The success or failure of health care depends upon the attitudes, perception and ethos of health workers and volunteers working in sub-centres. It is a matter of great dissatisfaction that health centres are not doing well and are showing poor performance. This may be attributed to lack of interest about them among union, state and district level health functionaries. Sub-centres are the pivot around which all important schemes revolve. At present, workers in these centres are highly dissatisfied resulting in bad delivery of primary health care services. Health centres can really communicate effectively with community, volunteers and the people.

In the new millennium, we must strengthen the health centres to reap the benefits of health care. World Health Organisation has also recommended it.[1]

The first line health workers are the major work force at the primary level. They provide a substantial part of the primitive and preventive components of the essential health care package. They also identify and refer complicated cases and emergencies. However, there are marked variations in their level of training among Member-States, with some workers being trained for only one and a half months. Appropriate training, proper deployment, and basic supplies and logistic support for the first line health workers are important for the delivery of essential health care.

The staffing pattern in peripheral health units is an important indicator of the effective functioning of PHC in basic health units, and shortages of personnel are reported from several countries. In the majority of countries of the region, auxiliary health workers are the main providers of care at the first level static health facilities. Medical officers are not usually posted to this level, except in DPR Korea and recently in Maldives.

To overcome the problem of limited access to static health facilities in some areas, many countries have organized outreach services through which health workers regularly visit communities to provide health care. Services commonly provided are immunizations, family planning, health education, growth monitoring and advice on nutrition, basic maternal care, vitamin A distribution, and treatment of common ailments such as diarrhoea and acute respiratory infection. Data on disease incidence and vital statistics are also collected during outreach visits in some countries.

I. RATIONALE AND PHILOSOPHY

During the Fourth Plan period, two committees viz., (1) Committee on Multi-purpose Workers (MPW) under Health and Family Planning Programme (also known as Kartar Singh Committee) 1972-73, and (2) Srivastava Committee, 1974 were constituted to suggest ways and means to improve the rural health services. The Kartar Singh Committee recommended establishment of a Sub-Centre for every 5,000 rural population and an integrated approach for delivery of health services through Multi-purpose Workers. The idea behind the Multi-purpose Health Worker Scheme launched in 1977 was that it would be more appropriate to provide a package of health and family planning services "through a single administrative set-up, rather than providing such services in a vertical manner through multiple agencies.

The number of Sub-centres has increased from 84376 in Sixth Plan (1981-85) to 144988 as on March 2006, (Refer Table 11.1), Table 11.2 reveals that out of 144988 sub-sentres, information is available for 144171 sub-centres. Out of these 69920, sub-centres are functioning in Government buildings, 57477 in rented buildings, 16774 in rent free buildings and 5141 sub-centres in buildings are under construction. There is a need of constructions 68848 buildings. Table 11.3 reveals that out of 144988 sub-centres, 7678 sub-centres are without ANMS, 5777 are without MPW (M), 4543 Sub-Centres are without both MPW, male and female.

The Sub-Centre is the most peripheral and first contact point between the primary health care system and the community. Each Sub-Centre is manned by one Auxiliary Nurse Midwife (ANM) and one Male Health Worker MPW(M). One Lady Health Worker (LHV) is entrusted with the task of supervision of six Sub-Centres. Sub-Centres are assigned tasks relating to interpersonal communication in order to bring about behavioural change and provide services in relation to maternal and child health, family welfare, nutrition, immunization, diarrhea control and control of communicable diseases programmes. The Sub-Centres are provided with basic drugs for minor ailments needed for taking care of essential health needs of men, women and children. The Department of Family Welfare is providing 100% Central assistance to all the Sub-Centres in the country since April 2002 in the form of salary of ANMs and LHVs, rent at the rate of Rs. 3000 per annum and contingency at the rate of Rs. 3200 per annum, in addition to drugs and equipment kits. The salary of the Male Worker is borne by the State Governments. Under the Swap Scheme, the Government of India has taken over an additional 39554 Sub-Centres from State Governments/Union Territories since April 2002 in lieu of 5434 number of Rural Family Welfare Centres transferred to the State Governments/Union Territories. There are 146026 Sub-Centres functioning in the country as on September 2005 as compared to 142655 in September 2004. This increased to 144988 on March 2006.

2. EXTENT, FUNCTIONS AND TRAINING

The MPW scheme aims at providing a package of health services to the rural population at their doorsteps. The main objective of this scheme is to ensure a minimum availability of public health facilities, which include preventive medicine, family welfare, nutrition and curative and referral services. The launching of this scheme marked the merger of the vertical programmes into an integrated health delivery system, thus lending additional strength to the Primary Health Centres.[2]

As per the norms, each Sub-centre is required to be manned by a trained Female Health Worker (ANM) and a trained Male Health Worker known as Multi-purpose Worker (Male). The Government of India had initiated a scheme of training and thereby converting the uni-purpose workers under various programmes to multi-purpose workers. However, because of the shortage of MPWs (Male) at Sub-centre level, a scheme of basic training for MPWs (Male) was initiated during the 7th Plan period. Under this scheme, 10th pass candidates are selected and trained for one year before they are inducted into services.[3]

"No one can really do first class work without a sense of function, without a measure of a crusading spirit, I am doing this, I have to achieve this as a part of great movement in a big cause.[4]

Job Responsibilities of Health Workers (M)

Malaria

Identify fever cases, make thick and thin blood films of all fever cases and send the slides for laboratory examination, Administer presumptive treatment to all fever cases, Record the results of examination of blood films, refer all cases of positive blood films to the health assistant (male) for radical treatment and Educate the community on the importance of blood film examination for fever cases, treatment of fever cases, insecticidal spraying of houses, larviciding measures, and other measures to control the spread of malaria.

Communicable Diseases

Identify cases of notifiable diseases, i.e. cholera, plague, poliomyelitis, and persons with continued fever, or prolonged cough, or spitting of blood,

TABLE 11.1

Establishment of Sub-Centres during Five Year Plans

Sl. No.	State/UT	Sub-Centres functioning at the end of					
		Sixth Plan [1981-85]	Seventh Plan [1985-90]	Eighth Plan [1992-97]	Ninth Plan [1997-02]	Tenth Plan Target	Sub-Centres Functioning[1] as on Sept. 2005
1.	Andhra Pradesh	6129	7894	10568	10568	0	12522
2.	Arunachal Pradesh	55	155	223	273	0	379
3.	Assam	1711	5109	5109	5109	0	5109
4.	Bihar	8299	14799	14799	14799	1210	10337
5.	Chhattisgarh					874	3818
6.	Goa	156	166	172	172	0	172
7.	Gujarat	4869	6834	7274	7274	0	7274
8.	Haryana	1591	2299	2299	2299	183	2433
9.	Himachal Pradesh	1299	1851	1980	2069	0	2068
10.	Jammu and Kashmir	609	1460	1700	1700	0	1879
11.	Jharkhand					0	4462
12.	Karnataka	4964	7793	8143	8143	0	8143
13.	Kerala	2270	5094	5094	5094	0	5094
14.	Madhya Pradesh[2]	6615	11910	11938	11947	0	8874
15.	Maharashtra	6391	9248	9725	9725	808	10453
16.	Manipur	301	420	420	420	0	420
17.	Meghalaya	172	272	377	413	51	401
18.	Mizoram	162	220	324	346	0	366
19.	Nagaland	133	244	244	302	23	394
20.	Orissa	4127	5927	5927	5927	447	5927
21.	Punjab	2602	2852	2852	2852	6	2858
22.	Rajasthan	3790	8000	9400	9926	461	10512
23.	Sikkim	82	132	147	147	0	147
24.	Tamil Nadu	5860	8681	8681	8682	0	8682
25.	Tripura	230	506	537	539	40	539
26.	Uttaranchal					240	1576
27.	Uttar Pradesh[1]	15653	20153	20153	20153	1944	20521
28.	West Bengal	6100	7873	7873	8126	2230	10356
29.	A & N Islands	32	84	96	100	0	107
30.	Chandigarh	12	12	12	13	0	13
31.	D & N Haveli	19	34	34	36	4	38
32.	Daman and Diu	14	14	21	21	0	21
33.	Delhi	42	42	42	42	148	41
34.	Lakshadweep	14	14	14	14	0	14
35.	Pondicherry	73	73	80	80	0	76
	All India	**84376**	**130165**	**136258**	**137311**	**8669**	**144988**

1. There is a reduction in the number of centres functioning as on March 2006 as compared to those functioning at the end of Ninth Plan due to the division of State.

TABLE 11.2

Building Position for Sub-Centres (As on March 2006)

Sl. No.	State/UT	Total Number of Sub-Centres functioning	Number of Sub-Centres for which information on building is available	Sub-Centres functioning in			Buildings under construction	Buildings requried' to be constructed
				Government Buildings	Rented Buildings	Rent Free Panchayat/ Vol. Society Buildings		
1	2	3	4	5	6	7	8	9
1.	Andhra Pradesh	12522	12522	4221	8301	0	0	8301
2.	Arunachal Pradesh	379	NA	NA	NA	NA	NA	NA
3.	Assam	5109	5109	2637	2472	0	0	2472
4.	Bihar	8858	8858	2483	4690	1685	73	66302
5.	Chhattisgarh	4692	4692	1458	0	3234	219	3015
6.	Goa	172	172	40	132	0	0	132
7.	Gujarat	7274	7274	5820	0	1454	264	1190
8.	Haryana	2433	2433	1499	0	934	6	928
9.	Himachal Pradesh	2069	2069	1262	14	793	72	735
10.	Jammu and Kashmir	1888	1888	654	1234	0	13	1221
11.	Jharkhand	3958	3958	1736	1948	274	0	2222
12.	Karnataka	8143	8143	4460	2893	790	0	3683
13.	Kerala	5094	5094	2986	1098	1010	19	2089
14.	Madhya Pradesh	8874	8874	3996	4878	0	489	4389
15.	Maharashtra	10453	10453	6964	750	2739	741	2748

(Contd.)

TABLE 11.2 (*Contd.*)

1 2	3	4	5	6	7	8	9
16. Manipur	420	420	230	168	22	15	175
17. Meghalaya	401	401	391	10	0	21	*
18. Mizoram	366	366	366	0	0	0	0
19. Nagaland	397	NA	NA	NA	NA	NA	NA
20. Orissa	5927	2927	2542	3385	0	242	3143
21. Punjab	2858	2858	1443	0	1415	0	1415
22. Rajasthan	10512	10512	8235	0	2277	340	1937
23. Sikkim	147	147	112	29	6	9	26
24. Tamil Nadu	8683	8683	6510	2113	60	0	2173
25. Tripura	539	539	278	202	59	7	254
26. Uttaranchal	1631	1631	562	1062	7	188	881
27. Uttar Pradesh	20521	20521	6581	13940	0	1693	12247
28. West Bengal	10356	10356	2236	8120	0	1000	7120
29. A & N Islands	108	108	108	0	0	0	0
30. Chandigarh	13	13	8	0	5	0	5
31. D & N Haveli	38	38	38	0	0	0	0
32. Daman and Diu	21	21	20	1	0	0	0
33. Delhi	41	NA	NA	NA	NA	NA	NA
34. Lakshadweep	14	14	8	6	0	0	6
35. Pondicherry	77	77	36	31	10	3	38
All India	**144988**	**144171**	**69920**	**57477**	**16774**	**5414**	**68848**

Notes: NA: Not available.

1. Required number = Total functioning—(Government Buildings + Under Construction) (ignoring excess)

* States having construction in excess of the number required to be constructed.

GRAPH 11.1

Building Position for Sub-Centres, March 2006

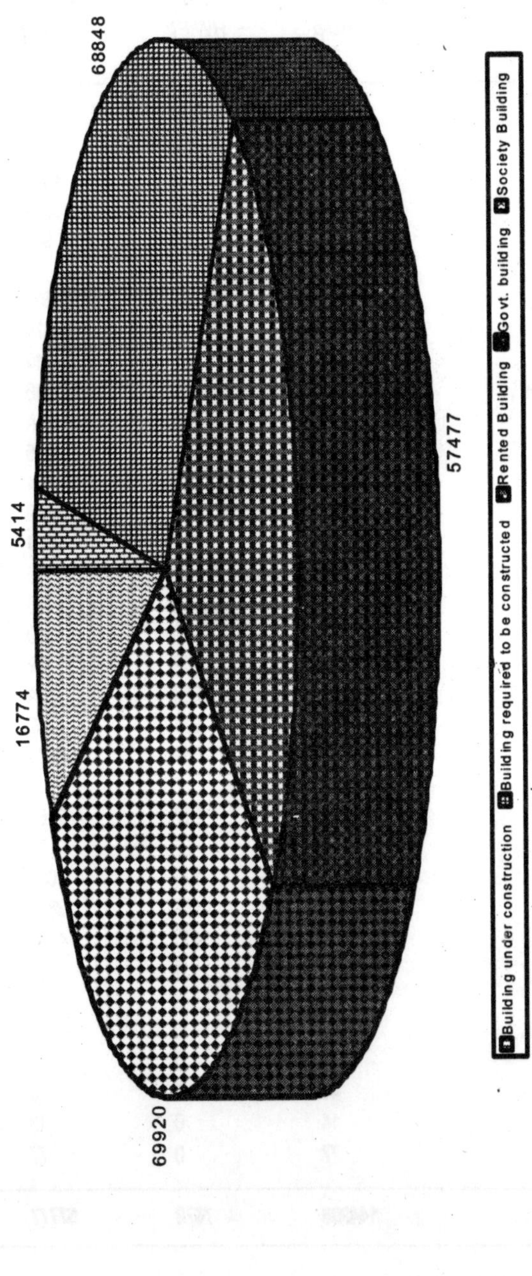

TABLE 11.3

Number of Sub-centres without ANMs or/and Health Workers [M] (As on Sept. 2005)

Sl. No.	State/UT	Sub-Centers Functioning	Without HW[F]/ ANMs	Without HW [M]	Without Both
1.	Andhra Pradesh	12522	460	6391	184
2.	Arunachal Pradesh	379	100	275	100
3.	Assam	5109	80	4997	80
4.	Bihar	8858	854	3564	854
5.	Chhattisgarh	4692	555	966	NA
6.	Goa	172	13	25	NA
7.	Gujarat	7274	421	1863	NA
8.	Haryana	2433	23	674	156
9.	Himachal Pradesh	2068	420	219	30
10.	Jammu and Kashmir	1888	29	16	NA
11.	Jharkhand	3958	NA	NA	NA
12.	Karnataka	8143	0	4955	0
13.	Kerala	5094	294	374	22
14.	Madhya Pradesh	8874	603	1539	0
15.	Maharashtra	10453	833	2024	740
16.	Manipur	420	20	49	12
17.	Meghalaya	401	0	123	0
18.	Mizoram	366	20	50	5
19.	Nagaland	397	59	59	59
20.	Orissa	5927	353	NA	NA
21.	Punjab	2858	264	762	167
22.	Rajasthan	10512	352	2701	178
23.	Sikkim	147	0	0	0
24.	Tamil Nadu	8682	817	7180	817
25.	Tripura	539	97	71	72
26.	Uttaranchal	1631	123	1015	634
27.	Uttar Pradesh	20521	431	12845	431
28.	West Bengal	10356	456	4804	NA
29.	A & N Islands	1078	1	108	1
30.	Chandigarh	13	0	5	0
31.	D & N Haveli	38	0	29	0
32.	Daman and Diu	21	0	4	0
33.	Delhi	41	0	0	0
34.	Lakshadweep	14	0	13	1
35.	Pondicherry	77	0	77	0
	All India[2]	**144988**	**7678**	**57777**	**4543**

Notes: NA: Not Available.

2 For calculating the overall percentages, the States/UTs for which manpower position is not available, should be excluded.

which he comes across during his home visits and notify the health assistant (male) and primary health centre about them and carry out control measures until the arrival of the health assistant (male). Educate the community about the importance of control and preventive measures against such communicable diseases including tuberculosis. Report the presence of stray dogs to the health assistant (male).

Environmental Sanitation

Chlorinate public water sources including wells at regular intervals, Educate the community on: (a) the method of disposal of liquid wastes; (b) the method of disposal of solid wastes; (c) home sanitation; (d) advantages and use of sanitary type of latrines; and (e) construction and use of smokeless chulhas and help the community in the construction of: (i) soakage pits; (ii) kitchen gardens; (iii) manure pits; (iv) compost pits; and (v) sanitary latrines.

Immunization

In the intensive area, administer DPT vaccination, BCG vaccination and wherever available, oral poliomyelitis vaccination to all children aged one to five years, in the twilight area, administer OPT vaccination, BCG vaccination and wherever available, oral poliomyelitis vaccine to all children aged zero to five years, assist the health assistant (male) in the school immunization programmes and—educate the people in the community about the importance of immunization against the various communicable diseases.

Family Planning

Utilize the information from the Eligible Couple Register for the family planning programme. Spread the message of family planning to the couples, in his area and motivate them for family planning individually and in groups and distribute conventional contraceptives to the couples. Provide facilities and help to prospective acceptors of vasectomy in obtaining the services and provide follow-up services to make family planning acceptors in the intensive area and all family planning acceptors in the twilight area, identify side-effects, give treatment on the spot for side-effects and minor complaints, and refer those cases that need attention by the physician to the PHC/Hospital, build rapport with the satisfied acceptors, village teachers and others and utilize them for promoting family welfare programmes and Establish male depot-holders in the intensive area and male and female depot-holders in the twilight area. Help the health assistant (male) and health assistant (female) in training them, and provide a continuous supply of conventional contraceptives to the depot holders. Identify the male leaders in each village in the intensive area and the male and female leaders in the twilight area and Assist the health assistant (male) in training the leaders in the community, and in educating and involving the community in family welfare programmes.

Medical Termination of Pregnancy

Identify the women in the twilight area requiring help for medical termination of pregnancy and refer them to the nearest approved institution and Educate the community on the availability of services for medical termination of pregnancy.

Maternal and Child Health (in the Twilight Area)

Identify and refer women with abnormal pregnancy to the health worker (female). Identify and refer women with medical and gynecological problems to the health worker (female). Immunize pregnant women with tetanus toxoid, Refer cases of difficult labour and newborns with abnormalities to the health worker (female) and Educate the community about the availability of maternal and child health services and encourage them to utilize the facilities.

Nutrition

Identify cases of malnutrition among pre-school children (one to five years) in the intensive area and refer them to Balwadis Primary Health Centre for nutrition supplements. Identify cases of malnutrition among pre-school children (zero to five years), in the twilight area and refer them to Balwadis/Primary Health Centre for nutrition supplements. Distribute iron and folic acid as prescribed to children from one to five years in the intensive area and to pregnant and nursing mothers, children from zero to five years, and family planning acceptors in the twilight area. Administer vitamin 'A' solution as prescribed to children from one to five years in both the intensive and the twilight areas and Educate the community about nutritious diet for mothers and children.

Vital Events

Enquire about births and deaths occurring in the intensive and twilight areas, record them in the births and deaths register and report them to the health assistant (male) and Educate the community on the importance of registration of births and deaths and the method of registration.

Record Keeping

Survey all the families in his area and collect general information about each village/locality in his area. Prepare, maintain and utilize family records and village registers, take assistance of the health worker (female) to prepare the Eligible Couple Register from the family records and maintain it up-to-date. Prepare and submit periodical reports in time to the health assistant (male) and prepare and maintain maps and charts for his area and utilize them for planning his work.

Primary Medical Care

Provide treatment for minor ailments, provide first-aid for accidents and emergencies, and refer cases beyond his competence to the primary health centre or nearest hospital.

Team Activities

Attend and participate in the staff meetings at primary health centre and Taluka Hospital. Coordinate his activities with the health worker (female) and other health workers, including the dais, in the twilight area and meet the health assistant (male) each week and seek his advice and guidance whenever necessary.

2. JOB RESPONSIBILITIES OF HEALTH WORKER (FEMALE)

Maternal and Child Health

Register and provide care to pregnant women throughout the period of pregnancy and test urine of pregnant women for albumen and sugar and estimate haemoglobin level during her home visits and at the clinic. Refer cases of abnormal pregnancy and cases with medical and gynaecological problems to the health assistant (female) or the primary health centre as well as conduct about 50 per cent of total deliveries in her intensive area and whenever called in the twilight area and supervise deliveries conducted by dais and assist them whenever called in. Refer cases of difficult labour and newborns with abnormalities and help them to get institutional care and provide follow-up care to patients referred to or discharged from hospital. Make at least three post-natal. visits for each delivery conducted in the intensive area and render advice regarding care of the mother and care and feeding of the newborn and assess the growth and development of the infant and take any necessary action. Help the medical officer and health assistant (female) in conducting MCH and family planning clinics at the sub-centre and educate mothers individually and in groups for better family health including MCH, family planning, nutrition, immunization, control of communicable diseases, personal and environmental hygiene and care of minor ailments.

Family Planning

Utilize the information from the Eligible Couple Register for the family planning programme and spread the message of family planning to the couples and motivate them for family planning individually and in groups. Distribute conventional contraceptives to the couples, provide facilities and help the prospective acceptors in getting family planning services, if necessary by accompanying them or arranging for the dais to accompany them to hospital and provide follow-up services to female family planning adopters, identify side-effects, give treatment on the spot for side-effects and minor complaints and refer those cases that need attention by the physician to the PHC/hospital. Establish female depot holders, help the health assistant (female) in training them, and providing a continuous supply of conventional contraceptives to the depot-holders and build rapport with acceptors, village leaders, dais and others and utilize them for promoting family welfare programmes, Identify women leaders and help the health assistant (female) to train them and participate in Mahila Mandal meetings, and utilize such gatherings for educating women in family welfare programmes.

Medical Termination of Pregnancy

Identify the women requiring help for medical termination of pregnancy and refer them to the nearest approved institution and educate the community of the availability of services for medical termination of pregnancy.

Nutrition

Identify cases of malnutrition among infants and young children (0 to 5 years), give the necessary treatment and advice and refer serious cases to the PHC and distribute iron and folic acid tablets as prescribed to pregnant and nursing mothers, infants and young children (0 to 5 years) and family planning acceptors. Administer vitamin 'A' solution as prescribed to children from 1 to 5 years and educate the community about nutritious diet for mothers and children.

Communicable Diseases

Identify cases of notifiable diseases, i.e. cholera, plague, poliomyelitis, and persons with continued fever or prolonged cough, or spitting of blood, which she comes across during her home visits and notify the health worker (male) about them.

Immunization

Immunize pregnant women with tetanus toxoid and Administer BCG vaccination to all newborn infants, and DPT vaccination, oral poliomyelitis vaccine (where available) and BCG vaccine (if not given at birth) to all infants (0 to 1 year).

Dai Training

List dais in the intensive and twilight areas and involve them in promoting family welfare and help the health assistant (female) in the training programme of dais.

Vital Events

Record births and deaths occurring in the intensive area in the births and deaths register and report them to the health worker (male).

Record Keeping

Register: (a) pregnant women from three months of pregnancy onwards; (b) infants zero to one year of age; and (c) women aged 15 to 44 years through systematic home visits in the intensive area and at the clinic.

Maintain the pre-natal and maternity records and child care records. Assist the health worker (male) in preparing the Eligible Couple Register and maintaining it up-to-date. Prepare and submit the prescribed periodical reports in time to the health assistant (female). Prepare and maintain maps and charts for her area and utilize them for planning her work.

Primary Medical Care

Provide treatment for minor ailments, provide first-aid for accidents and emergencies, and refer cases beyond her competence to the primary health centre or nearest hospital.

Team Activities

Attend and participate in staff meetings at primary health centre/ community development block or both. Coordinate her activities with the health worker (male) and other health workers including the health guides and dais. Meet the health assistant (female) each week and seek her advice and guidance whenever necessary. Maintain the cleanliness of the sub-centre. Participate as a member of the team in camps and campaigns.

An analysis of duties and responsibilities of Multipurpose workers Male and Female indicate very heavy schedule for them. Besides, the problems to be tackled are common, the interpersonal relationships and communications between the two workers need special attention to avoid duplication and wastage of efforts to ensure economy and efficiency. To achieve all these objectives, they need a good working environment, transport facilities and people's co-operation, as this is a challenging and arduous task. It requires determination, hard work, patience, communication skill, dedication on the part of multipurpose workers to achieve the goals.[5]

3. CRITICAL EXAMINATION

A critical examination of the performance of the scheme reveals dissatisfaction of the villagers. We may mention some of the important aspects which need analysis to improve the existing set-up.

1. Under Utilisation of time by Multipurpose Workers

Health services being labour-intensive, the effective delivery of primary health care services depends on the availability and efficient utilisation of the available manpower resources. To achieve the objectives of Health for all by the year 2000, through Primary Health Care approach, Sub-centre staff are expected to work at maximum efficiency to optimise physical resources.

Rapid population growth and limited resources have forced us to a greater recognition of the need to utilise the existing personnel and facilities in the health service system more effectively and efficiently.

Time utilization by health manpower, and their productivity, is expected to be influenced *inter alia* by their attitudes to the job, especially their perceptions of the objectives to be pursued; organisational inadequacies and other constraints; job-related tensions and job satisfaction, etc. The study of Rajneesh Goel found that the utilisation time of MPW (M) and MPW (F) in Karnataka was only 37.5 per cent.

We present here the results of some studies conducted earlier on time utilisation to support these findings.

1. A study of PHC staff Time Utilization pattern was undertaken in a PHC in Uttar Pradesh by S.K. Satpathy *et. at.* (1998). This study included only technical staff (excluding drivers, sweepers, etc.) and the technique followed was a non-participant observation of the staff for several days. From this study, it was found that the non-productive time of such staff was as high as 62%, Services time accounted for 27% and travel accounted for 11%.
2. A study on Cost Analysis of PHCs by M. Kataria and A.P. Srivastava (NIHFW, 1986) included the analysis of allocation of service time at PHC and sub-centre levels. The method used was observation (for field work) and work sampling (at PHC). Besides these two techniques, Delphi technique was also used for supplementing the information collected through the observations.

Three districts from two states (M.P. and U.P.) were selected; one PHC per district was selected. Thus, 3 PHCs from each state were selected and 12 sub-centres (2 from each selected PHC) were selected. The major findings of the study were:

- 50% of the activity time was spent on travelling and unproductive activities;
- Of the other 50% of productive time, 1/5th was devoted to 'Direct Services', the major activity being family planning followed by MCH services (by female workers) and control of communicable diseases (by male worker); and
- At PHC, direct services accounted for 47% (UP) and 49% (MP); supportive services accounted for 8% (UP) and 11% (MP); time spent on travel was 22% (UP) and 20% (MP). Thus, only 55-60% of total activity time was spent productively.

Johns Hopkins University conducted studies (1965-68) and came to the following conclusions:

- Only 1/6 of the total health centre effort went into direct service in Punjab, compared to 1/4 in Mysore. Further, in Punjab, supporting activities (33.3%) consumed more than twice as much time than service efforts (15.5%).

- More time was devoted in Punjab to the maintenance of records and preparation of reports than to the provision of services (16.3%), whereas in Mysore a mere 1/3 of the activity time was devoted to records and reports.

An analysis of the time utilization by service components showed that most of their service time was devoted to family planning activities (per cent of service time devoted ranged from 33-49%) followed by MCH services (22-27%), and immunization (5-15%).

Thus, all MPWs (male and female) were found to devote most of their service time on family planning activities. This could well be attributed to the government's emphasis on target achievement in the family planning programme. Since these workers are given a set target they are forced to spend more time on this activity, and thus neglect other important activities. However, the target approach has been abolished and we would see its impact in later studies.

The main purpose of the scheme was to devote more time on health education, nutrition, inter-sectoral co-ordination, people's participation, which, however, could not be attended to. There is a need to impart training to these workers to make them realise their true role. Only such understanding on their part can change health scene of rural India, otherwise, it would prove to be another institution with liabilities. The main function of MPW is to make people participate in Primary Health Care activities and get most of the functions performed by them. Besides, they need to devote more time for Inter-Sectoral Co-ordination, an essential Component of Primary Health Care.

The statement that "Time is money" sums up the significance of time management. Though most of the people in Government, Public Enterprises and Private Sector understand the implications of time management but in actual practice, we find that time is wasted and its importance is undermined. Most of the executives and workers in administration complain that they are too busy but still they while away a lot of their time in unnecessary activities. All other resources can be increased whenever required but not time as it is inelastic and therefore, we must make the best use of time. Just to illustrate the importance of time, many studies conducted revealed that persons in administration hardly devote 30 to 40 per cent of their time for the activities they have been engaged for. It means that if proper use is made of time, we can provide services with the existing infrastructure two to three times more and thus the process of development can be accelerated.

Thus, if all the services make the best use of time, we can accelerate the process of development and help the people of the country suffering from abject poverty, ill-health, illiteracy, unemployment, in leading a good standard of life. In developed countries, the most precious resource is time and that is why they are developed but in developing countries, time is unconsciously and consciously wasted in useless activities resulting in underdevelopment or backwardness.

Nation must be committed to utilise even a fraction of second for accelerating the tempo of development to usher in socio-economic democracy as enshrined in the preamble of the Indian constitution and further stressed in Fundamental Rights and Directive Principles of State Policy. How to go about it? How to ensure optimisation of time? How to make the best use of time? The answers to these questions are very simple, i.e. time management at all levels.

If our country can manage time, we can achieve in a year the work of a decade and thus can move fast towards modernisation and development and can say with pride that India occupies a prominent place as in the past in the comity of nations.

The aim of time management is not to turn workers into machines who work without interruptions or breaks, nor is it to develop rigid routines. Rather, the aim is to organise and arrange the use of time so that time pressures and overcrowded schedules and wastage are reduced, and that staff can have adequate rest periods without lowering work output.

If forced to work under continuous pressure, people devise means of escape such as by taking a few days off for illness or slowing down their pace and becoming inefficient. These ways of relieving pressure may be observed among staff in an average overcrowded department. It has been repeatedly shown in industry that regular breaks increase work efficiency and work output. We suggest the following methods to optimise time utilisation:

(i) Well Planned Time Table for field Visits

Many of the key personnel have to control a wide network of office. A part of it can be controlled through telephones, or reporting. But, there is a need of personal discussion among the headquarter and the field staff which involves the use of time in travelling and discussion. It has been seen that officials plan their visit in such a way that they waste most of the time in traveling and less in discussion. It is suggested that field/headquarter visits must be well planned so that the discussion can be pertinent and all the issues are discussed to avoid meetings off and on. The headquarter personnel must carry with them a well prepared schedule to guide them in the field while the field people must also come prepared with definite schedule to clarify the vague points.

(ii) Fixing of Time Schedule to Devote Time to Essential Work

Health workers need to design schedule of work to avoid wastage of time and concentrate on only the important items.

(iii) Providing Regular Time for Rest and Recreation to Avoid Fatigue

Health Workers are human beings and thus cannot work beyond their capacity. It is, therefore, suggested that they may observe regular rest periods to feel fresh. However, these rest periods may not be done at will but must be already notified to avoid difficulty to the people until and unless there are compelling reasons for it.

(iv) Brevity

Besides, the workers must learn to be brief and to the point and discourage relatives/friends to visit them in offices. Telephonic discussions must also be brief.

Time management would not only be beneficial to the workers but would also provide more opportunities to the people to share their ideas and views with the workers and this would be able to lay the solid foundations of people's participation, development and modernisation. It has been observed that workers in health system are not utilizing their time for the assigned job. They are wasting a lot of time in unnecessary activities which are non-productive. We must manage our time purposefully to build modern India otherwise we would remain an under-developed country as time and tide waits for none. We suggest that the health department should provide the following facilities to workers:

(a) We may provide vehicle facility to the workers to reduce time likely to be spent in visiting different places.

(b) We may reduce time spent on record-keeping by systematizing records management. We may even think of providing computers to ensure the supply of right information with less time consumption with ready-made software.

(c) There is a need to ensure quality supervision by PHC staff especially Health Assistants to ensure punctuality of health workers.

(d) There is a need for training to make the workers responsive and dedicated.

(e) There is a need to provide accommodation to workers with all facilities in the village to encourage them to stay near the sub-centre and improve rapport with the people.

(f) People may be motivated to come to the sub-centre rather than waiting for the workers visit at their door-steps, after initial meetings.

(g) Advance planning for a month schedule and its wide circulation can optimise time resource utilisation.

2. Low Job Satisfaction

The quality of the Health Institutions run by Government would be dependent to a great extent upon the quality of the employees engaged in their operation. Personnel run the health system. To quote Mrs. Indira Gandhi: "If Government has to do more for the people, its employees must play a more dynamic and more creative role as the instrument for implementing government policies and programmes."[5]

Among the three components required for developmental tasks-men, money and material-it is more the men (or the human element) than any other factor which determine the quantity and quality of the performance and output. After all, even the contribution of money and material to perfonnance depends substantially upon their manipulation by the men in an organisation.[6]

There is a general tendency in the organisations to lay more emphasis on materials and financial management to the utter neglect of the personnel. What are the consequences? It is observed that the process of development takes longer, sometimes even fails. Why?

The main reason for this is that we are not attending to the administration of personnel earnestly and forget that they are the real agents of development and ultimately the beneficiaries of the process of development.

According to Tead: "Personnel Administration is the utilisation of its best scientific knowledge of all kinds to the end that an organisation as a whole and the individuals composing it, shall find the corporate purpose and the individual purposes are being reconciled to the fullest possible extent, while the working together of these purposes realise also genuine social benefits."[7]

Dale Yoder defines personnel management as: "That phase of management which deals with the effective control and use of manpower as distinguished from other sources of power."[8]

Pigors and Myers defines it as:

> "A method of developing potentialities of employees so that they get maximum satisfaction out of their work and give their best efforts to the organisation."[9]

This dictum also applies to Multipurpose Workers who are the real providers of health care. When they would find job satisfaction or feel congruence with the goals of health for all, they would do their best to achieve the results. It may be made clear that job satisfaction is generated by an individual's perception of how well his job suits him. Job satisfaction may be different at different intervals of time or situations prevailing in an organisation.

The words of Ford are the best commentary on job satisfaction. According to him: "Job satisfaction mayor may not be tied to happiness. But we will know that, we are doing something right if we can change the conditions of job so that employees will stay on the work productively. For the older workers the best will be whether they are with us in spirit as well as in body. The way to achieve this end, for new or old employees, is not to confront them with demands, but to confront them with demanding, meaningful work." And the employees will always have the last word as to whether the work is meaningful."[10]

Strauss and Sayles have summarised the significance of 'job' and 'job satisfaction' in the following words:[11]

1. People want self-actualisation.

2. Those who do not obtain job satisfaction, never reach psychological maturity.
3. Those who fail to obtain job satisfaction, become frustrated.
4. The job is central to man's life.
5. Those without work are unhappy. People want to work, even when they do not have to.
6. Lack of challenging work leads to poor mental health.
7. Work-and-Leisure patterns spill into each other. Those with uncreative jobs engage in uncreative recreation.
8. Lack of job satisfaction and alienation from work leads to lower morale, lower productivity, and unhealthy society.

The subject of job satisfaction has been of keen interest for scientific investigation over the years. In the beginning, it was assumed that job satisfaction was related mainly to the amount of money earned. Workers at that time were regarded as part of the machinery to be managed in the most efficient way possible. But Hoppock conducted pioneer research on vocational satisfaction. He interviewed a cross-section of industrial workers and concluded that, 'job satisfaction could not be measured in terms of monetary rewards only. There were many other factors which contributed to job satisfaction, such as the individual's ability to adapt to the work situation, his ability to adapt to his co-workers, his relative status in the socio-economic hierarchy of the group, the nature of work in relation to his interest and abilities and his preparation for the job."[12]

He also conducted the first community-wide study of job satisfaction. He administered a questionnaire and computed an index of job satisfaction. The results indicated that 15% of the sample were not satisfied with their jobs. Robinson and Hoppock collated a number of studies reporting percentage of job satisfaction. They found that two-thirds of the studies revealed dissatisfaction by one-third workers.[13]

Job satisfaction does not depend on any single factor but many factors and situations congenial to employees. Conditions of services especially the pay is considered to be the best for job satisfaction.

According to Peter F. Drucker, "The carrot of material rewards has not, like the stick of fear, lost its potency."[14] Gellerman too regards money as an important motivator when he states, "money may well turn out to be the costliest motivator of them all, but money may also prove to be the most potent motivator of all, at least in certain circumstances, and when used on a sufficient scale."[15]

Many investigators have pointed out the relative unimportance of money as a motivating factor. Brown goes to the extreme by saying that "of all the incentives known to man, money is the least important."[16]

The Hawthorne experiments introduced the concept of human relations approach to the study of job satisfaction. These experiments highlighted the inter-relatedness of various elements of work, such as working hours, rest, fatigue, incentives, employer's attitudes, as well as formal and informal organisations.[17]

Mayo, concluded that the most important determinant of job satisfaction was group interaction. Mayo was the first author to consider the worker from the psychological perspective and to add the psychological dimension to job satisfaction.

Sajid Iqbal in his Article, "Money cannot buy me love for a job" in *Economic Times,* dated 16th August, 1999, says that: "Often managers are not happy with their pay packets because money is not a motivator but a sop for putting up with a rotten job. National Studies of the changing work force conducted by families and work institute, New York, in 1994, found that Open Communication was ranked highest by respondents when choosing their current jobs."[18] We discuss here the factors which can motivate Health Workers and improve their job satisfaction.

4. FACTORS RESPONSIBLE FOR JOB SATISFACTION

(i) Conditions of Service and Fringe Benefits

Money occupies the most important place in all contractual obligations. The very definition of work declares that it has to be paid for Haire *et al* have rightly pointed out that "pay in one form or another, is certainly one of the mainsprings of motivation in our society."[19]

An adequate and sound salary structure together with other working conditions is the *sine qua non* for the organisational efficiency and effectiveness. Otherwise, as the Administrative Reforms Commission aptly observes, it has been one of the major factors for strikes, agitations, inter-service tensions and rivalries, indifferent attitude to work, poor performance, frustration and low morale of the employees.

However, we must be clear that no compensation plan can satisfy all the employees. The true efficiency in an organisation can be promoted only through dedication and loyalty of its staff members. The Health managers must motivate the employees through no financial incentives. The quality of the health services depends more on the loyalty, the faith and the sense of mission which workers bring in the organisation than on the money expended on them.

(ii) Participation of Workers in Primary Health Care Delivery System

This can enhance their efficiency. We should encourage workers' participation in the achievement of primary health care goals. His participation would build his morale and ultimately his efficiency. An ILO document mentions that the individual worker "is not just a cog in the very big wheel, but that his personal effort is essential for the achievement of the overall production plan."[20]

The research theory in social organisational psychology has also suggested that participation in group decision-making enhances satisfaction among members and removes tensions. Michael R. Copper and Michael T. Wood have shown that satisfaction was greater where participation was complete than where it was partial.[21]

There is a need to practise 'Management by Objectives' to ensure fruitful participation. Management by Objectives shifts the focus to goals, to the purpose of the activity, supervisor and subordinate personnel of an organisation jointly identify its common goals and ensure performance. The PHC staff must encourage the development of such concepts among employees.

(iii) The PHC must Promote Effective Communication between the Workers and the PHC

It is not the official queries or the reservations in the confidential reports that earn staff loyalty. It is the extent that average staff member appreciates the objectives and purposes of the services rendered. The PHC staff should foster in the staff an 'esprit de corps', a spirit of togetherness and dedication to duty.

Changes in methods, organisation or physical facilities that should enhance substantial improvements in efficiency may result in drastically reduced efficiency, if the personnel are suspicious or resentful of the contemplated change. This type of resistance, sometimes referred to as organisational treason, must be anticipated. In order to administer an organisation in a manner designed to induce healthy attitudes among the workers towards the new changes, support should be obtained from the multipurpose workers before any change is injected. The PHC staff must encourage the workers to participate in developing solution. Under these conditions they will accept their responsibility to co-operate with others, and they will try to perform their assigned tasks in order to avoid a breakdown in the chain of interrelated functions. To quote Ted R. Brannen: "Only by an understanding of the individual, his habits, expectations, and beliefs, can the administrator know what is needed to induce his spontaneous co-operation for the benefit of the organisation."[22]

(iv) Nature of Job and Professional Growth

The greatest efficiency and productivity will flow from the efforts of those who find satisfaction in their work and conditions of service, who sense an awareness of usefulness of their function, who feel encouraged to move ahead and to meet new challenges, who perceive their working environment as one in which high standards of performance are maintained and rewarded and not one in which indolence and incompetence can be ignored or even protected and rewarded. Motivation can do miracles as a motivated worker can achieve more than an expert with no motivation. Health Managers must, therefore, devote considerable time and effort in planning for and achieving high levels of motivation and morale. In such a situation, we would achieve goal congruence, ie., identity between the multipurpose workers, goals and the Health organisational goals.

Living together is a beginning
Keeping together is progress
Working together is success.[23]

5. Co-operation and Support from Public

The people in Health Administration should have a sense of dedication, responsibility and be responsive and alert to the aspirations of the citizens. Citizens on the other hand should also provide meaningful co-operation to Health Administration. Under such an atmosphere, it would be very easy to implement the health tasks to ensure positive health for the people.

6. Participation of Beneficiaries

Multipurpose Workers (MPWs) must understand that they should learn the art and science of motivating the community to participate in their own health programmes. We mention here the following things to be achieved by MPWs:

(i) Creating will and determination among the members of the community for improvement of their present and future health.
(ii) Identification and development of the local resources, thereby generating self-reliance among the community.
(iii) Mobilising the available manpower for productive and useful activities.
(iv) Providing an open forum for the community to discuss its problems and find indigenous solutions which may be efficient and economical.
(v) To develop local leaders who can further educate and mobilise the people in the area.
(vi) Arranging extra-curricular activities to generate social awareness through well designed publicity.
(vii) Encouraging the people to develop themselves rather than depend upon the Government for all activities and thus become self-reliant which is the key to development.

To quote Brook Adams, "Administration is the capacity of coordinating many, and often conflicting, social energies in a single organism, so adroitly that they may operate as a unity."[24] Thus, community participation is the Pivot of the Rural Health Care System.

(vii) Effective Supervision

Under the new MPW scheme, supervision is regarded as the organic link between the PHC and the grass-root workers! beneficiaries. The major components of the supervisors work include planning and assessment of training needs, checking of records and public relations and supplies. Though most of these functions are carried out by almost all the supervisors, what is conspicuously missing is the sense of competence in the execution of these jobs. In particular, the component of 'assessment of training needs' leaves much to be desired. Also, it is disheartening to consider record checking and surprise field visits—a major method of supervision. Calculated guidance and meaningful monitoring ought to have been integral to their function. But these were not. Prominent among the problems that face the supervisors besides problems such as those relating to the logistics of fieldwork, supplies, transport incentives, etc., is the one relating to fixing up of work priorities and targets to be executed by MPWs. For example, those supervisors who in turn reported to the bosses who subscribed less to FP activities and more to their own specific work/discipline-oriented activities (malaria) or those whose bosses were primarily inclined towards FP invariably found their instructions conflicting in either case with the result that both the supervisors and MPWs, and their work suffered.

At other times, the supervisors themselves tended to exhibit bias in fixing work priorities that by and large reflected their parent departmental work/orientation (e.g. malaria) even at the cost of the other activities. However, the supervisors felt that the programme implementation was good.

The medical officers, regarded as the PHC Health Team Managers, were found suitable from the technical qualifications/work point of view but were found wanting in other equally critical dimensions of the work such as inspiring the staff reporting to them to perform qualitatively better, inculcate in the workers a good tradition of field work and establish rapport with the local population with a view to promoting preventive and rehabilitative health care.

(viii) Sound Logistic Support

1. Prompt and adequate drug supply,
2. Provision of a first aid kit,
3. Regular provision of necessary registers, and
4. Provision of transport facility, at least during emergencies and immunization camps.

(ix) Tapping the Potential

Health workers possess the potential which need be utilised Dr. Suresh Kant in his Article, "Tap That Potential" in the *Indian Express*, Dec. 15, 1999, Chandigarh, rightly suggests that Neuro Linguistic programming suggests that individual behaviour can be changed. Upgrading mental soft ware is the answer. Everyone has the requisite mental resources and potential to produce excellent outcome. The need is to properly optimise the potential of health workers by the leadership at primary health centres and district health system.

(x) Promoting Team Work

District health system should promote team work to avoid unnecessary duplication of effort, increase co-operation, develop ideas, maintain motivation, improve quality of health services and ensure satisfaction of the people. Aankur Uppal in his article, "The High Road" in the *Indian Express,* Dec. 1999, Chandigarh rightly suggests that in an organisation it is the team that operates. One has to have trust in that team and empower it to convert ideas into reality successfully. . . . There is no soft route. Hard work is the key to success. Making money should not be the only endeavour of a person.

5. RECENT DEVELOPMENTS

From April 1996, India's Family Welfare Programme has adopted a target free approach. This new approach is known as Reproductive and Child Health Programme (RCH). The RCH is considered to be equivalent to Family Planning + Child Survival and Safe Motherhood (CSSM) Programme + Prevention of RTIISTD and Aids + a client approach in providing Family Welfare and Health Care Services.[25]

In order to find out the impact of New Approach (Target Free) let us mention briefly the two studies undertaken by Population Research Centre in the Districts of Belgaum and Dharwad. At the instance of the Ministry of Health and Family Welfare, Government of India, New Delhi and as a part of monitoring and evaluation of the performance of the family welfare programme under the new target free approach, the Population Research Centre, J.S.S. Institute of Economic Research, Dharward, undertook a rapid survey in the rural areas of Belgaum District, Karnataka state during the last two weeks of December 1997 and first two weeks of January 1998. Using a simple and short questionnaire, the survey interviewed a total of 1,000 currently married women age 15-44, from 50 villages, at the rate of 20 women per village. The study found:

- Monitoring the weight and blood pressure, and urine tests were not carried out for the majority of women during their pregnancy by multipurpose workers females.
- Of the births that took place at home, the majority (62 per cent) were attended by untrained persons including relatives, friends and neighbours.
- Little less than one-quarter of women in the rural areas of Belgaum District have an unmet need for family planning, that is, they are not using contraception even though they do not want any more children.
- Among the three registers (Eligible Couple Register, ANC register, and Immunization register) examined, the EC register was found to be relatively more complete and accurate than the other two registers.[26]

In another study a rapid research survey was conducted in rural areas of Dharwad district in Karnataka during February-April, 1997 to check the coverage, quality of services and client satisfaction under the new strategy of 'target-free' approach.

The facility survey of 50 sub-centres showed that major problems are lack of housing accommodation for the ANMs (50 per cent), unoccupied official quarters (one-third of the cases), lack of adequate furniture, thermometer, BP apparatus, torch light, uristixl bendix solution and metronidazole tablets. On the other hand, ANMs reported a huge supply of IFA tablets. ANMs also complained about lack of supply of EC, ANC immunization and other registers. Some of the important policy recommendations emerging from the study are:

(a) Improve ANM services, especially make them visit women with unmet need for contraception, and past acceptors of sterilization.

(b) As a large number of sterilization acceptors complain about side effects, a special health campaign for sterilized men and women should be launched by multipurpose workers. In order to safeguard future levels of acceptance, past acceptors should be made to feel that they are looked after well by programme functionaries.

(c) It should be ensured that such Centres have adequate supply of drugs, and attempts should be made to reduce waiting time and provide free services at primary health centres. The guilty should be punished.

(d) A television set could be placed in PHC waiting room and also a VCP to disseminate information and messages on health and family welfare and facilities in sub-centres.

(e) Concerted attempts should be made to raise immunization levels by workers as they appear to have reached a point of stagnation before acquiring universality.[27]

6. FACTS AND SUGGESTIONS

We give here facts and suggestions to improve the functioning of sub-centres.

(i) Effective Logistic Support

There are enormous logistical problems like perennial shortage of medicines (e.g. wide spectrum antibiotics), non-availability of proper equipments (e.g. oxygen cylinder), storage facilities (cold and ordinary) and most important of all, inadequate transport facilities. For efficient and effective implementation of the MPW scheme, these critically important logistical problems need to be solved expeditiously.

(ii) Demarcating Smaller Areas

The population and the area MPW is supposed to cover intensively appears rather high. Hence, the authorities would do well if they could think of reducing this heavy size of population. This would certainly enhance the qualitative impact of the scheme in terms of greater client satisfaction, improved overall health conditions of the people and consequently, enhanced confidence of the people in the scheme.

(iii) Allocating Family Welfare Activities Exclusively to ANMs

It would be better if female MPWs (ANMs) alone were made to work for family planning and thereby, relieve the male workers of their FP responsibilities so that they can concentrate on their multipurpose work more rigorously and cover a larger number of clientele.

(iv) Refresher Courses to Create Confidence

Some of the workers, particularly the male, do not appear fully confident and professionally capable of conducting their duties in a manner desired by all. Hence, they need to be reoriented and given refresher/crash courses periodically.

Training is (a) an action process, (b) by which capabilities of the Health personnel can be improved, (c) to meet the Health workers needs in terms of their knowledge, skills, and attitudes required in performing tasks and functions, and (d) within relatively short period of time.

Training is the well articulated effort to promote competence in the Health service by imparting professional knowledge, by broadening of vision and adoption of correct patterns of behaviour among the Health employees with regard to their existing functional responsibilities. It also enables the Health employees to equip themselves for senior administrative positions in future.

Marshall suggests the development of the following ingredients to promote right and rational attitudes.[28]

(i) development of rational thinking,
(ii) development of objective thinking,
(iii) development of social understanding,
(iv) development of aesthetic responsiveness,
(v) development of practical abilities, and
(vi) development and placement of memory in action.

(v) Leadership Role of PHC

PHC doctors and supervisors should provide leadership and guidance to MPWs. This would hopefully help increase their interest in work.

According to Haimann, "Leadership is the process by which an executive or a manager imaginatively directs, guides and influences the work of others in choosing and attaining specified goals by mediating between the individual and the organisation in such a manner that both will obtain the maximum satisfaction."[29]

To quote Keith Davis, "Leadership is the ability to persuade others to seek defined objectives enthusiastically. It is the human factor which binds a group together and motivates it towards its goals."[30]

(vi) Decentralization of Authority

Towards vesting the privileges and powers with the PHC Medical officers for rewarding the subordinate staff or awarding punishment to them, conferment of authority and delegation of power to PHCs by the district and state level health bodies needs to be effected immediately. This would ensure effective control and supervision at PHC level.

(vii) Transport Facilities

Some transport facilities may be provided to MPWs so that they can save time for productive work especially during field campaigns.

(viii) Strengthening Supervisions

Supervision of Multipurpose Health workers needs to be strengthened as supervision is considered the link pin between PHC and the grassroot workers/present and potential users.

(ix) Financial Allocation as per Actual Need

The present method of uniformly allocating financial resources to the sub-centres irrespective of their size in terms of population served, disease profiles and geographical/locational consideration, should be changed and a rational method of financial allocation needs to be followed.

(x) Multipurpose Approach at all Levels

The Multipurpose Health Workers Scheme aims at as wide a coverage of health problems in as much as it envisages totality of health via integration of both programmes/activities and services. Hence, the role of the MPW is considered pivotal. However, the purported multipurpose orientation appears to be confined to the MPWs alone as if they alone mattered exclusively. But, what is required is multipurpose orientation at all levels. However, such a development is rarely found in the implementing agencies beyond the PHC/SC level. The legacy of the uni-purpose health work philosophy and its erstwhile practitioners tends to manifest itself in a variety of forms. For example, at the district level unipurpose-oriented and programmes departments continue to exist. Similarly, the erstwhile Unipurpose Health Coordinators/Supervisors continue to exhibit biases that smack of their parental discipline orientation. For example, those who work in the area of malaria tend to emphasise the component of malaria work more than the others in the multipurpose work with the result that, willy nilly conflicting and counter-productive instructions are issued. Therefore, one needs to carefully re-examine the concept of multipurpose work as also reorient both the office and field-based staff to the new requirements and the philosophy of the MPW scheme.

P.H. Rayppa and N. Bhaskara Rao in their study found that there was no proper integration of work under this scheme at the state and district levels. Even at the periphery level, health workers tended to think generally in terms of unipurpose activities rather than multipurpose work.[31]

(xi) Displaying the List of Available Medicines

The wonders of modern medicine serve no purpose when people have no access to the drugs and vaccines that relieve suffering and prevent death.

Femandos Rntegana in his article, "Action For Equity" in *World Health* (March-April, 1992, p. 7) rightly stresses that primary health care can only be more effective if even the most remote health centres can rely in receiving regular supplies of affordable drugs of good quality and if health workers are trained in their use. If medicines are not available at health centre, people loose confidence in the whole system and will seek other remedies, usually from sources unqualified to diagnose or prescribe.

In view of the perennial shortage of medicines at the PHCs and SCs, the doctors/MPWs should arrange to display on information boards about availability of medicines. This would help to erase the wrong notions that people have about the integrity of the PHC/SC staff *vis-a-vis* availability.

(xii) Strengthening of Sub-centers

In view of the limited reach ability of PHCs (the servicing zone being by and large confined to a radius of three to five kilometers), there is a strong need to strengthen the sub-centres that MPWs are available for most part of the day and night.

(xiii) Building Morale and Motivation of Multipurpose Workers

Morale has an individual as well as a group or institutional aspect. It is a self-stimulating incentive within the minds and hearts of the multipurpose workers. A whole some morale stimulates loyalty, generates cooperation and encourages team work. At these are essential for the achievement of the goals of sub-centre and primary health care system. Planning and Scheduling of Work under the multipurpose workers' scheme, health workers provide integral health services based on targets and directives from district and PHC levels. Health workers at sub-centres need to schedule their day-today planning activities for the whole month. The work schedule for health workers is thus a simple management tool that will help deliver better primary health care to the rural areas of India.

(xiv) Providing Congenial Organisational Climate

It would be of utmost significance to stress that organisation is not merely a structure; in fact, it embraces a structure as well as the human beings who man and run it in order to realise the pre conceived objectives.

We must always strive through administrative improvements and reforms to remove the irritants which creep into the organisations to ensure an effective organisational climate. We may ensure the following:

(a) Clear definition of objectives.
(b) Systematic grouping of related activities.
(c) Maximum delegation of authority.
(d) Minimum layering.
(e) Proper conditions of work.
(f) Provision for easier communications.[32]

(xv) Creating Ethical Values of Service Among MPWs

Workers must be imbued with the ideal of service. It was rightly held by the Gamer that "No society can reach heights of greatness unless in all fields critical to its growth and creativity there is an ample supply of dedicated men and women." The ideals of ethics enshrined in the valuable scriptures of all religions must be imbibed by MPWs to make Health Care a success. Swami Vivekananda has put beautifully the ideals of service which must be practised by MPWs with interest and dedication:

"It is a great privilege
for all of us to be allowed
to do anything for the world
in helping the world.
We really help ourselves.

In brief, we can suggest the following very important remedies:

(1) Prompt and adequate drug supply.
(2) Provision of a first aid kit.
(3) Regular provision of necessary registers.
(4) Provision of transport facility, at least during emergencies and immunization camps.
(5) More effective training programmes.
(6) Job Satisfaction.
(7) Recognition of good work.
(8) Promotional opportunities.

We may conclude by saying that the Health Department should give top priority to remove bottlenecks at the sub-centre level and infuse ethical and moral values among MPWs to make a success of the dream of Health for All.[33]

Notes and References

1. WHO: SEARO, Health Situation in South-East Asia Region, 1994-97, New Delhi, 1997, pp. 184-85.
2. Annual Report, 1996-97, Ministry of Health and Family Welfare, Government of India, p. 33.
3. *Ibid.*, p. 34
4. Jawahar Lal Nehru and Public Administration, *IJPA*, New Delhi, 1975, p. 88.
5. Presidential Address by Mrs. Indira Gandhi delivered on October 22, 1971, at the Annual Meeting of *IJPA*, New Delhi.
6. S.L. Goel, Personnel Administration and Management, New Delhi, Sterling, 1996, p. 6.
7. Ordway Tead: The Art of Administration, New York, McGraw Hill, 1951, p. 145.
8. Dale Yoder, Personnel Management and Industrial Relations, New Delhi, Prentice Hall of India, 1972, p. 6.
9. P. Pigor and C.A. Myers: Personnel Administration, Tokyo, McGraw, Kogakusha, 1961, p. 11.
10. Robert N. Ford, Motivation Through the Work Itself, American Management Association, New York, 1969, p. 199.
11. George Strauss and Leonard R. Sayles, Personnel: The Human Problems of Management, Prentice Hall of India, New Delhi, 1971, p. 26.
12. R. Hoppock, Job Satisfaction, Harper and Row, New York, 1935, p. 252.
13. H.A. Robinson and R. Hoppok, Job Satisfaction Resume of 1951, *Occupation*, 10(2), 1952, p. 594.
14. Quoted in S.L. Goel, Personnel Administration and Management, New Delhi, Sterling, 1996, p. 364.
15. Quoted in S.L. Goel, Personnel Administration and Management, New Delhi, Sterling, 1966, p. 304.
16. A. Kornhouser, Psychological Studies of Employee Attitudes, *J. Consult Psycho*, 8, 1944, p. 132.
17. J.A.C. Brown, Social Psychology of Industry, Pelican, London, 1969, p. 193.
18. *The Economic Times*, New Delhi, 16 August, 1999, p. 7.
19. Haire Mason *et al.*, Psychological Research on Pay, An Overview, *Industrial Relations*, 3(1), 1963, p. 3.
20. ILO: International Labour Conference, 33rd Session, Provisional Records, p. 34.
21. Micheal R. Cooper and T. Micheal Wood, Member Participation and Commitment in Group Decision-making on Influence Satisfaction and Decision Riskness", *Journal of Applied Psychology*, Vol. 59, No. 2, April, 1974.
22. Ted R. Brannen, The Organisation as a Social System, a paper presented at the Midwest Regional Members Conference of the College on Oct. 23, 1958, on Kansas city, Missourie.
23. S.L. Goel, Personnel Admn. and Management, New Delhi, Sterling, 1997, p. 323.
24. Brook Adams, The Theory of Social Revolution, New York, 1913.
25. Ministry of Health and Family Welfare, Government of India (No date) Manual on Target Free Approach in Family Welfare Planning, New Delhi.
26. B.M. Ramesh, S.B. Ganiger and D.G. Satishal, "Family Welfare Programme Under Target Free Approach, A Rapid Survey in Belgaum District, Karnataka, 1998, Population Research Centre, J.S.S. Institute of Economic Research, Dharwad, pp. 56-58.
27. P.N. Marl Bhal, Target Free Approach to Family Planning Programme, A Rapid Survey in Dharwad District in Karnataka, 1997, Population Research Centre, SSS Institute of Economic Research, Dharwad, pp. i-vi.

28. Hames L. Marshal, Development Teaching, New York, 1949, pp. 190-306.
29. Haimann, Professional Management, Eruasia, New Delhi, 1966, p. 440.
30. Keith Davis, Human Relations at Work, McGraw Hill, New Delhi, 1967, pp. 96-97.
31. P.H. Rayppa and N. Bhaskara Rao: Multipurpose Health Workers' Scheme in Karnataka, A Study of Malur and Dibbur Primary Health Centres in Kolar District, Bangalore, ISEC, 1982, Mimeo.
32. S.L. Goel, Personnel Administration and Management, *op. cit.*, p. 324.
33. John W. Gardner, Excellence, New York, 1961, Harper and Brothers, p. 154.

12

CHAPTER

Working of Primary Health Care

A Case Study of Punjab

INTRODUCTION

We now examine working of Primary Health Care with the help of a case study, i.e. "Primary Health Care in Punjab." Before we discuss about Primary health care, let us examine the demographic profile, health infrastructure and current health status in Punjab State.

DEMOGRAPHIC PROFILE

Punjab is one of the richest states of Indian Union consisting of 20 districts. It is situated in the North-Western region of the country, approximately between 29"32' and 32"32' latitude and 73"54' and 76"56' E longitude. It is bound in the North by Jammu and Kashmir, in the East by Himachal Pradesh, in the South by Haryana and in the West by Pakistan. The river Ravi marks the Western boundary of the state with Pakistan. The state covers an area of 131,015 Sq. Kms. with a population of 24358999 (2001 census). The percentage of rural population to total population is 66.1%.

Administrative Structure

Divisions	3
Districts	20
Sub-Divisions	55
Tehsils	55
Sub-Tehsils	69
Blocks	136
No. of inhabited villages	12,352
No. of towns	120

MAP I

Map of Punjab

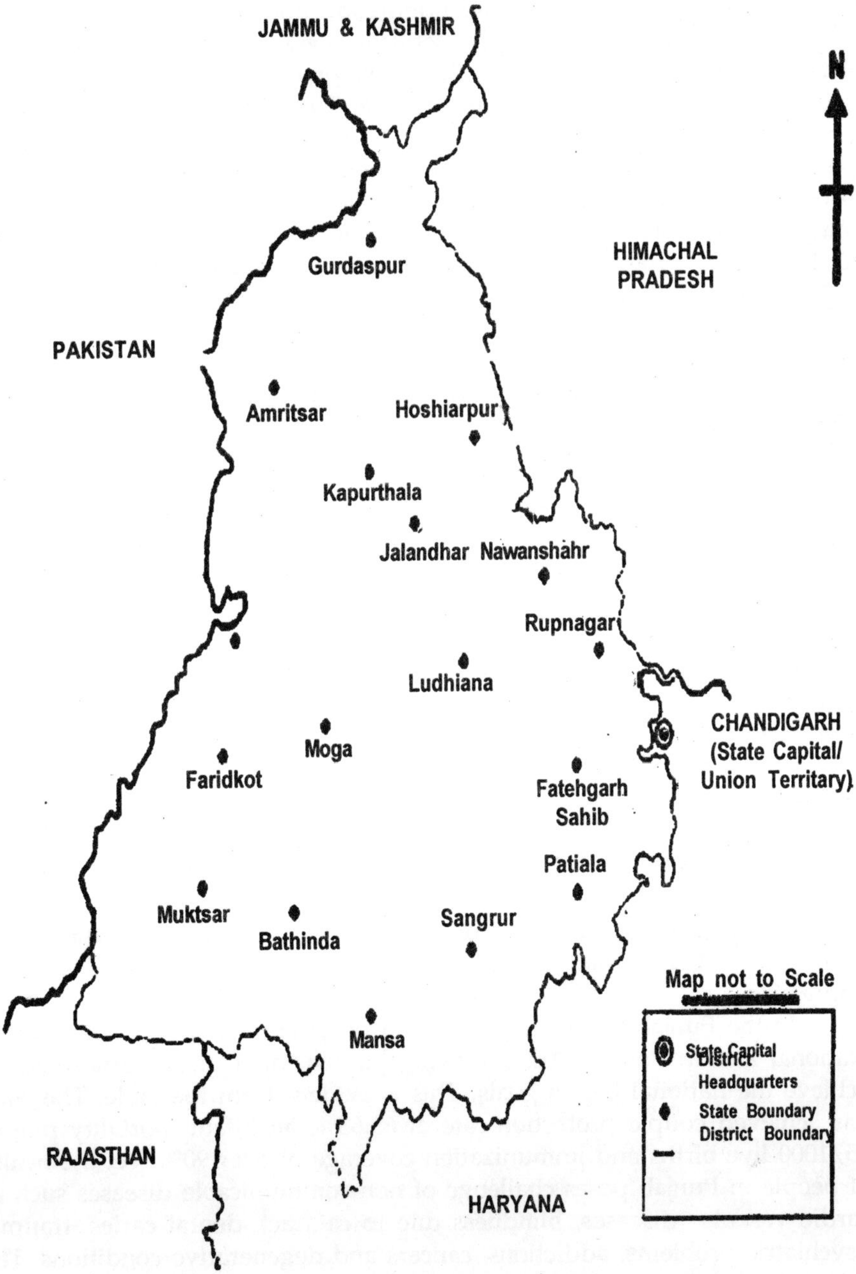

One of the significant things that happened during the Sixth Plan was the adoption of National Health Policy. Health Care Programmes were restructured and reoriented for achieving objectives of the policy. Priority was given to extension and expansion of rural health infrastructure through net work of Community Health Centres, Primary Health Centres and Sub-Centres on a liberalised population norm. Efforts were made to develop promotive and preventive services along with the curative services. High priority has been given to the development of Primary Health Care located as close to the people as possible. The approach and strategy for developing health care delivery system in rural areas initiated in the Sixth Plan was pursued vigorously during the 7th Plan to consolidate the health infrastructure and making up the deficiencies in training of personnel, equipment and other physical facilities. Coordinated efforts are being made under various programmes to provide effective and efficient rural health services to the people.

Current Health Situation

We present in brief the current health status of the people in Punjab in Table 12.1.

TABLE 12.1

No. of Villages	12673
Total Population	24358999
Rural Population	66.1
Population Density	483 persons/sq.km
Birth Rate	18.7
Death Rate	6.4
Infant Mortality Rate	45
Expectation of Life at birth	68.39 (2000)
Females of Life at birth	71.4 (2000)

Source: Panjab Government

Analysis of the Table 12.2 reveals that the health status of the people of Punjab is better than the all India Average. However, it is still not impressive.

In the Punjab State, all polices and programmes as laid down in the National Health Policy 2002, are being implemented in all earnestness to achieve the national health goals. This is evident from the table. The state has achieved couple protection rate of 65.63%, an infant mortality rate of 45/1000 live births and immunization coverage of over 90%. Yet the health of people in Punjab poses challenge of non-communicable diseases such as cardio vascular diseases, blindness due to cataract, dental caries, trauma, psychiatric problems, addictions, cancers and degenerative conditions. The infant deaths are largely due to neonatal causes, while maternal mortality still is a cause of concern.

TABLE 12.2

Rural Health Infrastructure of Punjab as on March 2006

Sub-Centres	2858 (March 2006)	1415 Without building	
Primary Health Centres	484 (March 2006)	74 Without building	
Community Health Centre	126	NA	
Multipurpose worker (Female)	*Total*	*In Position*	*Shortfall*
Female (ANM) at Sub-Centre	2858	2290	568
Multipurpose worker Female (ANM) at PHC's and Sub-Centre	3342	2515	827
Health Workers Male MPW at Sub-Centres	2858	1375	1483
Health Assistant Female (LAV) at PHC	484	264	220
Health Assistant Male at PHC	484	208	276
Doctors at PHC	484	350	134
Surgeons at CHC	126	62	64
Obstetricians and Gynecologists	126	41	85
Physicians	126	44	82
Pediatricians	126	'30	96
Hospital Specailists at PHC	504	177	327

Source: Panjab Government.

TABLE 12.3

Basic Statistics of Punjab

Item	*Number*
Areas	50,362 sq.km.
Divisions	4
Districts	17 likely to be 18 on Basakhi
Sub-division	72
Tehsils	72
Sub-Tehsils	81
Blocks	140
Towns (Census 2001)	143
Cities (Census 2001)	14
Inhabited Villages (Census 2001)	12673

Source: Ibid.

TABLE 12.4

Target of Health Indicators by 2000 A.D.

S. No.	Indicators	Target	Current Status India	Current Status Punjab
1.	Birth Rate	21.00	28.06	25.00
2.	Death Rate	9.00	9.	7.6
3.	Infant Mortality Rate	Below 60	73	53.0
4.	Expectation of life at Birth (1960-96)			
	Male	64.00	60.6	66.6
	Female	64.00	61.7	66.6
5.	Percentage of eligible couples effectively protected upto 31st March 1995	60.00	45.5	65.63
6.	Annual growth rate of population	1.2	2.39	2.08
7.	Family Size	4.3	5.6	5.1
8.	Immunization Status			
(i)	TT Pregnant Mothers	100%	69	91.3%
(ii)	DPT	85%	82	90.9%
(iii)	BCG	85%	89	88.2%
(iv)	Polio	85%	82	90.4%

Source: Ninth Year Plan, 1997-2000, Government of Punjab, pp. 256-57.

The Health development is the process of continuous progressive improvement of the health status of the population. Its outcome is the rising level of human well- being, not only by reduction in the burden of the disease but also by the attainment of positive, physical and mental health related to satisfactory economic functioning and social integration. Health is both an input and output and is linked with development. Inspite of this realization, the people, especially those in rural areas, are not getting facilities of modern medicine. The state of hopelessness and frustration among people is not because of lack of professional knowledge or competence, but due to poor administration of health services."

Based on the recommendations of expert committees, Alma Ata Declaration and the National Health Policy, a Primary Health care system was developed and diversified to make health services accessible and available to people near their living places. As a result of these developments, by March 2001, there were established 1,37,311 sub-centres, 22,842 PHCs, and 3043 CHCs in the country. However, these institutions of Primary Health care are not being utilized by the people as anticipated. This is also evident from the fact that the improvement in health status has not been commensurate with the expansion of health services infrastructure and functions. The population growth rate continues to be high, morbidity rates for women and children are distressingly high, nutritional status is low, infant mortality rate is high, communicable diseases and non-communicable diseases are still to be controlled, negligible population have access to safe-drinking water and basic sanitation facilities. Further, diseases like blindness, leprosy, TB, diarrhoea, etc. continue to have high incidence, lowering the health status of the people.

HEALTH INFRASTRUCTURE

Punjab has a vast network of Public Health care facilities comprising of 217 hospitals, including 126 Community Health Centres excluding three tertiary level hospitals, 484 primary health centres and 1462 subsidiary health centres, dispensaries and 2858 sub-centres. The tertiary care facilities in Punjab consists of three Government Medical Colleges, at Amritsar, Patiala and Faridabad two private medical colleges, i.e. Dayanand Medical College and Christian Medical College, Ludhiana and a prestigious Regional Post-Graduate Institute of Medical Education and Research (PGIMER), Chandigarh.

OBJECTIVE OF THE POLICY PROVIDING PRIMARY HEALTH CARE

The National Health Policy aims at providing Primary Health Care for all by the year 2000 A.D. The National Health Policy lays stress on Primary Health Care, which ensures essential Health Care to be made accessible to the community in an acceptable and affordable manner and with the community participation. Accordingly, the perspective long-term plan of the Health Department has been proposed, which *inter alia* aims at:

(1) Correcting the existing imbalance in the availability of medical facilities and manpower between Urban and Rural areas.
(2) Providing total health coverage to the rural population.
(3) To provide more and better medical facilities in urban areas to remove regional imbalance.

To achieve these objectives, the long-term health plan envisages die provision of following health infrastructure facilities:

Rural Areas

In rural areas at the village level, there are some voluntary village health functionaries such as trained indigenous Dais and Health Guides. They function as contact persons between the Health Department staff and the village community. In addition, they are providing certain basic health services to the village community under the guidance and support of local MPWs stationed at the sub-centres. Primary Health Care Services in the rural areas of the State are provided through a net work of Medical Institutions comprising of Sub-Centres (2852), SHCs (1462), PHCs (484), Rural Hospitals (53), Urban Slum Area Dispensaries (252) and CHCs (104). In addition 40 Mobile Dispensaries have been provided for Intensive Health

Care to serve the population living within 16 Kms of the International Borders of the State.

Table 12.5 examines the comparative picture indicating the national norms and level of achievements by Punjab

TABLE 12.5

Health Department

S. No.	Parameters Indicators	National Norms	Level of Achievements
1.	Trained Dais	Atleast one for each village	22276 Dais trained 0.5 villages covered by each dai
2.	Village Health Guide	One for each village on 1000 population	One for 1135 population Total 11657. Trained VHG i.e. 1196 female and 10561 males
3.	Population served health workers (M & F)	M 3000-5000 F 3000-4500	5545 approx. 4638 approx.
4.	Ratio of HA (M) to HW (M)	1:6	1:5:4
5.	Ratio of HA (F) to HW (F)	1:6	1:4:8
6.	Population covered by Sub-Centres	3000-5000	4648
7.	Population covered by PHC/SHC	20,000-30,000	6499
8.	Population covered by Community Health Centres	About 1 lakh	1.94 lakh
9.	No. of sub-centres for each PHC	6 sub-centres	6 sub-centres PHC at 30,000 Population
10.	No. of PHCs for Community Health Centres	4 PHCs	6 PHCs S

Source: *Ibid.*, p. 255.

An analysis of the Table indicates that Punjab still lags behind the norms. For Example, a Community Health Centre should cover a population of 1 lakh, while in Punjab, it is 1.94 lakh. There is deficiency in many indicators.

The State Government should expand its health services to fulfil the norms. Table 10.5 discusses the norms for setting up these institutions and the finances required for setting up and running these institutions.

Primary Health Care in Urban Slums

Opening of New Dispensaries in Urban Slum Areas

The purpose of opening new dispensaries in Urban Slum Areas and other suitable places is to provide medical facilities to the growing urban population and to take-off the work load from the bigger hospitals, so that staff working there could spend more time in attending to serious cases. Such dispensaries are opened in those parts of the towns which are predominately inhabited by poor working class economically weaker sections of the society on the recommendation of District Planning's Boards, so that people living in such localities may derive maximum benefit from such Institutions. Opening of such dispensaries will also help in providing medical facilities to the slum-dwellers near their home.

CRITICAL APPRAISAL

We have examined the primary health care system in Punjab, based on personal discussions with the staff working at CHC, PHC, SC, Health Guide and TBA on random basis and also soliciting the views of beneficiaries. Besides, the discussions with District and State headquarter health staff was also held to get their view points. In addition, the study of documents relating to health in Punjab was also undertaken. We give here the facts and suggestions, which can help in providing decent primary health care in the new millennium.

I. Insufficient and badly Maintained Buildings

Despite rapid expansion, majority of Institutions are without proper buildings. Table 12.2 examines the shortage of buildings. Besides shortage, the existing buildings:

(a) are not properly maintained
(b) are not adequate
(c) are not adequate

Infrastructural Facilities in PHCs

The infrastructural facilities available in five PHCs, selected at room, were tabulated and their availability *vis-a-vis* the need brings out the following issues:

1. Insufficient buildings for PHCs and poor maintenance.
2. Inadequate amenities like flush latrines, pipe water supply, electricity, etc.
3. Non-availability of good residential accommodation, in rural areas.
4. Inadequate supply of medicines and equipment.
5. Poor sanitation arrangements.
6. Ineffective inspection and supervision by District Health System.
7. No coordination with local private practitioners.
8. Inpatient capacity in PHCs not utilized.
9. Vacant posts in PHCs affect their functioning.
10. Administrative training not imparted to medical staff.

Utilization of PHCs by Beneficiaries

Accessibility and acceptance of health services depends on availability of manpower, facilities and services, the consumer costs for service, other factors affecting the consumer-provider relationship and the need for health services. The "acceptance" of health services, that is actual utilization of health services and the expressed demand for services by the consumers, is found to be low. In order to ascertain the reasons, 100 respondents from PHC samples were interviewed on random basis. They have listed the following factors for low utilization of health services:

1. PHC staff not punctual and are generally absent.
2. Non-availability of medical equipment in working order.
3. Long waiting time for medical examination.
4. Patients not satisfied with medical examination.
5. Discourteous behaviour of PHC staff.
6. Non-availability of required medicines.
7. No arrangements for ISM.
8. Preventive health aspect is neglected.
9. People not involved in Health care exercise.
10. Referral system does not exist.

2. Lack of Effective Training of Medical and Paramedical Staff

It is observed that after basic professional training. Officers/Officials have not been exposed to reorientation courses for improving their knowledge and updating their skills, there is also dire need for imparting induction training to the Medical Officers and the para-medical staff at the time of their first entry into Government Service, In order to cover this gap, it is proposed to provide reorientation training to all medical/para medical staff after every 3/5 years of service in the State Training Institution, Mohali and Health Family Welfare Training Research Centre. Amritsar. We suggest below the need of training for various categories of personnel.

A. Medical Officers' Training

(i) Fresh medical graduates may be given induction training for a period of at least three months with special emphasis on field training before posting them to Primary Health Centres.

(ii) As apart of undergraduate medical education curriculum, management training programme comprising of financial management, materials management and personnel management, in particular, may be incorporated.

(iii) Periodic in-service training programmes may be instituted.

(iv) Training in medico legal aspects for medical graduates may be duly stressed.

(v) Training of interns at Primary Health Centre may be done through a well conceived programme based on practical and field experiences. Interns may be posted to Sub-centres to enable them to learn the management of a Sub-centre Independently under an overall composite supervision of Primary Health Centre Medical Officer and members of the faculty from medical, surgical, obstetrics and Gynaecology and paediatrics disciplines of medical colleges.

(vi) Appropriate training to develop proper and positive aptitude towards primary health care may be imparted to medical faculty as a part of training to trainers' programme.

(vii) VOs/NGOs may also be involved in such training programmes by making use of training material and journals produced by them.

(viii) Adequate physical and residential facilities for trainees may be created so that they are ensured of a place to stay in Primary Health Centres for training.

(ix) Medical officer should be trained at P.S.M. Department for implementation of national health programme at least one week in every year.

(x) Medical Officers should be trained in the process of planning, control and monitoring.

B. *Training of Para-Medicals*

(A) MPW

(i) New recruitment training must be done at PHC level and that should be done mainly through field orientation training.

(ii) There should be on the spot refreshing of knowledge of female MPW at the time of supervision by medical officer/block extension educator as well during monthly and sector meeting.

(iii) They should be given training in the art and science of People's participation.

(iv) They should be trained at in the Sectoral co-ordinations processes.

(v) Multipurpose Worker (MPW) should be taken for field practice in Primary Health Centre areas, as the present training is more hospital-oriented.

(vi) MPW training manual does not have a chapter on "understanding the community." This may be got included.

(B) Supervisor

(i) Training must be practical and field-oriented rather than class-oriented training, at least three months field training should be done before promotion.

(ii) Supervisors should refresh their knowledge from time to time during supervision.

(iii) Supervisor should be trained in the art of interpersonal relationships.

Policy regarding training of Supervisors needs to be modified because at present Supervisors and Male Health Workers receive the same training. Being of a different level, Supervisor requires a separate curriculum of training. Training in education methodology and techniques of supervision is to be given. Supervisors have to be trained in problem-solving techniques and not indulge in fault finding.

(C) V.H.G. and DAI

V.H.G. and dai should be oriented about their work at least five days every three months. It should be done seriously.

(D) Training Tutors

Refresher training of tutors of training school should be organized and it should be practical training.

In Resolution WHA 37.31, Member-States were urged to support universities in conducting the education and training of workers in health and related fields towards the attainment of health for all. Universities were invited to provide the kind of education and training for students and post-graduates in the health and related disciplines that will prepare them technically and attune them socially to meet the health needs of the people they are to serve. They were also encouraged to conduct biomedical, epidemiological, technological, social, economic and behavioural research required to prepare and carry out strategies for health for all.

Medical and health professions have increasingly been required to break out of their traditional boundaries to encompass emerging developments: increased emphasis on the humanization of care, integrated care, more consumer participation, equal access to care, assessment of technology, cost containment, consideration of the population perspective in planning health care, protection of the environment, promotion of health lifestyles, etc.

Advances in the patterns of health development cannot proceed unless the human resources that lead, plan, staff, monitor and evaluate health-related services and programmes are enlightened and enabled to define and respond to societal needs. Given the evolving understandings of health problems and the changing dynamics of health system development, there must be a close and continuous interaction between educational, research and health system development to ensure relevance of education to need.[1]

Too often, the training of health personnel follows a pattern of yesterday's view of health care, or even of only the clinical care, and falls seriously short of meeting today's and tomorrow's requirement for personnel who can lead or participate in effective health services responding to people's needs.[2]

3. Lack of Intra-Sectoral Coordination

Health is not the sole concern of health personnel, but there are several related sectors, namely, water supply, and sanitation, nutrition, education, economy and information whose cooperation is equally important but these are never taken care of by Primary health care system in Punjab. Has the Public Health Department of Punjab ever discussed the nutrition content of our food, inspite of the fact that the major problem in Punjab is nutritional deficient and malnutrition, although the food is available in plenty.

The International Conference on Nutrition in Rome in 1992 crystallized awareness about the causes and consequences of malnutrition, and of the ways in which the international community can combat them. It stressed the importance of incorporating nutrition objectives into development programmes and issued recommendations on seven major nutrition strategies. These include: improving household food security; protecting consumers through improved food quality and safety; caring for the poor and nutritionally vulnerable; preventing and managing infectious diseases; promoting appropriate diets and healthy lifestyles; preventing specific micro-nutrient deficiencies; and assessing and monitoring nutritional status.[3]

Shri B.K. Chaturvedi, Former Secretary, Department of Women and Child Development in his article 'Malnutrition: An Obstacle to National Development' in *Hindustan Times*, dated 3rd September 2000 advocated that time has now come for all agencies working in the development sector to launch a multipronged strategy to eradicate malnutrition. We realise that it is complex public health problem, resulting from a combination of factors such as poverty, Illiteracy, superstition, social custom and lack of awareness. We already have a National Nutrition Policy which covers all aspects relating to malnurition with sound prescriptions for combating this problem. We must implement it in full measure. To achieve quicker and more permanent results, malnutrition must be addressed inter-generationally namely through ensuring proper nutritional care of the infant from 0-2 years, adolescent girl and the pregnant and lactating mother.

Some Consequences of Malnutrition:

- Higher Child mortality,
- Impaired brain growth and development in children.
- Higher maternal mortality,
- Life long physical disability,
- Compromised immunity, easy suceptibility to infections, and
- Increased risk of chronic diseases.

What we can do—

- Nutrition advocacy, sensitisation, capacity building and awareness generation, especially at the grassroot level.
- Preventing onset of malnutrition among 0-2 year old children by promoting complementary feeding of infants at six months, using home-based foods.
- Preventing low birth weight of the newborns and breaking the inter-generational cycle of malnutrition by addressing the nutritional needs of the girl child, adolescent girls, pregnant and lactating women.
- Preventing Calorie and micronutrient malnutrition by promoting community-based production of low cost nutritious foods, and consumption of fruits and vegetables.
- Involvement of women's groups in advocating and practising proper nutritional practices.

Present understanding of inter-sectoral coordination invariably means only what the other sector does for the health sector, not what health sector does for the other sectors. It should be understood in the proper perspective to achieve mutual coordination.

4. Lack of Community Participation

In some states of the Indian Union like Karnataka, planning, implementation and evaluation of primary health care has been entrusted to Panchayati Raj Institutions. However, in Punjab, there is still the control of bureaucracy over primary health care system. In such a situation, how the people can participate in this process?

Therefore, there is a need to empower the people, so that rural population can participate effectively in the affairs affecting their lives. One of the major problems of primary health care is the absentism and lack of punctuality among the health personnel. People are highly agitated over the non-availability of health personnel to provide health services. Realising the feelings of people, the Punjab Government passed an order that the Panchayats would mark the attendance of the doctors. There was great agitation and resentment among health and medical staff. They resorted to strike. As a result, the Government had to withdraw its order. It is high time that the people, especially the disadvantaged sections of the society, should be empowered to usher in true democracy.

Under such an ideal atmosphere, the Government through health experts, can motivate the local people to help in mobilising resources for improving primary health care system. WHO suggests the ways and means of mobilising resources. To quote:[4]

The resources available for health care, particularly in developing countries, are limited. Community involvement in primary health care makes it possible to mobilize community resources that might otherwise remain unused. Examples of such involvement are given below:

- *Action by the people*: This could include the provision of physical labour for building a health centre or constructing a safe well or sanitary latrine; the provision of transport, to take a woman in labour or a sick person to hospital; the organisation of a special day for immunization and for identification of children at special risk.
- *Provision of facilities*: A building owned by the community might be allocated to the community health worker for treating patients or storing medicines and records.
- *Provision of goods and materials*: The following could be provided: food such as grain, fruit, and fish for cooking demonstrations or for distribution to malnourished children; agricultural implements to boost community food production; or building materials, such as wood and bricks, to be used in self-help construction schemes.
- *Money or contributions*: Money donated for primary health care in a community may be used to purchase medicines, to purchase equipment such as agricultural implements, or to pay the community health worker. Methods of obtaining financial resources are many and varied; examples include:
- A fixed payment for each service provided.
- Payment for each service, depending on ability to pay.
- Payment that varies according to the type of service provided.
- Payment for drugs or a prescription, which may vary according to the type of drug and/or ability to pay.
- Payment through an insurance scheme, in which individuals or families make continued regular payments to provide for services when they are sick.
- Donations for services, the amount depending on the patient's willingness or ability to pay.
- Payment through an insurance scheme covering preventive and promotive activities as well as individual illnesses in the community.
- Periodic donations (for example, by the local cooperatives).
- Periodic fund-raising campaigns, which may include athletic or cultural activities organized by communities.

Partnerships with the community involve attitudinal changes and a new approach to health development. Health care providers need to be convinced that illiterate communities are not unintelligent or uncreative. They need to understand that the problems affecting the poor are best understood by the poor; that, therefore, the community must be involved in conceptualizing, planning, implementing, monitoring and evaluating health care. In this respect, NGOs and voluntary sectors have a better record than the public sector.[5]

5. Low Utilization of Primary Health Care Services Inspite of Good Availability and Accessibility

Utilization of services or actual coverage is expressed as the proportion of people in need of a service, who actually receive it in a given period, usually a year; for example, the proportion of children at risk who are immunized, or the proportion of pregnant women who receive antenatal care or have their deliveries supervised by a trained attendant. In some cases facilities exist but lack of drugs or poor quality care results in the people not using the services. Other reasons for non-utilization are that facilities may be opened at hours of the day when people will not come because they are occupied in the fields or factories. Also, people may be attracted by the prestige of a more distant hospital, and may use it for care that could have been provided by local primary health care facilities.[6]

The utilisation of primary health care services is very low because of the following reasons:

(i) Lack of interest and enthusiasm among health functionaries.
(ii) Lack of infrastructural facilities and public health facilities.
(iii) Non-availability of drugs and medical equipment.
(iv) Lack of faith of the people in the rural health system.
(v) Lack of effective supervision and control.

Thus, we have to introduce reforms at all levels to ensure the optimum utilisation of health services, otherwise it would become an example of clear-cut wastage of resources collected from the hard earned money of the people through various taxes.

6. Lack of Availability of Potable Water Supply and Sewerage Disposal System

Sanitation is a composite concept, which involves waste disposal system, water supply, sewerage and prevention of environmental pollution. It has been variously described by different sanitation experts to finally settle down to the concept of human waste disposal.[7]

Safe drinking water has been one of the felt needs of the people. While making development plans, it was, however, not adequately realised that the absence of sanitary conditions may cause as much harm to health as can polluted water, which is now being contaminated by effluents and chemicals discharged into water. No wonder, sanitation has been given a low priority. Sanitation is not only the problem of keeping clean; it is a development issue without which a healthy society is not possible. It is the problem of raising production and productivity. In India alone, 15 lakh children below the age of five years die each year of diarrhoeal diseases. As many as 50 diseases are caused due to lack of proper sanitation. And over 80 percent of sickness is caused by human excreta and water-related diseases. The most common of these are intestinal parasitic infections, diarrhoea, typhoid and cholera. Very clearly, major causes of deaths in poor countries are sanitation-related diseases, while cancer is the prime killer in the West.[8] Let us mention the various diseases due to insanitation:

By Bacteria

- Cholera
- Diarrhoea
- Bacillary dysentry
- Typhoid and para-typhoid

By Protozoa

- Amoebic dysantry

By Virus

- Infective Hepatitis
- Poliomyelitis

By Intestinal Worms .

- Hook worm
- Round worm
- Thread worm
- Tape worm, etc.

By Polluted Air

- Eye diseases
- Respiratory diseases
- Skin and hair problems

By Liquid Waste and Stagnant Water

- Malaria
- Kalazar
- Filaria
- Dengue
- Japanese encephilis
- Skin diseases
- Eye problems

By Airborne Micro-organism

- Chicken Pox
- Measles

- Deptheria
- Pneumonia
- Whoopnia
- T.B.
- Mumps, etc.
- Other respiratory diseases

Reasons for Unsatisfactory Sanitation Status in Urban Slums

- Overcrowding
- Lack of safe drinking water
- Insanitation due to open defecation, stagnate water, dirty heap of garbage
- Lack of awareness and facilities regarding Health, Hygiene and Sanitation
- Poverty and unemployment
- Make shift shelter and uncertainty about habitat ownership.

Let us discuss the potable water supply situation in Punjab:

There are 12673 villages in the state according to 2001 census, out of which 8579 are identified as problem villages as per the criteria laid down by GOI for this purpose. The details of criteria laid down by GOI for identification of problem villages are as under:

(i) Those not having an assured source of drinking water within reasonable distance (0.05 km) or within the depth of 15 meters.

(ii) Which suffer excess of salinity, iron, flouride or other toxic elements hazardous to health.

(iii) Where sources of water are liable to risk of cholera or guinea worm infestation.

Broadly speaking, the State of Punjab has two types of scarcity. Firstly, where the existing drinking water sources in the villages are health hazards, i.e. where the water contains flourides, total solids, hardness in excess of the permissible limits prescribed by Government of India. Most of such villages are located in the districts of Patiala, Mansa, Moga, Muktsar, Sangrur, Bathinda, Faridkot, Ferozepur and a part of Amritsar district. In the second category the existing drinking water sources are either deeper than 16 meters (50 ft.) or are situated beyond a distance of 0.05 km from the population. Such problem villages are mostly located in the sub-montaneous areas in the districts of Ropar, Hoshiarpur, Nawashahar and Gurdaspur. In the case of first category the water is provided after treatment through slop and filters or by installing deep tubewells where there is under ground deeper strata yield potable water. In the second category, i.e. where the existing source of deep water is at a distance, the schemes are based either on tubewells or percolation.

As far sanitation is concerned, the position is highly unsatisfactory, as only negligible number of villages are covered under the sewerage disposal programme.

Reasons for unsatisfactory sanitation status in rural set-up:

- Lack of sufficient political and administrative will.
- Lack of priority to sanitation and health.
- Absence of uniform administrative structure in states and lack of uniform code and guidelines to NGOs.
- Lack of community perception in sanitation.
- Inadequate information and dissemination to rural folks.
- Absence of awareness regarding health, hygiene and sanitation.
- Lack of involvement of target groups like women, youth, school teachers and students, panchayats and NGOs.
- Lack of options for sanitation measures and local trained personnel.

There is no denying the fact that inadequacy of safe drinking water, improper disposal of human excreta, solid and liquid waste leading to unfavourable environmental conditions and lack of personal food hygiene in the rural areas have been the major causes of many killer diseases. According to an estimate, more than 1.7 lakh children are affected by polimyelitis, 2.5 lakh die of tetanus and 15 lakh die of diarrhoea and dehydration every year. This high infant mortality rate is attributed largely to poor sanitation.

7. Maternal and Child Health Services not Effective

It is estimated that each year, at least half a million women die from causes related to pregnancy and childbirth. Over 99% of the maternal deaths take place in developing countries, which account for 86% of the world's births. In the poorest countries of the world, when a woman becomes pregnant, her chances of dying as a result are between 100 and 200 times higher than those of a pregnant woman of affluent countries.

In India, women in the reproductive age groups and young children contribute about 62% of the population. These groups of the population are also regarded as most vulnerable because of special health problems. Despite our efforts over the last 35 years, the attention given to pregnant mothers, to mothers post-natal and to children has not been adequate to reduce mortality and morbidity.

The average woman in India can expect to have around 5 to 6 live births and may have 7 to 8 pregnancies. Her lifetime chance of dying from pregnancy related causes is about 1 in 20. Some of the important causes of maternal mortality are sepsis, hemorrhage, taxaemia, illegal abortion, malnutrition and repeated childbirths. The important causes of deaths among infants and young children are prematurely, tetanus neonatorum, diarrhoea, malnutrition and respiratory infections. Several factors, such as inadequate care of mothers at risk, poor maternal health, lack of referral services, etc. contribute to this mortality.

Respondents Contact with Health Worker and Perceptions about Government Services: A Study of 100 Respondents in Ropar District

One of the important functions of the health workers is to provide health care services to the people in their homes. About 36 per cent of respondents were visited by health workers at home. Among them, about 85 per cent of the respondents were visited by ANMs, 37 per cent by male health workers and 5 per cent by anganwadi workers in rural areas. Majority of the respondents (63.5 per cent) were satisfied with the time spent by ANM in discussions with women respondents about their health problems. However, only 22.5 per cent respondents reported that ANM counselled their unmarried adolescent girls and not even a single respondent received Iron and Folic Acid tablets for their adolescent girls.

Currently married women in 15-44 age group, who had visited a government health facility like Hospital, Community Health Centre (CHC), Primary Health Centre (PHC) or Sub-Centre (SC) were asked whether they were satisfied with the services provided and the way the facilities functioned. Twenty-six per cent of them reported that they were satisfied with the services and would recommend it to others. An equal proportion of women reported that the working time of the facilities and their locations are convenient. Staff explains how to take prescribed medicines and are friendly with patients. However, women felt no waiting time (26.5 per cent) treatment free (30.3 per cent) and treatment at centre effective (40.3 per cent) as positive factors.

We mention the following problems which need the attention of the persons responsible for primary health care. Knowledge of the female multipurpose worker is poorer than expected. Female multipurpose worker does not use her kit during field visits. Female M.P.W. does not visit all the villages regularly and does not visit some villages at all because they are not approachable. Antenatal care through sub-centres is roughly 15 to 20 percent, and internatal and postnatal services are also poor. Multipurpose supervisors knowledge is the same as that of male and female M.P.Ws., so they are not in a position to check work and train them in field situations. Supervision by them is also very irregular.

Medical officers did not visit the sub-centres, nor are they interested in national health programmes other than family planning. Moreover, M.O. does not have adequate administrative powers to take action against workers, who are slack or defaulting. Information education communication (J.E.C.) material supplied to P.H.C. is not utilized usually at sub-centres. Health education posters are usually made for the literate. Illiterate persons are not able to understand messages contained in the posters.

8. Lack of Effective Supervision and Control

Considering the rise in population size, the continuing constraint of resources and the pressure for higher priority to develop other sectors of the national economy, it appears absolutely essential to make the fullest and most efficient use of the available allocations, ensuring against underutilisation, misutilisation and diversion of resources. This objective can be achieved through appropriate administrative reforms, devolution of decision-making power and introduction of relevant managerial techniques. Bimal Jalan says that "the most important organisational reform that deserves to be implemented is to decentralise delivery of government health services." Centralisation of financial powers is a major cause of delay and inefficiency as even the slightest deviation in specification of drugs or service requires approval of a number of departments, with several layers of bureaucracy at state headquarters.

Decentralisation of financial powers with performance monitoring can greatly improve the health care delivery system in rural areas and strengthen accountability of local institution.[10]

Recommendations

(i) Medical officer and supervisor must pay regular visits to sub-centre and supervise working pattern of M.P.W. as well as support TBAs.

(ii) Block extension educator should devote maximum time on training and reorientation of workers and TBAs.

(iii) Registration of infants should be a continuous process; it should not be done on a fixed month of the year. There should be the same register for infants and for immunization.

(iv) Community must know that dai is not a government servant; she should get compliments from community.

(v) There should not be rigidity in working time of worker; it should be modified according to the availability of the villagers in the houses.

(vi) All administrative powers should be delegated to block medical officer.

Most maternal and infant deaths are preventable, provided M.C.H. and family planning programme are given equal status and importance. supported by, I.E.C. activities for demand generation and community participation at sub-centre level and below through TBAs.

9. Lack of Effective Evaluation and Monitoring

Monitoring is the process of measuring, coordinating, collecting, processing, and communicating information to assist management in decision-making. The sources of information used in monitoring health activities include monthly, quarterly and annual reports from health centres and hospitals, data on notifiable diseases, and special surveys. Good information systems are required for effective monitoring. There is a practice to collect unnecessary information resulting in wastage of human and material resources. It must be emphasized that the problem is not a shortage of data. However, there is often too much data, but the fact that little useful information can be gleaned from them.

We suggest the following to achieve evaluation:

1. Primary health care in Ministry and Secretariat should have a separate cell to coordinate the activities of nodal officers connected with primary health care, namely, Maternal and Child Welfare, Immunization, Health Education, etc.
2. Independent evaluation must be done in every State to improve the quality of services.
3. Improvement in existing information system is needed.
4. Lessons must be learnt from successful NGOs.
5. Services of medical colleges may also be utilised to perform independent evaluation.
6. Every Primary Health Centre should develop one model Sub-centre and one model Primary Health Centre in every district and these should serve as examples for other sub-centres and Primary Health Centres to follow.

10. Limited Coverage of Health Activities

At present, primary health care services are not available to all because of mismanagement and lack of available resources. There is a need of optimisation of available resources to spread planned health care to all. We suggest the following to achieve this:

(i) The preparation of daily work/tour plan should be done at PHC with participation of the medical officer, block extension educator, supervisor and workers for a month so that all are clear. This programme should be given to all at sub-centre as well as in each village so that everyone in PHC knows when the worker is visiting the village. Both male and female workers should visit a village on the same day to have full impact.

(ii) Unapproachable village should be covered by four team members (2 supervisors and 2 M.P.W.s), at least once a month. Medical officer should check implementation of plan during monthly meeting as well as a surprise check. Vehicles should be provided for this purpose.

(iii) Workers may identify 3 to 4 informants who are influential in each village and give responsibility of some exceptional families to them. They will give back information to M.P.W. on their visit, like antenatal case, child birth, death, immunization problem, so that worker need not visit each house every time.

(iv) All the national health programmes should be treated equally. More attention should not be given to family planning. Even in family planning attention may be given to sterilization.

(v) Detailed history of patients is to be taken immediately after registration so that the worker can identify high risk cases. This needs sufficient educational training of workers.

(vi) Urine examination, haemoglobin and weight record must be done at sub-centre during antenatal clinic.

11. No Provision for Educating the Community about Health For All

How can one provide rational choices to people in order to modify their health care behaviour and practices? In 1997 the RF came up with a communication strategy focusing on group discussions, and Communications Needs Assessment (CNA), aimed at designing and developing a community-based primary health care model of 'Health For All'. To quote the report:

This model uses the concept of social marketing. We organized training workshops for Rural Health Communicators and Primary Health Workers, who put up 96 performances of street plays, 'nautankis', puppet shows, folk songs, 'qawaalis', and 'kajari' in 32 villages of Amethi Tehsil. Through these performances, the RHCs disseminate information about primary health care and services available to the community. Mobile health vans provide services like maternal and child health care, immunisation, and treatment of common diseases and injuries, at the doorstep. The community's awareness of hygiene, sanitation, safe drinking water, communicable diseases, diarrhoea, STDs/AIDS and immunistion has been greatly increased, and more people do not know the benefits of family planning and birth spacing. The success of the pilot project has encouraged us to continue and expand it all over Amethi Tehsil to achieve the goal of 'Health For All'.

12. Insufficient Funds and Encouragement for Indian System of Medicine

True primary health care involves self-sufficiency and empowerment in the long-run. The RGF encourages traditional health practices with a view to making primary health care services available in rural areas in Anantapur District, Andhra Pradesh. Forty Community Health workers have been trained in traditional methods of treatment with ayurvedic and herbal medicines. They have established Health Centres in their villages, selling herbal medicines such as Aloe Jelly, Ashta Churan, Neem Ointment, and Sctropaladi, favoured by villagers because they are low cost and have no side effects. We hope not only to promote traditional methods based on local material and expertise, but to document and publish this valuable knowledge. Punjab should try such experiments.

13. Doctors and Paramedical Staff Display Bureaucratic Culture

P.D. Sharma in his article, "Administrative Culture" in *IJPA*, July to September, 1990 (pp. 620-21) rightly says that medical doctors and para-medical staff in all cultures have to work and behave like professionals.

This professional culture implies a professional comraderie and professional ethics with a high sense of professional skills and pride. The Indian doctors are fairly competent and knowledgeable about their job, but it is a sad commentary on their professional ethic that they behave like 'medical feudals' in the hospital wards and glory in bossing over nurses and attendants. The District Collector or the Superintendent of Police is their, 'power model' and the Indian society also evaluates their professional competence in terms of private practice money, which they mint by abusing the public facilities in government hospitals. They seldom find time to read or conduct their own researches. Obviously, they exploit popular ignorance and refuse to share their outdated knowledge or its absence with their colleagues, juniors, patients and society at large.

The general democratic culture of American society keeps the medical professionals constantly on their toes and often showing them their place also. They work under constant surveillance of the legal profession and face social audit in the press. Money minting does not earn a special kind of social status for the American doctor. Rather, the professional competition keeps pushing the fake ones out of circulation. No wonder, my doctor George was a mere doctor. He was George to us all, because he won't not a Doctor Sahib. The nurse could disagree with him in the open and he won't mind sitting on the patient's bed and tasting a sample of food from the hospital kitchen. As a professional, he enjoyed tremendous reputation, but he will come to his patients in utter humility, confessing that his treatment was an experiment, based on certain hunches and researches on which the patient should also reflect and comment.

CONCLUSION

More than 30 years after the health-for-all policies and strategies were adopted, it was realized that it was not possible to reach the goal unless concerted efforts were made to reorient the provision of health care through appropriate reforms. This involved a complex process of change in health sector policy and institutional arrangements which needed to be carefully initiated by analysing the present situation, the future goals and how these goals could be reached.

The following points should be kept in mind while suggesting health reforms based upon facts and observation:

(1) In view of the differences in the socio-economic and overall health status in different states of the Indian union, health sector reforms should be initiated with the overall national development framework as well as within the framework of the explicit national health policies, which provide the fundamentals such as health for all, equity, social justice and partnership.

(2) The organisation of managerial changes in the health systems need to be appropriately monitored and evaluated in order to identify the implications of these changes, not only in terms of efficiency, quality and sustainability, but also in terms of equity.

(3) We should explore effective strategies for the political and administrative management of the process and content of health sector reforms and to make such reforms changes known to policy-makers, health care providers and the general population.

(4) We should make full use of national institutions and other mechanisms, including WHO collaborating centres, to plan and manage health sector reforms effectively.

(5) Efforts should be made to promote and exchange experience on health sector reforms through appropriate consultations, documentation, use of information technology, including use of technical forums, with a critical assessment of the positive and negative impact of reforms.

(6) Government of India should provide technical and other support to States to pursue their own health sector reform measures and to coordinate with other research institutions in pursuing and supporting national efforts for health sector reforms.

(7) Existing human resources for health may require reorientation to new goals and tasks in pursuit to the PHC approach. The majority of existing health workers do not possess the appropriate skills or conceptual awareness of the PHC approach. The training they received often emphasized clinical skills, rather than work within communities. Then, too, the skills required for PHC at all levels go well beyond technical competence. For example, if health is understood in broader terms, health workers will be able to identify the social and economic factors that are the main contributors to ill-health in a given situation or among particular groups, for example, young children of families in certain occupational groups. They should be able to communicate with community leaders and other sector professionals in the search for solutions. Skills are required in management, community development, and epidemiology, as well as in integrating different programme tasks.

(8) Primary Health Care Planners and Policy-makers should achieve the following to make a success of PHC programme:

(i) To reduce gaps between health status of haves and have not by ensuring the following:

(a) create adequate infrastructure,

(b) train the local support manpower,

(c) extend the outreach of various health programmes to remote areas, and

(d) ensure availability of health functionaries at service point.

(ii) Encourage the practice of getting feedback from the field workers and the community and acting on it.

(iii) Emphasize the health education and IEC activities and educate regarding available services and its utilization by the community.

(iv) Organise leadership and team training for PHC and sub-centre health teams.

(v) Provide incentive for teamwork rather than an individual performance.

(vi) Introduce system of performance analysis and development rather than performances appraisal.

(vii) Build strong inter-sectoral ordination at all levels with those services agencies which have direct bearing on health status of the community.

(viii) Overcome the resistance to the acceptance of primary health care approach by building a strong referral support and liberating specialists from treating the minor health problems.

(xi) Initiate new strategies to educate professionals regarding HFA leadership initiative and accepting health as a value.

(x) Innovate alternate strategies of health services delivery suited for the area using appropriate health care technology.

Shri K.K. Bakshi, former Secretary, Health, in his Welcome Address to the delegates of Sixth Conference of Central Council of Health and Family Welfare, April 8-10-1999, New Delhi has rightly mentioned that the need to improve the efficiency and effectiveness of the basic health delivery system so that the poor, particularly in the rural areas, gain adequate, prompt and timely access to the health care facilities is of utmost importance. Though over the years we have built up an impressive rural health infrastructure consisting of Sub-Centres, Primary Health Centres and Community Health Centres. However, due to various reasons the functioning of these centres leaves much to be desired. One of the major problems is the chronic absenteeism and non-availability of qualified professionals, paramedics and other health functionaries.

Shri K.C. Pant, the then Deputy Chairman, Planning Commission, in his Inaugural Address to the delegates of Sixth Conference of Central Council of Health and Family Welfare, April 8-10-1999 stated that nearly 30% of India's population lives in urban areas. In many towns and cities the health status of urban slum-dwellers is worse than that of the rural population. There is either non-availability or substantial underutilisation of available primary care facilities along with an over-crowding at secondary and tertiary care centres. This problem should be sorted out by appropriate reorganisation and restricting of existing institutions and redeployment of existing manpower. These should be linked with existing secondary and tertiary care institutions in the same geographically delineated areas for referral. India perhaps has the largest primary health care network manned by professionals and para-professionals. However, there are substantial differences between the states and between districts in the same state in the availability and utilisation of the health care services and health indices of the population. It is a matter of concern that the gaps in functional infrastructure are widest in the districts where the health care needs are greatest and private sector health care services are not readily available. The emphasis in the coming years should be to optimise the coverage and quality of care by identifying and rectifying the critical gaps in existing infrastructure, manpower, equipment, essential diagnostic reagents and drugs. Efforts will have to be directed to improve functional efficiency of the health care system through training and deployment of health manpower with requisite professional competence, and skill upgradation of all categories of health personnel, through structured continuing education.[11]

The structure of the Primary Health Care Services provided by the government is impressive. However, the government has not been able to provide and maintain critical infrastructure, adequate resources in terms of manpower, finances and equipment, a sound administrative set-up, accountability and responsiveness of the system and commitment of the Health Department. This half-hearted approach fails to satisfy the people and cannot provide job satisfaction to the providers of Community Health Care. All these problems also emanate from the fact that Government has been rapidly expanding the number of health institutions, without focusing on improving the Physical facilities in the existing institutions. There is a need to consolidate existing infrastructure to ensure proper facilities in the existing institutions.

Mr. A.J. Phillip in his Article, "Public Health Care in Punjab a Sham", in *The Tribune,* datd Feb. 2006 observes: It is not for want of resources that the poor patients in Punjab have to suffer. For instance, most PHCs have pucca buildings constructed at enormous cost. It is doctors and igi paramedical staff who are lacking at these centres. A study found that 39 per cent of doctors and 14 per cent of medical staff are absent on any given day in Punjab.

On paper, things are hunky-dory as this quote from the Human Development Report, prepared by the Punjab Government in 2004, suggests: "The reach of health institutions is very good in Punjab. The average population covered by any medical institution is around 10,000-11,000. In terms of access, the average radius served per institution is 2.68 km. There has been a four-fold increase in the number of PHCs servicing rural Punjab since 1980, covering the entire state."

However, a World Bank report published in the same year is nearer to truth: "A recent perception survey by the Public Affairs Centre places Punjab in eleventh place in the quality of service delivery across 16 major Indian states."

Notes and References

1. WHO: SEARO: Declaration on Health Development in the South-East Asia Region in the 21st Century, New Delhi, 1997, p. 45.
2. *Ibid.*, p. 33.
3. WHO: Primary Health Care Concepts and Challenges in a Changing World, Geneva, 1996. p. 15 (E. Tarimo and E.G. Webster).
4. WHO: Towards a Healthy District, Geneva, 1991, pp. 62-65.
5. Declaration on Health Development, *op. cit.*, p. 44.
6. WHO: Development of Indicators for Monitoring Progress Towards Health For All by the Year 2000, Geneva, 1981, p. 27.
7. Padam Bhushan and Bindeshwar Pathak, Rural Sanitation Programme NGO's in *Kurukshetra*, October 1992, p. 25.
8. *Ibid.*
9. *Ibid.*, p. 26.
10. Quoted in R.K. Sapru, Health Care Policy and Administration in India, in *IJPA*, July to Sept. 1997, pp. 746-47.
11. Ministry of Health and Family Welfare, DGHS, GOI, Sixth Conference of Central Council of Health and Family Welfare, held April 7 to April 10, 1999.

ANNEXURE I

Declaration of Alma-Ata

The International Conference on Primary Health Care, meeting in Alma-Ata this twelfth day of September in the year Nineteen hundred and seventy-eight, expressing the need for urgent action by all governments, all health and development workers, and the world community to protect and promote the health of all the people of the world, hereby makes the following Declaration:

I

The Conference strongly reaffirms that health, which is a stage of complete physical, mental and social well-being, and not merely the absence of disease or infirmity, is a fundamental human right and, that the attainment of the highest possible level of health is a most important world-wide social goal whose realization requires the action of many other social and economic sectors in addition to the health sector.

II

The existing gross inequality in the health status of the people particularly between developed and developing countries as well as within countries is politically, socially and economically unacceptable and is, therefore, of common concern to all countries.

III

Economic and social development, based on a New International Economic Order, is of basic importance to the fullest attainment of health for all and to the reduction of the gap between the health status of the developing and developed countries. The protection of the health of the people is essential to sustained economic and social development and contributes to a better quality of life and to world peace.

IV

The people have the right and duty to participate individually and collectively in the planning and implementation of their health care.

V

Governments have a responsibility for the health of their people which can be fulfiled only by the provision of adequate health and social measures. A main social target of governments, international organisations and the whole world community in the coming decades should be the attainment by all peoples of the world by the year 2000 of a level of health that will permit them to lead a socially and economically productive life. Primary health care is the key to attaining this target as part of development in the spirit of social justice.

VI

Primary health care is essential health care based on practical, scientifically sound and socially acceptable methods and technology made universally accessible to individuals and families in the community through their full participation and at a cost that the community and country can afford to maintain at every stage of their development in the spirit of self-reliance and self-determination. It forms an integral part both of the country's health system, of which it is the central function and main focus, and of the overall social and economic development of the community. It is the first level of contact of individuals, the family and community with the national health system bringing health care as close as possible to where people live and work, and constitutes the first element of a continuing health care process.

VII

Primary health care:

1. reflects and evolves from the economic conditions and socio-cultural and political characteristics of the country and its communities and is based on the application of the relevant results of social, biomedical and health services research and public health experience;
2. addresses the main health problems in the community, providing promotive, preventive, curative and rehabilitative services accordingly;
3. includes at least, education concerning prevailing health problems and the methods of preventing and controlling them; promotion of food supply and proper nutrition; an adequate supply of safe water and basic sanitation; maternal and child health care, including family planning; immunization against the major infectious diseases; prevention and control of locally endemic diseases; appropriate treatment of common diseases and injuries; and provision of essential drugs;

4. involves, in addition to the health sector, all related sectors and aspects of national and community development, in particular, agriculture, animal husbandry, food, industry, education, housing, public works , communications and other sectors; and demands the coordinated efforts of all those sectors;
5. requires and promotes maximum community and individual self-reliance and participation in the planning, organisation, operation and control of primary health care, making fullest use of local, national and other available resources; and to this end develops through appropriate education the ability of communities to participate;
6. should be sustained by integrated, functional and mutually-supportive referral systems, leading to the progressive improvement of comprehensive health care for all, and giving priority to those most in need; and
7. relies, at local and referral levels, on health workers, including physicians, nurses, midwives, auxiliaries and community workers as applicable, as well as traditional practitioners as needed, suitably trained socially and technically to work as a health team and to respond to the expressed, health needs of the community.

VIII

All governments should formulate national policies, strategies and plans of action to launch and sustain primary health care as part of a comprehensive national health system and in coordination with other sectors. To this end, it will be necessary to exercise political will, to mobilize the country's resources and to use available external resources rationally.

IX

All countries should cooperate in a spirit of partnership and service to ensure primary health care for all people since the attainment of health by people in only one country directly concerns and benefits every other country. In this context the joint WHO/UNICEF report on primary health care constitutes a solid basis for the further development and operation of primary health care throughout the world.

X

An acceptable level of health for all the people of the world by the year 2000 can be attained through a fuller and better use of the world's resources, a considerable part of which is now spent on armaments and military conflicts. A genuine policy of independence, peace, detente and disarmament could and should release additional resources that could well be devoted to peaceful aims and in particular to the acceleration of social and economic development of which primary health care, as an essential part, should be allotted its proper share.

The International Conference on Primary Health Care calls for urgent and effective primary health care throughout the world and particularly in developing countries in a spirit of technical cooperation and in keeping with a New International Economic Order. It urges governments, WHO and UNICEF, and other international organisations, as well as multilateral and bilateral agencies, non-governmental organisations, funding agencies, all health workers and the whole world community to support national and international commitment to primary health care and to channel increased technical and financial support to it, particularly in developing countries. The Conference calls on all the aforementioned to collaborate in introducing, developing and maintaining primary health care in accordance with the spirit and content of this Declaration.

Annexure II

Alma-Ata Recommendations

1. Interrelationships between Health and Development

The conference recognizing that health is dependent on social and economic development, and also contributes to it:

Recommends that governments incorporate and strengthen primary health care within their national development plans with special emphasis on rural and urban development programmes and the coordination of the health-related activities of the different sectors.

2. Community Participation in Primary Health Care

The Conference, considering that national and community self-reliance and social awareness are among the key factors in human development and acknowledging that people have the right and duty to participate in the process for the improvement and maintenance of their health:

Recommends that governments encourage and ensure full community participation through the effective propagation of relevant information, increased literacy and the development of the necessary institutional arrangements through which individuals, families and communities can assume responsibility for their health and well-being.

3. The Role of National Administrations in Primary Health Care

The conference, noting the importance of appropriate administrative and financial support at all levels, for coordinated national development, including primary health care, and for translating national policies into practice: Recommends that governments strengthen the support of their general administration to primary health care and related activities through coordination among different ministries and the delegation of appropriate responsibility and authority to intermediate and community levels, with the provision of sufficient manpower and resources to these levels.

4. Co-ordination of Health

The Conference, recognizing that significant improvement in the health of all people requires the planned and effective coordination of national health services and health-related activities of other sectors:

Recommends that national health policies and plans take full account for the inputs of other sectors bearing on health: that specific and workable arrangements be made at all levels—in particular at the intermediate and community levels—for the coordination of health services with all other activities contributing to health promotion and primary health care; and that arrangements for coordination take into account the role of the sectors dealing with administration and finance.

5. Content of Primary Health Care

The Conference, stressing that primary health care should focus on the main health problems in the community, but recognizing that these problems and the ways of solving them will vary from one country and community to another:

Recommends that primary health care should include at least: education concerning prevailing health problems and the methods of identifying, preventing, and controlling them; promotion of food supply and proper nutrition, an adequate supply of safe water, and basic sanitation; maternal and child health care, including family planning; immunization against the major infectious diseases; prevention and control of locally endemic diseases; appropriate treatment of common diseases and injuries; promotional of mental health and provision of essential drugs.

6. Comprehensive Primary Health at the Local Level

The Conference, confirming that primary health care includes all activities that contribute to health at the interface between the community and the health system:

Recommends that, in order for primary health care to be comprehensive, all development-oriented activities should be inter-related and balanced so as to focus on problems of the highest priority as mutually perceived by the community and health system, and that culturally acceptable, technically appropriate, manageable, and appropriately selected interventions should be implemented in combinations that meet local needs. This implies that single-purpose programmes should be integrated into primary health care activities as quickly and smoothly as possible.

7. Support of Primary Health Care within the National Health System

The Conference, considering that primary health care is the foundation of a comprehensive national health system and that the health system must be organized to support primary health care and make it effective:

Recommends that governments promote primary health care and related development activities so as to enhance the capacity and determination of the people to solve their own problems. This requires a close relationship between the primary health care workers and the community and that each team be responsible for a defined area. It also necessitates reorienting the existing system to ensure that all levels of the health system support primary health care by facilitating referral of patients and consultation on health problems; by providing supportive supervision and guidance, logistic support, and supplies: and through improved use of referral hospitals.

8. Special Needs of Vulnerable and High-risk Groups

The Conference, recognizing the special needs of those who are at least able, for geographical, political, social or financial reasons, to take the initiative in seeking health care, and expressing great concern for those who are the most vulnerable or at greatest risk:

Recommends that as pan of total coverage of populations through primary health care, high priority be given to the special needs of women, children, working populations at high risk, and the under-privileged segments of society, and that the necessary activities be maintained, reaching out into all homes and working places to identify systematically those at highest risk. To provide continuing care to them, and to eliminate factors contributing to ill-health.

9. Roles and Categories of Health and Health-related Manpower for Primary Health Care

The Conference, recognizing that the development of primary health care depends on the attitudes and capabilities of all health workers and also on a health system that is designed to support and complement the frontline workers:

Recommends that governments give high priority to the full utilization of human resources by defining the technical role, supportive skills, and attitudes required for each category of health worker according to the functions that need to be carried out to ensure effective primary health care, and by developing teams composed of community health workers, other developmental workers, intermediate personnel, nurses, midwives, physicians, and, where applicable, traditional practitioners and traditional birth attendants.

10. Training of Health and Health-related Manpower for Primary Health Care

The Conference, recognizing the need for sufficient numbers of trained personnel for the support and delivery of primary health care:

Recommends that governments undertake or support reorientation and training for all levels of existing personnel and revised programmes for the training of new community health personnel; that health workers, especially physicians and nurses, should be socially and technically trained and motivated to serve the community; that all training should include field activities; that physicians and other professional health workers should be urged to work in under-served areas early in their career; and that due attention should be paid to continuing education, supportive supervision, the preparation of teachers of health workers, and health training for workers from other sectors.

11. Incentives for Service in Remote and Neglected Areas

The Conference, recognizing that service in primary health care focused on the needs of the under-served requires special dedication and motivation, but that even then there is a crucial need to provide culturally suitable rewards and recognition for service under difficult and rigorous conditions:

Recommends that all levels of health personnel be provided with incentives scaled to the relative isolation and difficulty of the conditions under which they live and work. These incentives should be adapted to local situations and may take such forms as better living and working conditions and opportunities for further training and continuing education.

12. Appropriate Technology for Health

The Conference, recognizing that primary health care requires the identification, development, adaptation and implementation of appropriate technology:

Recommends that governments, research and academic institutions, non-governmental organisations, and especially communities, develop technologies and methods that contribute to health, both in the health system and in associated services; are scientifically sound, adapted to local needs, and acceptable to the community; and are maintained by the people themselves, in keeping with the principle of self-reliance, with resources the community and the country can afford.

13. Logistic Support and Facilities for Primary Health Care

The Conference, being aware that the success of primary health care depends on adequate, appropriate and sustained logistic support in thousands of communities in many countries, raising new problems of great magnitude:

Recommends that governments ensure that efficient administrative, delivery and maintenance services be established, reaching out to all primary health care activities at the communities level; that suitable and sufficient supplies and equipment be always available at all levels in the health system. in particular to community health workers; that careful attention be paid to the safe delivery and storage of perishable supplies such as vaccines; that there be appropriate strengthening of support facilities including hospitals, and that governments ensure that transport and all physical facilities for primary health care be functionally efficient and appropriate to the social and economic environment.

14. Essential Drugs for Primary Health Care

The Conference, recognizing that primary health care requires a continuous supply of essential drugs; that the provision of drugs accounts for a significant proportion of expenditures in the health sector; and that the progressive extension of primary health care to ensure eventual national coverage entails a large increase in the provision of drugs:

Recommends that governments formulate national policies and regulations with respect to the import, local production, sale and distribution of drugs and biologicals so as to ensure that essential drugs are available at the various levels of primary health care at the lowest feasible cost; that specific measures be taken to prevent the over-utilization of medicines; that proved traditional remedies be incorporated; and that effective administrative and supply systems be established.

15. Administration and Management for Primary Health Care

The Conference, considering that the translation of the principles of primary health care into practice requires the strengthening of the administrative structure and managerial processes: Recommends that governments should develop the administrative framework and apply at all levels appropriate managerial processes to plan for and implement primary health care, improve the allocation and distribution of resources, monitor and evaluate programmes with the help of a simple and relevant information system, share control with the community and provide appropriate management training of health workers of different categories.

16. Health Services Research and Operational Studies

The Conference, emphasizing that enough is known about primary health care for governments to initiate or expand its implementation but also recognizing that many long-range and complex issues need to be resolved, that the contribution of traditional systems of medicine calls for further research, and that new problems are constantly emerging as implementation proceeds:

Recommends that every national programme should set aside a percentage of its funds for continuing health services research; organize health services research and development units and field areas that operate in parallel with the general implementation process; encourage evaluation and feedback for early identification of problems; give responsibility to educational and research institutions and thus bring them into close collaboration with the health system; encourage the involvement of field workers and community members; and undertake a sustained effort to train research workers in order to promote national self-reliance,

17. Resources for Primary Health Care

The Conference recognizing that the implementation of primary health care requires the effective mobilization of resources bearing on health:

Recommends that, as an expression of their political determination to promote the primary health care approach, governments, in progressively increasing the funds allocated for health, should give first priority to the extension of primary health care to under-served communities; encourage and support various ways of financing primary health care; including, where appropriate, such means as social insurance, cooperatives and all available resources at the local level, through the active involvement and participation of communities; and take measures to maximize the efficiency and effectiveness of health-related activities in all sectors,

18. National Commitment to Primary Health Care

The Conference, affirming that primary health care requires strong and continued political commitment at all levels of government, based upon the full understanding and support of the people:

Recommends that governments express their political will to attain health for all by making a continuing commitment to implement primary health care as an integral part of the national health system within overall socio-economic development, with the involvement of all sectors concerned; to adopt enabling legislation where necessary; and to stimulate, mobilize and sustain public interest and participation in the development of primary health care.

19. National Strategies for Primary Health Care

The Conference, stressing the need for national strategies to translate policies for primary health care into action: Recommends that governments elaborate without delay national strategies with well-defined goals and develop and implement plans of action to ensure that primary health care be made accessible to the entire population, the highest priority being given to under-served areas and groups, and reassess these policies, strategies and plans for primary health care; in order to ensure their adaptation to evolving stages of development.

20. Technical Cooperation in Primary Health Care

The Conference, recognizing that all countries can learn from each other in matters of health and development:

Recommends that countries share and exchange information, experience and expertise in the development of primary health care as part of technical cooperation among countries, particularly among developing countries.

21. International Support for Primary Health Care

The Conference, realizing that in order to promote and sustain health care and overcome obstacles to its implementation there is a need for strong, coordinated, international solidarity and support, and welcoming the offers of collaboration from United Nations organisations as well as from other sources of cooperation:

Recommends that international organisations, multilateral and bilateral agencies, non-governmental organisations, funding agencies, and other partners in international health acting in a coordinated manner should encourage and support national commitment to primary health care and should channel increased technical and financial support into it, with full respect for the coordination of these resources by the countries themselves in a spirit of self-reliance and self-determination, as well as with the maximum utilization of locally available resources.

22. Role of WHO and UNICEF in Supporting Primary Health Care

The Conference, recognizing the need for a world plan of action for primary health care as a cooperative effort of all countries: Recommends that WHO and UNICEF, guided by the declaration of Alma-Ata and the recommendations of this conference, should continue to encourage and support national strategies and plans for primary health care as part of overall development. Recommends that WHO and UNICEF, on the basis of national strategies and plans, formulate as soon as possible concerted plans of action at the regional and global levels that promote and facilitate the mutual support of countries, particularly through the use of their national institutions, for accelerated development of primary health care.

Recommends that WHO and UNICEF continuously promote the mobilization of other international resources for primary health care.

BOOKS BY THE SAME AUTHOR

1. International Administration: WHO South East-Asia Regional Office (New Delhi, 1977), Sterling Publishers
2. Principles, Problems and Prospects of Co-operative Administration (New Delhi, 1979), Sterling Publishers (Co-Author Dr. B.B. Goel)
3. Administration of Personnel in Co-operative (New Delhi, 1979), Sterling Publishers (Co-Author Dr. B.B. Goel)
4. Health Care Administration: Ecology, Principles and Modern Trends (New Delhi, 1980), Sterling Publishers
5. Health Care Administration: Policy-making and Planning (New Delhi, 1980), Sterling Publishers
6. Health Care Administration: Levels and Aspects (New Delhi, 1980), Sterling Publishers
7. International Civil Service: Principles, Problems and Prospects (New Delhi, 1984), Sterling Publishers
8. Public Health Administration (New Delhi, 1984), Sterling Publishers
9. Public Personnel Administration (New Delhi, 1984), Reprint 1987, Sterling Publishers
10. International Civil Services—Principles, Problems and Prospectives (New Delhi, 1984), Sterling Publishers.
11. Social Welfare Administration: Theory and Practice (Vols. I and II) (New Delhi, 1988), Deep & Deep Publications Pvt. Ltd.
12. Hospital Administration and Management (ed.) Co-Author Dr. R. Kumar in 3 volumes (New Delhi, 1989), Deep & Deep Publications Pvt. Ltd.
13. Policy and Administration: Family Planning & Beyond (New Delhi, 1990), Deep & Deep Publications Pvt. Ltd.
14. Modern Management Techniques (Revised and Reprinted) (New Delhi, 1990), Deep & Deep Publications Pvt. Ltd.
15. Development Planning and Administration (ed.) S. Bhatnagar (Co-editor) (New Delhi, 1992), Deep & Deep Publications Pvt. Ltd.
16. Financial Administration and Management (New Delhi, 1993), Sterling Publishers
17. Advanced Public Administration (New Delhi, 1993), Sterling Publishers

18. Personnel Administration and Management
(New Delhi, 1994), Deep & Deep Publications Pvt. Ltd.
19. Educational Policy and Administration
(New Delhi, 1994), Deep & Deep Publications Pvt. Ltd.
20. Slum Improvement Through Participatory Urban Based Community Structures
(New Delhi, 1999), Deep & Deep Publications Pvt. Ltd.
21. Distance Education in 21st Century
(New Delhi, 2000), Deep & Deep Publications Pvt. Ltd.
22. Health Care System and Management: Organisation and Structure
(New Delhi, 2000), Deep & Deep Publications Pvt. Ltd.
23. Health Care System and Management: Policies and Programmes
(New Delhi, 2000), Deep & Deep Publications Pvt. Ltd.
24. Health Care System and Management: Management and Administration
(New Delhi, 2000), Deep & Deep Publications Pvt. Ltd.
25. Heath Care System and Management: Primary Health Care Management
(New Delhi, 2000), Deep & Deep Publications Pvt. Ltd.
26. Management Techniques: Principles and Practices
(New Delhi, 2001), Deep & Deep Publications Pvt. Ltd.
27. Encyclopaedia of Disaster Management in 3 Volumes
(New Delhi, 2001), Deep & Deep Publications Pvt. Ltd.
28. Management of Hospitals: Hospital Core Services
(New Delhi, 2002), Deep & Deep Publications Pvt. Ltd.
29. Management of Hospitals: Hospital Supportive Services
(New Delhi, 2002), Deep & Deep Publications Pvt. Ltd.
30. Management of Hospitals: Hospital Preventive and Promotive Services
(New Delhi, 2002), Deep & Deep Publications Pvt. Ltd.
31. Management of Hospitals: Hospital Managerial Services
(New Delhi, 2002), Deep & Deep Publications Pvt. Ltd.
32. Public Personal Administration
(New Delhi, 2002), Deep & Deep Publications Pvt. Ltd.
33. Public Financial Administration
(New Delhi, 2002), Deep & Deep Publications Pvt. Ltd.
34. Urban Development and Management
(New Delhi, 2002), Deep & Deep Publications Pvt. Ltd.
35. Public Administration: Theory and Practices
(New Delhi, 2003), Deep & Deep Publications Pvt. Ltd.
36. Advanced Public Administration (Revised and Enlarged Edition)
(New Delhi, 2003), Deep & Deep Publications Pvt. Ltd.

37. Panchayati Raj in India
(New Delhi, 2003), Deep & Deep Publications Pvt. Ltd.
38. Encyclopedia of Higher Education in 21st Century: Organisation and Structure
(New Delhi, 2004), Deep & Deep Publications Pvt. Ltd.
39. Encyclopaedia of Higher Education in 21st Century: Quality and Excellence
(New Delhi, 2004), Deep & Deep Publications Pvt. Ltd.
40. Encyclopedia of Higher Education in 21st Century, Extension Education Services
(New Delhi, 2004), Deep & Deep Publications Pvt. Ltd.
41. Stress Management and Education: An Indian Perspective
(New Delhi, 2004), Deep & Deep Publications Pvt. Ltd.
42. Human Values and Education:
(New Delhi, 2004), Deep & Deep Publications Pvt. Ltd.
43. Public Health Policy and Administration
(New Delhi, 2004), Deep & Deep Publications Pvt. Ltd.
44. Administration and Management of NGO's: Text and Case Studies
(New Delhi, 2004), Deep & Deep Publications Pvt. Ltd.
45. Nursing Services: Management and Administration
(New Delhi, 2005), Deep & Deep Publications Pvt. Ltd.
46. Population Policy and Family Welfare Administration
(New Delhi, 2005), Deep & Deep Publications Pvt. Ltd.
47. Human Resource Development in 21st Century
(New Delhi, 2005), Deep & Deep Publications Pvt. Ltd.
48. Encyclopaedia of Disaster Management (3 Volumes)
(New Delhi, 2006) Deep & Deep Publications Pvt. Ltd.
49. School Health Education
(New Delhi, 2007), Deep & Deep Publications Pvt. Ltd.
50. Health Education: Theory and Practices
(New Delhi, 2007), Deep & Deep Publications Pvt. Ltd.
51. Good Governance: An Integral Views
(New Delhi, 2007), Deep & Deep Publications Pvt. Ltd.
52. Right to Information and Good Governance
(New Delhi, 2007), Deep & Deep Publications Pvt. Ltd.
53. Disaster Management: Text and Case Studies
(New Delhi, 2007), Deep & Deep Publications Pvt. Ltd.
54. Hospital Administration: Theory and Practices
(New Delhi, 2007), Deep & Deep Publications Pvt. Ltd.
55. Environmental Health Values and Education,
(New Delhi, 2008), Deep & Deep Publications Pvt. Ltd.

56. Administrative and Management Thinkers: Revelvance in New Millennium
(New Delhi, 2008), Deep & Deep Publications Pvt. Ltd.
57. Principles and Practices of Human Values
(New Delhi, 2008), Deep & Deep Publications Pvt. Ltd.
58. Distance Education: Principles, Potentialities and Perspectives
(New Delhi, 2008), Deep & Deep Publications Pvt. Ltd.
59. Educational Administration and Management: An Integral View
(New Delhi, 2008), Deep & Deep Publications Pvt. Ltd.
60. Women Health Education
(New Delhi, 2008), Deep & Deep Publications Pvt. Ltd.
61. Health Care System and Hospital Administration
Vol. 1 (Organisational Structure)
(New Delhi, 2008), Deep & Deep Publications Pvt. Ltd.
62. Health Care System and Hospital Administration
Vol. 2 (Resources: Human, Finance and Material)
(New Delhi, 2008), Deep & Deep Publications Pvt. Ltd.
63. Health Care System and Hospital Administration
Vol. 3 (Policy-making and Programmes)
(New Delhi, 2008), Deep & Deep Publications Pvt. Ltd.
64. Health Care System and Hospital Administration
Vol. 4 (Emerging and Thrust Areas)
(New Delhi, 2008), Deep & Deep Publications Pvt. Ltd.
65. Health Care System and Hospital Administration
Vol. 5 (Primary/Rural Health Care)
(New Delhi, 2008), Deep & Deep Publications Pvt. Ltd.
66. Health Care System and Hospital Administration
Vol. 6 (Secondary and Tertiary Health Care)
(New Delhi, 2008), Deep & Deep Publications Pvt. Ltd.
67. Health Care System and Hospital Administration
Vol. 7 (Management Techniques and Good Governance)
(New Delhi, 2008), Deep & Deep Publications Pvt. Ltd.
68. Education of Lifestyle and Lifetime Diseases
(Deep & Deep Publications Pvt. Ltd.)
69. Health Education Administration—From International Level to Village Level
(Deep & Deep Publications Pvt. Ltd.)
70. Education for Healthy Urban Cities
(Deep & Deep Publications Pvt. Ltd.)
71. Rural Health Education
(Deep & Deep Publications Pvt. Ltd.)

Bibliography

Acton Society Trust, Hospitals and the State: Hospital Organisation and Administration under the National Health Service Series, London: Action Society Trust, 1956, 54p.

Acton Society Trust, Hospitals and the State: Hospital Organisation and Administration under the National Health Service, London: The Trust, 1959, iii, 80p.

Andhra Pradesh, Health and Local Administration Department Panchayats Executive Officers Regulations relating to Recruitment, etc., Hyderabad: The Author, 1956, l6p.

Bannington, B.G., English Public Health Administration, 2nd ed., London: P.S. King, 1929, 325p.

Berkov, Robert, The World Health Organisation: A Study in Decentralized International Administration, Geneva Droz, 1957, 173p.

Better Health by Community Projects Administration, Planning Commission, New Delhi: Community Projects, Planning Commission, n.d., 32p.

Blum, Henrik L., Public Administration: A Public Health Viewpoint, N.Y.: Macmillan, 1963, 532p.

Hugh Flanagan and Peter Spurgeon, Public Sector Managerial Effectiveness: Theory and Practice in the National Health Service, Buckingham: Open Univ. Press, 1996, 128p.

Freeman, Ruth B., Administration of Public Health Services and Edward M. Holmes, Philadelphia: Saunders, 1960, 507p.

Goddard, H.A., Principles of Administration Applied to Nursing Service by H.A. Goddard, Geneva: World Health Organisation, 1958, 106p.

Goel, Rajneesh, Community Health Care, New Delhi: Deep & Deep Publications Pvt. Ltd., 2004, 403p.

Goel, S.L., Health and Care Administration: Policy-making and Planning, Delhi: Sterling, 1980, 288p.

Goel, S.L, Health Care Administration: Ecology, Principles and Modern Trends, Delhi: Sterling, 1980, 233p.

Goel, S.L., Health Care Administration: Levels and Aspects, Delhi: Sterling, 1980, 245p.

Goel, S.L., Health Care System and Management, New Delhi: Deep & Deep Publications Pvt. Ltd., 2004, 4 Vols.

Goel, S.L., International Administration: WHO South-East Asia Regional Office, Delhi: Sterling, 1977, 344p.

Goel, S.L., Population Policy and Family Welfare: Reproductive and Child Health Administration, New Delhi: Deep & Deep Publications Pvt. Ltd., 2005, 526p.

Goel, S.L., Public Health Administration, Delhi: Sterling, 1984, 472p.

Goel, S.L, Public Health Policy and Administration, New Delhi: Deep & Deep Publications Pvt. Ltd., 2005, 651p.

Graduate Study in Public Administration: A Guide to Graduate Programs by Office of Education, Department of Health, Education and Welfare, Washington: United States Government Printing Office, 1961, 158+p.

Greenfield, Margert, State-Local Service for Mental Health, Bureau of Public Administration, Berkeley: The Bureau, 1955, 93p.

Guangde, Sun, Health Care Administration in China, Westport: Greenport, 1993, pp. 53-62.

Handbook on Human Services Administration, edited by Jack Rabin and Marcia B. Steinhauer, New York: Marcel Dekker, 1988, 604p.

Health Policy Research in South Asia: Building Capacity for Reform, edited by Abdo S. Yazbeck and David H. Peters, Washington, D.C.: World Bank, 2003, 428p.

Heaver, Richard, Managing Primary Health Care: Implications of the Health Transition, Washington, D.C.: World Bank, 1995, 41p.

Health Status of the Underprivileged, New Delhi: Centre for Urban Studies, Indian Institute of Public Administration, 1991, 225p.

Indian Institute of Public Administration, Centre for Urban Studies, Urban Health System, edited by P.K. Umashankar and Girish K. Misra, New Delhi: Reliance and IIPA, 1993, 259p.

Institute for Training in Municipal Administration, Administration of Community Health Services, Chicago: ICMA, 1961, 560p.

Johnston, Timothy, Investing in Health: Development Effectiveness in the Health, Nutrition, and Population Sector, Washington, D.C.: World Bank, 1999, 69p.

Khandewale, Shreekant V., Health Administration and the Weaker Sections in an Indian Metropolis, Delhi: Devika, 1996, 231p.

Klinoubol, Kriengkrai, Public Health Development and Administration: A Study of Developing Economy, Delhi: Deep & Deep Publications Pvt. Ltd., 1989. 436p.

Local Self-Government Administration in States of India, 1956, New Delhi: Ministry of Health, 1956, 149p.

Local Self-government Administration in States of India, 1962, Ministry of Health, Delhi: The Manager of Publications, 1962, 161+p.

Legislature Committee on Local Administration by Health, Education and Local Administration Department, Madras, Madras: Health, Education and Local Administration Department, 1958, 5 Parts.

Morden, Margaret Gorsuch, Cooperative Health Administration in Metropolitan, Los Angeles: The Bureau, 1949, 52p.

Panchayat Manual, Madras: Health, Education and Local Administration Department, 1956, 368+p.

Papers in Public Administration, No. 6, Ann Arbor: The Bureau, 1950, 85p.

Public Services M.B.A. Induction Module: India-U.K. context (August-September, 1999: Indian Institute of Public Administration, New Delhi), Gender-related Issues (course material), New Delhi: Indian Institute of Public Administration, 1999, vp.

Report of the Regional Training Seminar on Social Security Administration, New Delhi: Regional Office for Asia and Oceania, 1979, 75p.

Rowbottom, R., Hospital Organisation: A Progress Report on the Brunel Health Services Project, London: Heinemann, 1973, 314p.

Survey of Research in Public Administration, 1980-90, edited by V.A. Pai Panandiker, Delhi: Konark, 1997, 631p.

Tebow, Hilda P., Staff-Development as an Integral Part of Administration, Washington, D.C.: Department of Health, Education and Welfare, 1959, 33+p.

The Indo-US Symposium on Community Mental Health at National Institute of Mental Health and Neuro Sciences, Bangalore: National Institute of Mental Health and Neuro Sciences, 1992, 520p.

Weaver, Jerry L., Conflict and Control in Health Care Administration, Beverly Hills: n.p., 1975, 197p.

Welfare Administration and Social Welfare Around the World, by Department of Health, Education and Welfare, United States, Washington: Government Printing Office, 1963, 9p.

Wishwakarma, R.K., Health Status of the Underprivileged, New Delhi: Centre for Urban Studies, Indian Institute of Public Administration, 1993, 283p.

Index

Abrams, H., 154
Accelerated Social Health Activists, 58
Advising People, 113
Alma-Ata Declaration, 21
Alma-Ata Recommendations, 311
Appropriate Research for;
  Primary Health Care, 157
Appropriate Technology, 150
ASHA (Accredited Social Health Activist), 40
Aspects of CHC Services;
  OPD Functions, 187
Availability of Medicine, 19
Azad, R.N., 86

Bajpai, P.K., 96
Bankowaski, Zbigniew, 142
Bhore Committee, 208
Block Extension Educator, 226
  Duties, 241
  Responsibilities, 241

CDP (Community Development Programme), 85
Community Health Centres, 174, 178
  Equipment, 185
  Facilities, 185
  Norms of Services, 185
  Functions, 186
  Vacant Posts, 199
Community Health Workers;
  Exploitation, 33
  Insufficient Training, 32
Community Leaders, 143
Community Link Worker, 43
Community Ownership, 44
Community Participation; 104
  Methods to Ascertain Participation, 162
  Obstacles, 104
  and Health Development, 90
  Meaning, 91
Converging Sanitation and Hygiene under NRHM, 60
Curative Services, 132

Dai Training Programme, 166
Dayal, Ishwar, 147
Decentralized Planning, 41
Declaration of Alma-Ata, 307
Declaration on Health Development, 3
Deodhar, N.S., 34
Devashyam, M.G., 109
Developing Social Networks, 118
Dilution of Services;
  Undue Expansion, 131
District Health Plan, 60
DRDA (District Rural Development Agency), 86

Effective Public Relations, 110
Effective Supervision, 270
Environmental Sanitation, 244, 257

Family Planning, 257
Family Welfare, 245
Fendall, N.R.E., 8
Financial Administration for;
  Primary Health Care, 125
Funding Arrangements, 66

General Development;
  Closer Links, 25

Hassouna, W.A., 157
Health Assistant (Female), 246
Health Education, 232
Health Experts Lack Commitment, 30
Health Infrastructure, 285
Health Manpower Development, 19
Health Programmes;
  Process of Community Participation, 100
Health Promotion;
  Inter-sectoral Co-ordination, 73
Health Services;
  Availability, 21
  Accessibility, 21
  Acceptability, 21
Health Trust of India, 63

Health Workers (Male);
  Job Responsibilities, 251
Health Workers (Female),
  Maternal and Child Health, 259
  Family Planning, 259
  Medical Termination of Pregnancy, 260
  Nutrition, 260
  Communicable Disease, 260
  Immunization, 260
  Dai Training, 260
  Vital Events, 260
  Record Keeping, 260
  Primary Medical Care, 261
  Team Activities, 261

ICDS (Integrated Child Development Services), 86
Immunization, 47
Importance of TBA, 169
Inadequate PHC Buildings, 232
Indian System of Medicine;
  Insufficient Funds, 301
India;
  Primary Health Care, 29
Indoor Beds, 233
Insufficient Supply of Drugs, 35
Integrated Rural Development Programme, 86
Inter-sectoral Co-ordination;
  Essentials, 81
Institutional Mechanisms, 62
IRDP (Integrated Rural Development Programme), 86

Janani Suraksha Yojana, 49
Job Satisfaction;
  Factors, 268
Johansen, Kirsten Staehr, 155

Kala-Azar, 50

Lalitha, N.V., 107
LMO (Lady Medical Officer), 225
Learning about Community, 120
Low Job Satisfaction, 265

Mahler, H., 99, 174
Mainstreaming AYUSH, 65
Maternal and Child Health, 247
Medical Officer;
  Duties and Resposibilities, 238
Medical Officers' Training, 288
Medical Record Keeping;
  Poor Quality, 194
Medical Termination of Pregnancy, 247
MMR (Maternal Mortality Ratio), 166
MSG (Mission Steering Group), 41
Mutalik, Gururaj, 1

Nair, C. Madhavan, 1
National Rural Health Mission, 55, 71
NCMP (National Common Minimum Programme), 38
  Goals, 38
Ndeki, Sidney, 131
New Health Financing Mechanisms, 61
Nossal, Gustav, 160
NRHM, 38
  Role of State Governments, 64
  Progress, 45
  Monitoring and Evaluation, 42
  Partnership with NGOs, 42
  Capacity Building, 42
  Institutional Arrangements, 41

OPD;
  Problems, 187
Osuntokun, B.P., 159

PAC (Public Accounts Committee), 86
Panchayati Raj Institutions, 65
Paramedical Staff;
  Lack of Effective Training, 288
Pediatric Care, 189
Personnel Administration;
  For Primary Health Care, 136
Personnel Communication, 116
Pharmacist, 228
PHC;
  Organisational Structure, 224
  Leadership Role, 274
Pillai, Sivathanu, 25
Polio Eradication Programme, 48
Poor;
  Empowerment, 117
Prevention of Diseases, 18
Primary Health Care;
  Appropriate Technology and Research, 150
  Comparative Cost of Training Health Workers, 138
  Roots, 4
  Need, Meaning and Scope, 4
  Nature, 10
Primary Health Care Development;
  General Principles, 23
Primary Health Centres;
  Organisation and Working, 206
Primary Health Infrastructure;
  Strengthening, 44
Primary/Rural Health Care;
  Administration, 1
Program Management Support Centre, 63

Provision of Rural Health, 207
Public Health Facilities, 232
Public-Private Partnership for Public Health Goals, 61

Quality of Behaviour, 192

Ray, C.N., 111
Record Keeping, 258
Resources;
  Ineffective Utilisation, 132
Responsive Administration, 109
Ross, Murray G., 90
Rural Health Issues;
  Reorienting Health/Medical Education to Support, 62

Sachs, Jeffrey D., 50
Senior Health Assistants;
  Detailed Duties, 243
Singapore Scheme, 52
Smith, Brain Abel, 125
State of Public Health, 55
Strengthening CHCs for First Referral Care, 59
Strengthening Disease Control Programmes, 60
Strengthening Primary Health Centres, 59
Sub-centres;
  Organising and Working, 249

Topping the Potential, 271
TBAs (Trained Birth Attendants), 164
  Need and Activities, 169
Taure, Madion, 118
Trained Birth Attendants;
  Low Status, 170
  Inadequate Training, 170
  Trainees Lack Interest, 171
Training Tutors, 290
Transport Facilities, 275

Understanding Public Needs, 112
Urban Basic Services Scheme, 82
Urban Primary Health Care, 9
Urban Slums;
  Primary Health Care, 286

Vajpayee, Atal Bihari, 111
Village Health Guide Scheme, 29

Ward, 188
Women's Health, 84
Working of Primary Health Care, 280

X-Ray Facilities, 190

Yadav, Jadambi Prasad, 11
Yoder, Dale, 266